Galileo's Visions

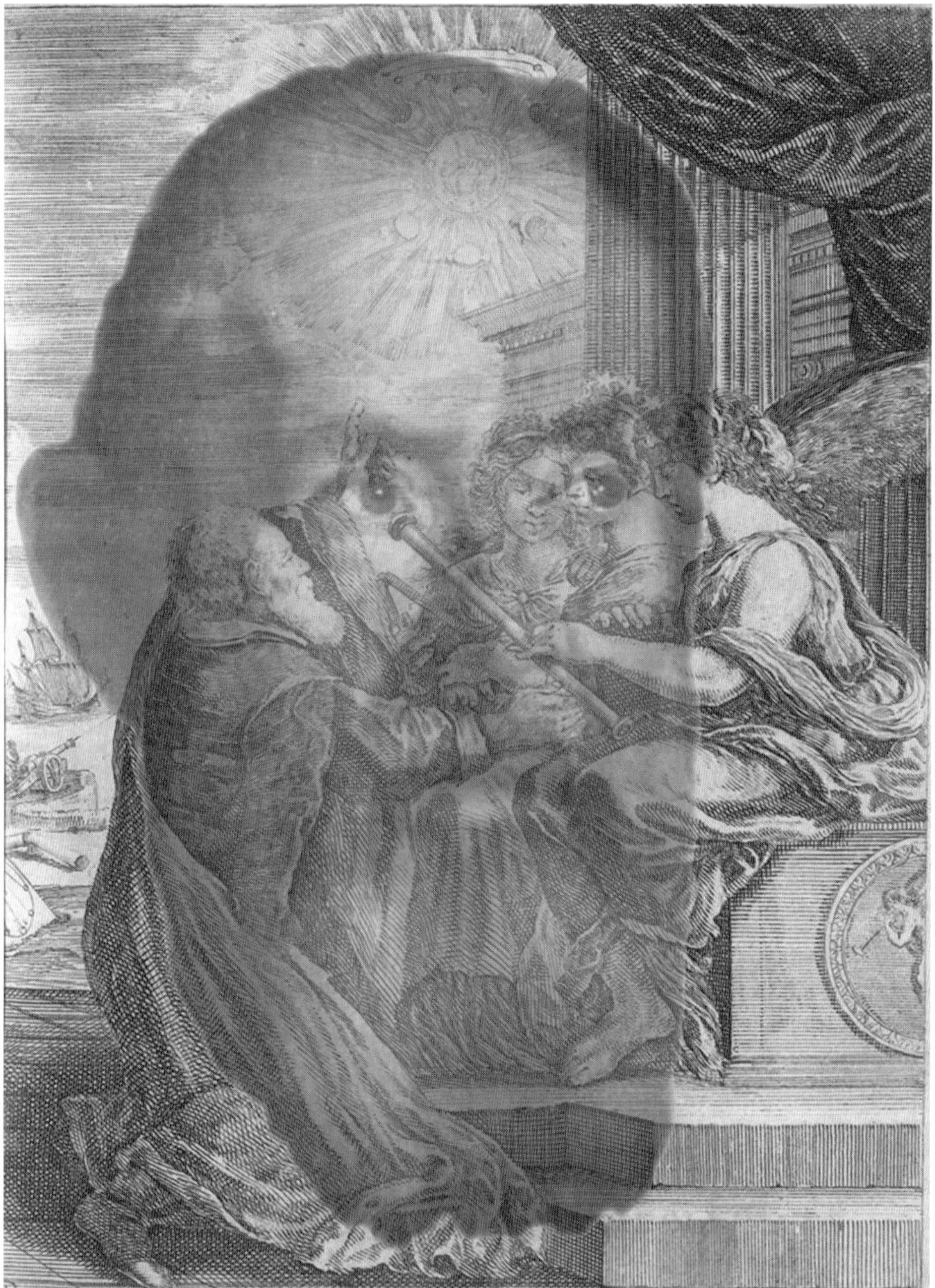

Frontispiece *Galileo's allegory* by Nicholas Wade. Galileo is represented twice. First in the engraving (from the frontispiece of *Opere di Galileo Galilei* directing his listeners to observe the heavens with the telescope. Secondly, in the large portrait (derived from the Pisa painting) with his right eye connecting the telescope and the pointing hand.

Credit: Frontispiece of 'Opere di Galileo Galilei', published in Bologna in 1656 (engraving) (b/w photo), Italian School, (17th century) / Bibliotheque Nationale, Paris, France / Archives Charmet / The Bridgeman Art Library.

Galileo's Visions
Piercing the spheres of the heavens by eye and mind

Marco Piccolino and Nicholas J. Wade

OXFORD
UNIVERSITY PRESS

OXFORD
UNIVERSITY PRESS

Great Clarendon Street, Oxford, OX2 6DP,
United Kingdom

Oxford University Press is a department of the University of Oxford. It furthers the University's objective of excellence in research, scholarship, and education by publishing worldwide. Oxford is a registered trade mark of Oxford University Press in the UK and in certain other countries

First Edition published in 2014

Impression: 1

Published in the United States of America by Oxford University Press
198 Madison Avenue, New York, NY 10016, United States of America

British Library Cataloguing in Publication Data
Data available

Library of Congress Control Number: 2013948632

ISBN 978–0–19–955435–5

Printed and bound by
CPI Group (UK) Ltd, Croydon, CR0 4YY

To Anna Maria and Christine

Preface

The endeavour of a book is necessarily connected to the encounter it may facilitate between those who read and those who write, or better, have written. This is because of the magic property of written words, capable—as they are—of maintaining an enduring possibility of communication, of potentially reaching persons distant in time and space. In this way written words differ from spoken words which once pronounced immediately fade away. The magic of the written word cannot be better praised than with the concluding sentences of the First Day of Galileo's *Dialogue concerning the two chief world systems*:

> But surpassing all stupendous inventions, what sublimity of mind was his who dreamed of finding means to communicate his deepest thoughts to any other person, though distant by mighty intervals of place and time! Of talking with those who are in India; of speaking to those who are not yet born and will not be born for a thousand or ten thousand years; and with what facility, by the different arrangements of twenty characters upon a page!
>
> Let this be the seal of all the admirable inventions of mankind and the close of our discussions for this day.

There are other aspects of the encounter, too, like that between the writers and their subjects, which can occur through a multiplicity of (often unpredictable) paths. In addition, when there are several authors the book will be influenced by the ways in which they encountered one another. In our case the project centres on Galileo, his science and especially his reflection on the senses. We can locate the origins of the book to a meeting we organized at the Villa di Corliano near Pisa, in the summer of 2006. The themes of the meeting, expressed in its title, *Galileo's Walks: Art, Science and Vision*, led us to deepen the knowledge of the work of Galileo, from a point of view that has rarely been dealt with in the current, very rich, literature on the Pisan scholar: that of the importance of his reflections on the senses in his endeavour that led to one of the greatest intellectual revolutions in Western civilization.

Both of us are interested in visual science from an experimental point of view (although from slightly different perspectives) but we were surprised to discover the extent to which Galileo's interest in the senses, and particularly in vision and its fallacies, was a recurring theme in his writings and how it was applied as a formidable intellectual tool in his discoveries, particularly those concerning astronomy. To our eyes, Galileo seemed to reveal himself in a novel light distinct from the many, and sometimes conflicting, representations accumulated in the course of history (great mathematician and astronomer, physicist and engineer, master in rhetoric and writer, hero, victim of religious intolerance or saint, philosopher or theologian, critic of arts or artist, practised courtesan or astrologer, plagiarist or liar).

Although conscious, as Michel de Montaigne wryly remarked, that Homer was unlikely to have said all the things attributed to him by subsequent interpreters, we hope that readers will feel that this unexpected image of Galileo as a physiologist (and also a philosopher) of the senses is justified.

Galileo loved to deal with science without any 'strictness' and we will follow his interests in the senses and science in the same spirit. We will make every effort to present our arguments with the support of Galileo's own words so that readers can come into direct contact with some of the most beautiful passages of European literature.

An editorial consequence of our choice will be that we will keep bibliographic reference to a minimum in the main part of the book. Only in the last chapters will we discuss in some detail the antecedents of Galileo's sensory science, trying to situate his endeavour within a definite historical context, with the consequence of a more scholarly treatment of the matter.

As we hope our book will make clear to readers, the interest of Galileo in senses, and particularly in vision, was tightly connected to all his science and philosophy. In particular it was an essential aspect of his reflection on the mechanisms by which humans acquire a knowledge of the world around them, and thus, a necessary step in their walk towards new visions of this world and a new situation within it.

M. Piccolino
N. J. Wade
September 2013

Acknowledgements

The authors wish to express their gratitude to their colleagues and friends who have contributed in various ways, with their discussions and help, to this book. Among them in particular, Michele Camerota, Giovanni Niccoli, Andrea Frova, Libero Sosio, Daniela Basile, and Giandomenico Giarnella. A special thanks to all the librarians and institutions that have helped us in the search of ancient and rare texts and especially to Livia Iannucci of the University of Pisa and Alessandra Lenzi of the Museum Galileo of Florence.

Contents

Bibliographic abbreviations

BNF GAL (followed by item number and folium number with the indication "r" or "v" for recto or verso respectively):	Galileo's manuscripts from the database of the Biblioteca Nazionale Centrale of Florence.
COMETE:	Galileo, G. & Guiducci, M. (1619). *Discorso delle comete di Mario Guiducci*. Firenze, Cecconcelli. English translation by S. Drake, *Discourse on the comets*, from *The controversy of the comets of 1618*. S. Drake & C. D. O'Malley eds. (1960) Philadelphia, PA, University of Pennsylvania Press, pp. 21–65.
DIALOGO:	Galilei, G. (1632). *Dialogo... sopra i due massimi sistemi del mondo Tolemaico, e Copernicano*. Firenze, Landini. English translation: Galilei, G. (1967). *Dialogue concerning the two chief world systems, Ptolemaic & Copernican*. S. Drake trans. Berkeley, CA, University of California Press.
ISTORIA:	Galilei, G. (1613). *Istoria e dimostrazioni intorno alle macchie solari e loro accidenti comprese in tre lettere scritte all'illustrissimo signor Marco Velseri*. Roma, Mascardi. English translation: Reeves, E. A. & Van Helden, A. (2010). *On sunspots*. Chicago, IL, University of Chicago Press.
LNB (followed by the volume number):	Leonardo da Vinci (1970). *The notebooks of Leonardo da Vinci/compiled and edited from the original manuscripts by Jean Paul Richter*. New York: Dover Publications.
MACULIS:	Scheiner, C. (1612). *Tres epistolæ de maculis solaribus: scriptæ ad Marcum Velserum*. Augustae Vindelicorum, Ad Insigne Pinus. English translation in: Reeves, E. A. & Van Helden, A. (2010). *On sunspots*. Chicago, IL, University of Chicago Press.
MAURI:	Galilei, G. *Considerazioni d'Alimberto Mauri sopra alcuni luoghi del discorso di Ludovico delle Colombe intorno alla stella apparita 1604*. Firenze, Caneo. English translation: *Consideration of Alimberto Mauri on some places of the discourse of Lodovico delle Colombe about the star which appeared in 1604*; from: Drake, S. (1976). *Galileo against the philosophers in his Dialogue of Cecco di Ronchitti (1605) and Considerations of Alimberto Mauri (1606)*. Los Angeles, CA, Zeitlin & Ver Brugge, pp. 73–130.
OG (followed by the volume number):	Galilei, G. (1890–1909). *Le opere di Galileo Galilei. Edizione nazionale*. A. Favaro ed., 20 vols. Firenze, Barbèra.
OPTICA:	Kepler, J. (1604). *Ad Vitellionem paralipomena, quibus astronomiae pars optica traditur....* Francofurti, Apud Claudium Marnium & Haeredes Ioannis Aubrii. English translation: Kepler, J. (2000). *Optics: Paralipomena to Witelo & optical part of astronomy*. W. H. Donahue ed. Santa Fe, NM, Green Lion Press.
PENSIERI:	Sarpi, P. (1996). *Pensieri naturali, metafisici e matematici*. Luisa Cozzi & Libero Sosio eds. Milano, Ricciardi.
RONCHITTI:	*Dialogo de Cecco di Ronchitti da Bruzene in perpuosito de la stella nuova*. Padova, Tozzi. English translation in: *Dialogue concerning the new star by Cecco di Ronchtti of Brugine* from: Drake, S. (1976). *Galileo against the philosophers in his Dialogue of Cecco di Ronchitti (1605) and Considerations of Alimberto Mauri (1606)*. Los Angeles, CA, Zeitlin & Ver Brugge, pp. 33–53.

SAGGIATORE:	Galilei, G. (1623). *Il Saggiatore…* Roma, Mascardi. English translation by S. Drake: *The assayer*; from *The controversy of the comets of 1618*. S. Drake & C. D. O'Malley eds. (1960) Philadelphia, PA, University of Pennsylvania Press, pp. 51–336.
SIDEREUS:	Galilei, G. (1610). *Sidereus nuncius…* Venezia Baglioni. English translation in: Galilei, G. (1989). *Sidereus nuncius, or, The Sidereal messenger*. A. Van Helden ed. Chicago, IL, University of Chicago Press.
TOO (followed by the volume number):	Brahe, T. (1913). *Tychonis Brahe Dani Opera omnia*. J. L. E. Dreyer, ed. Hauniæ, in Libraria Gyldendaliana.

January ten, sixteen ten:
Galileo Galilei abolishes heaven.

(Bertolt Brecht, *Life of Galileo*)

Introduction

History, at the levels of human groups as well as of individuals, is made up of episodes involving the predictable and the unexpected. The protagonist of this book, a professor of 'mathematics' in Padua, was a brilliant scientist with an aversion to formalism and an attraction to literature and art. For such a person, it was likely that he would make some important scientific discoveries in his chosen fields of experimental physics, and particularly mechanics and motion. As normally happens in science, his discoveries and theories would become submerged in 'the vast ocean of universal science' (as an astute Spanish neuroanatomist put it) and his name would be lost forever, except for a few specialists and perhaps a few historians of science.

A longsighted butterfly arrives to Venice

Nothing like that happened to Galileo, nothing at least after an event, around the middle of 1609, which created a stir between Venice and Padua. Venice was then the chief town of the *Serenissima* republic to which Padua belonged and Galileo frequented it with some assiduity, enjoying its splendours and stimulation. He was welcomed in its intellectual society because of his intelligence and witty conversation and was a guest in many of the magnificent palaces along the Grand Canal. What happened in 1609 was the arrival of an optical instrument consisting of two lenses mounted at the extremities of a rather long tube so that 'one can see far away up to 25 and 30 miles so clearly, that things appear as if they were present in front of us—as they say'.

Despite the excitement caused in Venetian society by this instrument, its properties were perhaps not so extraordinary as they transpired from the words (just quoted) from a note sent to the Court of Florence by the secretary of the Tuscan ambassador in Venice. In a letter written about one month earlier by a Venetian scholar, father Paolo Sarpi of the Order of Servites, the instrument was deemed of no particular practical application, even if it was to be admired 'for the beauty of the invention and for the dignity of the art'.

The amazing instrument (given a variety of names like *occhiali in canna*, *cannone*, etc.) attracted the attention of Sarpi's friend, Galileo, who improved its functions, mainly through an intense technical work aimed at improving the optical quality of the lenses (an endeavour undoubtedly favoured by the great experience of Venetian craftsmen in working glass). Eventually, Galileo pointed his instruments toward the sky.

Like the flutter of butterfly wings, said to be capable of producing a hurricane in distant places, the arrival of the *occhiali in canna* in Venice and Padua became the crucial event that changed the life of this brilliant but obscure university professor. Galileo was then 45, having been born in 1564 Pisa, the town with the famous leaning tower. By using the telescope between autumn 1609 and the first months of the next year, he was able to make a series of amazing astronomical discoveries which changed the course of his life. Moreover, they projected him onto the world's stage, where he has remained centuries after his death never to be forgotten. It could be said that the events following Galileo's first astronomical use of the telescope changed the history of the world.

To have an idea of the interest aroused by Galileo's small book (entitled *Sidereus nuncius*) published in Venice on 13 March 1610, which described the initial discoveries made with his new instrument it suffices to say that it sold out very rapidly, with copies rapidly reaching all the centres of European culture. On the very day of its publication a copy was sent by the English ambassador in Venice, Sir Henry Wotton, to King James. The diplomatic parcel contained an accompanying letter addressed to Sir Robert Cecil, Count of Salisbury, where Wotton commented on the discoveries announced in the book that he had been reading with the alacrity and rapidity generally devoted to extremely urgent and important diplomatic affairs, the pages still smelling of the fresh ink:

> Now touching the occurrents of present, I send herewith unto His Majesty the strangest piece of news (as I may justly call it) that he has ever yet received from any part of the world; which is the annexed book (come abroad this very day) of the Mathematical Professor at Padua, who by the help of an optical instrument (which both enlargeth and approximateth the object) invented first in Flanders and bettered by himself, hath discovered four new planets rolling around the sphere of Jupiter, besides many other unknown fixed stars; likewise the true cause of the Via Lactea [Milky Way], so long searched; and lastly that the moon is not spherical but endued with many prominences, and, which is strangest of all, illuminated with the solar light by reflection from the body of the earth, as he seemeth to say. So as upon the whole subject, he hath overthrown all former astronomy [...] And the author runneth a fortune to be either exceeding famous or exceeding ridiculous. By the next ship your Lordship shall receive from me one of the above instruments, as it is bettered by this man. (Smith, 1907, pp. 486–487)

Even though expressed with some diplomatic caution, the discoveries announced by Galileo were indeed amazing, and—if true—capable of upsetting 'all former astronomy'. For several months some harsh arguments were set against the astronomical novelties announced in *Sidereus*, and centuries were needed before the physical and philosophical implications of the astronomical revolution fostered by Galileo's discoveries were accepted by the most conservative institutions (and particularly by the Catholic Church). This notwithstanding, what happened was that 'the author runneth a fortune to become exceedingly famous', to paraphrase Sir Henry's words.

This was because these discoveries, and particularly 'the four new planets rolling around the sphere of Jupiter', the fact that 'the moon is not spherical but endued with many prominences, and, which is strangest of all, illuminated with the solar light by reflection from the body of the earth' (together with other subsequent surprising observations, like those concerning the appearance of Venus and the presence of spots on the surface of the sun) really were such to have 'overthrown all former astronomy' and perhaps not only astronomy.

Changing life's agenda

Galileo seemed to have only a modest interest in astronomy in the first part of his scientific life but he soon grasped the implications of his telescopic observations. They supported the revolutionary and 'upsetting' conception of the world presented by the Polish astronomer Nicolaus Copernicus in 1543. Against the traditional cosmological doctrine of Aristotle and Ptolemy based on the centrality of the earth, Copernicus had developed a model in which the centre of the world was occupied by the sun and the earth and other planets were supposed to revolve around it. However, despite several astronomical observations made since the second half of the sixteenth century against geocentric cosmology, the Copernican system had been enjoying only modest success. By many it was considered only as a mathematical tool, useful for predicting the movement of planets, but without any real implications for the true constitution of the world. This was mainly because it was difficult to account for a series of objections against the movement of earth, a fundamental implication of the Copernican theory and a crucial difference with respect to old cosmology. If earth were to move—it was argued—we should perceive the effects in various ways. Birds or clouds would be transported toward the west due to the rapid eastward motion of earth; in an analogous way, a stone dropped from the top of a tower would fall in a westward direction; finally because of the centrifugal consequences of the motion, objects would tend to leave the ground and rise up toward the sky with ruinous effects for animals and buildings.

The reasons why Galileo was strongly attracted by the news about the *occhiali* coming from Flanders, and was then ready to realize the revolutionary implications of his telescopic observations were related to his ongoing studies on motion. In the previous years he had been finalizing a theory of motion based on the principle of inertia which allowed him to account for why a terrestrial observer would be insensitive to the motion of earth, even if this was moving at a fast speed as implied by the Copernican model. As Galileo proceeded with his investigations he became increasingly interested in astronomy even though he had some reluctance to deal with this field in public; he was reluctant to express the Copernican option he had been adopting probably since an early age. Following the appearance of a new star in October 1604, he published two astronomical pamphlets under pseudonyms; they were strongly critical of the traditional cosmological model while expressing some cryptic and ambiguous preference for the model of Copernicus.

As we shall see in Chapter 2, in many respects Galileo's telescopic observations had deep revolutionary implications with respect to traditional astronomy. They were not only undermining a long-established theory but they also implied a radical revision of the relationship between humans and the world.

With the publication of *Sidereus nuncius*, Galileo's scientific life and the propagation of his ideas changed dramatically. In order to develop his new programme, he left Padua and moved to Florence, placing himself under the protection of the Grand Duke of Tuscany. He could dedicate himself entirely to scientific investigations free from the heavy academic engagements of Padua.

Galileo had soon realized that a conception like the cosmology of Aristotle and Ptolemy, which had been retained for millennia despite the relatively poor correspondence between its astronomical predictions and the actual observations of planetary motions, could not be overturned simply by providing new scientific data in support of the Copernican system. What was needed was also a philosophical reflection on human psychology. This should focus on the mechanisms of knowledge acquisition and on the reasons why humans tend to establish theories based on faith rather than on sensory appearances and evidence from scientific experiments and logical reasoning.

Besides obliging Galileo to deepen his philosophical reflection on these themes, the new agenda generated an important change in his communication strategies. One was the use of Italian, a language that certainly he mastered better than Latin (the language of *Sidereus nuncius* and of his academic texts) and which allowed him to address his intellectual elaborations outside the rather restricted circles of academic and official culture. In 1612, he justified this decision with reference to his first letter on sunspots written in Italian, and also to a recently published short treatise on floating bodies: 'I have written it in the common tongue because I have the need that every person could read it, and for the same reason I have written in the same idiom this last small treatise of mine' (OG XI, p. 327). This was—he added—because also persons unacquainted with Latin 'could see that nature, in the same way has given them the eyes to see its own works, has also given to them the brain to intend and understand them, and this not only to *filuorici*' (a term in the dialect of Padua meaning philosophers, and used here with a clear pejorative connotation).

The use of Italian allowed Galileo to raise the level of his prose, an important aspect of his communication strategy which was instrumental for the diffusion of the fruits of his intellectual work to a large audience. Another dimension of this strategy was the use of the dialogue form in his writings. This would be explicit in his two main masterpieces, the *Dialogo sopra i due massimi sistemi del mondo* (*Dialogue concerning the two chief world systems*), published in 1632, and the *Discorsi e dimostrazioni matematiche intorno a due nuove scienze* (*Discourses and mathematical demonstrations concerning two new sciences*) published in 1638.

In both these works the dialogue is between three people, two of whom bear the name of Galileo's friends. One is Filippo Salviati, a Florentine gentleman who plays the role of the supporter of the new science, and is in fact the spokesman of the author. The other is Giovanfrancesco Sagredo, a Venetian aristocrat, open to the new ideas as well as being intelligent and intuitive. The third person plays the role of the defender of the traditional science, and particularly of the doctrines of Aristotle and his followers. Although possibly inspired by a contemporary, his allusive name, Simplicio, was derived from that of a famous commentator of Aristotle's works, Simplicius of Cilicia, who lived between the fifth and sixth century AD.

In addition to being more attractive for the reader, the dialogue form had a didactic valence and allowed Galileo to elaborate about the reasons for the resistance to the new science and for the uncritical acceptance of ancient doctrines. In an implicit or explicit way dialogues were present in some other works, starting with two pamphlets published in 1605 and 1606 in a pseudonymous form, in his dissertational letters on sunspots published in 1613, in *Saggiatore* ('Assayer') published 10 years later, in the *Discorsi e dimostrazioni matematiche*, and also in his last scientific work, the letter on the lunar candour published in 1640 (two years before his death). The *Dialogue* and *Saggiatore* are texts of great relevance for the main theme of our book, that of Galileo's interest in the senses, and we will discuss them in some detail in the next chapters.

This theme also emerges in Galileo's private correspondence, and particularly from a letter he sent in September 1611 to Christoph Grienberger, professor of mathematics in the Collegium Romanun (the University of Jesuits), which we also consider in detail in this book. As we shall see, this poorly studied document is perhaps the text in which Galileo develops his more acute reflection on the meaning and limits of vision.

Although vision was the main theme of reflection within Galileo's elaboration on senses, his interest was not limited to visual mechanisms. It was more general and involved a 'philosophical' reflection on the relationship between the senses and the external world. This reflection, expounded in some important pages, implied a profound transformation of the sensory centrality of humans with respect to the world.

For Aristotle, and for the prevailing philosophical conceptions of the classical era, the world was continuously sending sensory messages in forms particularly adapted to senses. In other words, sensations like colours, odours, sounds are objective realities that exist in the external world and finalized to senses generally, and to human senses in particular. This was an important aspect of the general finalism of Aristotelian philosophy, which in the Middle Ages was incorporated in the idea of a providential God, governing the world for the salvation of humankind. However, finalism was not the principle of all classical philosophy. Among those who denied it (and rejected the idea of providential Deities interested in human destiny) the atomists were particularly important. That is, the Greek and Roman philosophers who saw the world as due to the encounter of minute elements continuously moving under the agency of more or less casual forces. Lucretius expounded his particular atomistic view in a poetic form through his masterwork *De rerum natura*. It is no surprise therefore if, in his effort to substitute the classical human-oriented cosmos with an entirely new vision in which humans would occupy a more peripheral position, Galileo would make recourse to atomism. This conception, which was judged deeply heretical by the Church, would play a fundamental role in the scientific revolution of the seventeenth century. It would also be the background for the revolution operated by Galileo in the 'philosophy' of senses, an important, although neglected, aspect of the scientific revolution of the seventeenth century.

No wonder that the deep philosophical (and theological) implications of Galileo's intellectual revolution eventually led to a conflict with the religious authorities. This was together with his decision to write in Italian, addressing a vast readership beyond the restricted limits of the academic and scientific circles, also by using a style of high literary level in order to achieve this. It was the basis of the so-called 'Galileo's affair', perhaps the event in Galileo's life that attracts the attention of laymen. The words that Galileo wrote on the relation between science and religion are still topical because there remains conflict between scientific knowledge and the power of the religious authorities.

Coming to the main theme of our book, we could say (pursuing the theme of the butterfly capable of producing hurricanes) that the arrival in Venice from Flanders of the *occhiale*, not only led to the overthrow of the old astronomy, but it also upset the traditional vision of the senses, laying the foundations for modern sensory physiology.

Chapter 1

Approaching Galileo's science through a fable

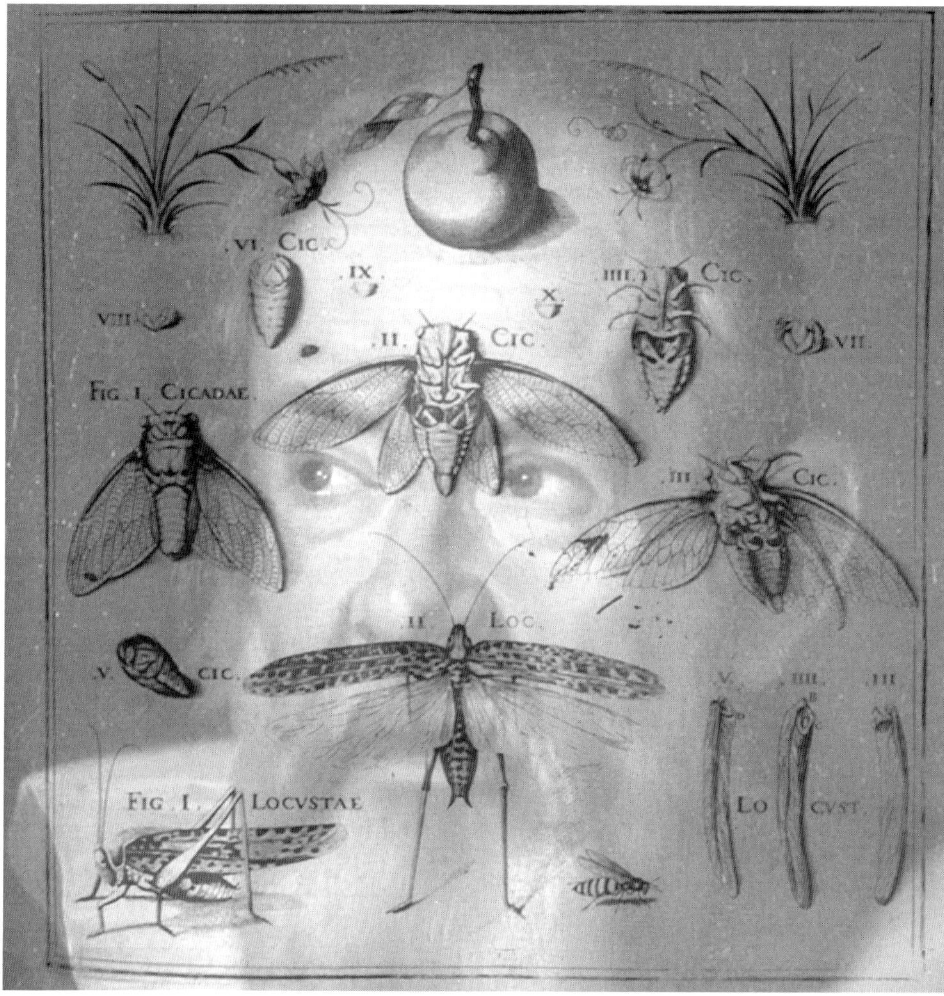

Figure I *The lure of the locust* by Nicholas Wade. Galileo's portrait is derived from the Pisa painting and is combined with an engraving of sound-producing insects from *De vocis auditusque organis historia anatomica* published in 1600 by Giulio Casseri. For some of the illustrated insects the anatomical structures supposedly responsible for the generation of sound are shown. Casseri, a student of Fabricius ab Aquapendente (and later a rival, and like him—and also Galileo—a professor in Padua), was particularly interested in the larynx and the other organs involved in the production of sounds in humans and animals; he developed the analogy between these physiological processes of sound production and the functioning of musical instruments.

1.1 Comets, balances, masques, and apple cores

Before commencing on the specific theme of our book, in this first chapter we would like to present an image of the ways Galileo deals with science which are, in our view, largely unexpected. We will present this through some of Galileo's more beautiful texts, where his approach reveals some of the charm and passion of the scientific endeavour.

In addition to a short quotation from his masterpiece, *Dialogue concerning the two chief systems of the world*, published in 1632 (from now on referred to simply as the *Dialogue*), we will present some selections from his polemic pamphlet, *Il Saggiatore* ('The assayer'), the title page of which carries Galileo's portrait in Figure 1.1. Galileo published *Saggiatore* in 1623 in response to attacks from the Jesuit, Horatio Grassi, in his *Libra astronomica ac philosophica* ('Astronomical and philosophical balance',[1] published in 1619: Grassi, 1619b). The controversy, which had its origins before publication of Grassi's *Libra*, would continue well after Galileo's *Saggiatore* was printed. It concerned the nature of comets and was stimulated by the observation of three comets in the second

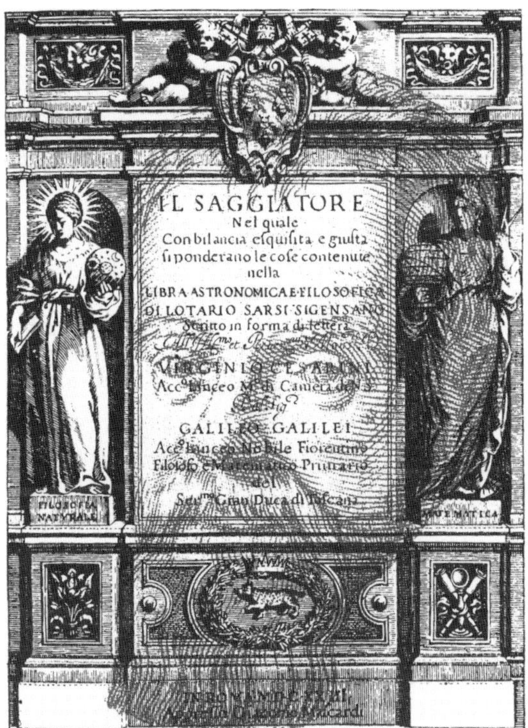

Figure 1.1 *Galileo's Assayer* by Nicholas Wade. Galileo's portrait is derived from the painting by Francesco Villamena and is framed by the frontispiece of Galileo's *Il Saggiatore*. In this book he developed the philosophical background for the new approach to the senses.

Credit: Frontispiece of 'The Assayer' by Galileo Galilei, 1623 (engraving), Villamena, Francesco (1566–1624) / Private Collection / Photo © Christie's Images / The Bridgeman Art Library.

[1] The word *Libra* meaning principally the balance by which pondering, in a metaphorical way, astronomical and philosophical arguments also alluded to the constellation of Libra, which was implied in the discussion between Galileo and Grassi.

half of 1618; these were considered by many to herald sad tidings for Europe which was troubled by a long series of fierce and bloody wars.

Galileo had been urged by various members of his circle to reply to Grassi, who wrote the *Libra* under the pseudonym Lothario Sarsi Sigensano (an imperfect anagram of Horatio Grassio Salonensi, the last term containing a cryptic allusion to Savona, the town near Genoa where the Jesuit was born in 1583). Galileo was, however, reluctant to do that. There were certainly political reasons for his reluctance, because some years earlier the chief of the Holy Office, Cardinal Bellarmino, had discouraged him from treating astronomical matters publicly. There was also the problem that Galileo had not studied the 1618 comets in the detail he would have wished. This was mainly due to health problems which had prevented him from undertaking the long and painstaking observations necessary for a thorough analysis of these intriguing celestial events.

In point of fact, the hypothesis expounded in *Saggiatore* is largely erroneous; it assumed that comets were not material bodies and that their appearance was due to some sort of optical illusion. That is, Galileo considered that it was a visual phenomenon similar to those responsible for the aurora borealis, various kinds of iridescences, or the luminescence appearing at sunrise and sunset due to the reflection of the sun on the wavy surface of the sea.

Despite the flawed character of Galileo's hypothesis on the nature of comets, *Saggiatore* remains one of his most interesting texts and one undoubtedly capable of exerting a strong attraction on readers. This is due partly to the power of its polemical style, which oscillates between polite irony and pitiless sarcasm. It is particularly important for the clear enunciation of a new way to conduct science and especially for the pages in which Galileo develops a critical analysis of the senses as sources of knowledge; this he does by distinguishing between two attributes of the sensory world which were later characterized as primary and secondary qualities of sensation (see Chapter 10).

Galileo's Italian prose is rich and lively, quickly moving from one stylistic device to another; this accounts in large measure for the literary charm of *Saggiatore*. His prose contrasts with the pedantic Latin of the propositions in Grassi's *Libra*. These are reported serially and confuted one by one, in a contrapuntist movement, which anticipates the dialogues of Galileo's masterpieces. There is, moreover, the rhetorical mastery with which Galileo succeeds in unmasking the tangled ploys of his antagonist, and of a science still based on the authority of ancients and on the arguments of a logic incapable of confronting reality.

There is also Galileo's sophisticated adoption of the game of roles, according to a custom typical of a world characterized by baroque rituals. It is a game he uses to extend from inside the intellectual range of his age. Galileo does not direct his cutting remarks to Horatio Grassi, but he addresses him indirectly through Virginio Cesarini, a young Roman aristocrat and fellow of the Accademia dei Lincei. This was the intellectual society founded at the beginning of the century by Federico Cesi to promote a scientific, cultural, and moral renewal of Catholicism. Cesarini was also an important Vatican prelate, very close to Pope Urban VIII. Galileo's choice of Cesarini as interlocutor in the polemic with Grassi was intended to place *Saggiatore* under the Pope's protection. As a matter of fact, in 1623, the year of publication of *Saggiatore*, Maffeo Barberini ascended to the papal throne; he was a Tuscan from a merchant family of Florence, and a great admirer of Galileo. His arrival encouraged hope for a relaxation of the conservative climate dominating the scientific and cultural vision of the Church, particularly in the field of astronomy (and especially in connection with the censorship on discussions of the Copernican system).

The game of roles developed by Galileo in *Saggiatore* is indeed very elaborate and refined. Despite the authorial pseudonymity of *Libra*, Galileo knows who his antagonist is, and he overtly admits his supposition that Lothario Sarsi is only a mask hiding some important scholar. However, in *Saggiatore* he never names Grassi directly and writes that he wishes to adopt this attitude in order to avail himself 'of the privilege accorded in masquerades' to 'deal with them freely', without the restraint and reserve required when speaking face to face with distinguished people. Indeed, in his personal copy of Grassi's *Libra*, Galileo had written the following marginal note: 'Having Sarsi wear a masque will be a big prejudice for him; this is because in masquerades one can throw small apples and apple-cores [*meluzze e torsi*] even though they are princes' (SAGGIATORE p. 9; transl. p. 170). As we shall see, in *Saggiatore* Grassi will be the target of much worse than '*meluzze e torsi*'.

1.2 The 'fable of sounds': Nature's many manifestations

The 'fable of sounds' is one of Galileo's most enchanting and famous texts. Perhaps it should be said that it is famous among the circle of those who have really read Galileo, a circle certainly more restricted than those who pretend to speak about him, several philosophers in particular.[2] Among the readers of this fable was Pope Urban VIII who was so fascinated by this text that it was his wish to hear it read to him several times a day. In the nineteenth century, among the interested readers was Giacomo Leopardi, one of the greatest Italian poets, who inserted Galileo's fable in his anthology of literary and scientific texts, the *Crestomazia italiana*, first published in 1827.

Galileo's fable is replete with suggestions and motifs, as is often the case with great literature, and it is open to many different interpretations. Before presenting it we should outline the richness of Galileo's style. It is capable of moving across different registers—from scientific treatise to an open dialogue between science and literature, to the polemical discourse which is dominant in *Saggiatore*, but also present in many of his texts.

Inserted in the tissue of *Saggiatore*, among the lively and sometimes very harsh attacks on Grassi, the fable of sounds also performs the literary function of reducing the reader's tension. With the variation of the narrative rhythm it creates, it surprises readers and takes them far away from the polemic pages of a controversy on comets (and on other aspects of science), towards the territory of fairy tales. We are stimulated to follow the singular voyage of 'a man endowed by nature with a very perspicacious mind and an extraordinary curiosity' (*un uomo dotato da natura d'uno ingegno perspicacissimo e d'una curiosità straordinaria*), who tries to understand the various ways in which sounds are generated, starting from the 'delicate' sound emitted from the instrument played by a shepherd boy and ending with the 'very strident sound' (*altissimo stridore*) produced by a cicada (Figure 1.2).

From *Saggiatore*:

> Long experience has taught me that with regard to intellectual matters, this is the status of mankind: The less people know and understand about such matters, the more positively they attempt to reason[3] about them, and on the other hand the number of things known and understood renders them more cautious in passing judgement about anything new.
>
> There once lived,[4] in a very solitary place, a man endowed by nature with a very perspicacious mind and an extraordinary curiosity. He raised many birds as a hobby, much enjoying their songs, and he used to observe with great admiration the happy contrivance by which they would transform at will the very air they breathed into a variety of very sweet songs. It happened one night that close to his house

---

2 Among them is the German philosopher Edmund Husserl who dedicates a large part of his book *Krisis* to a criticism of Galileo, based on a very superficial and largely indirect knowledge of his writings.

3 In Galileo's prose the original term *discorrere* has a variety of meanings and connotations. It means 'to speak, to talk', but also—and mainly—'to reason', 'to argument', and sometimes even 'to demonstrate'.

4 The start of the narration, as also the beginning in the next sentence ('It happened one night') serves to introduce the reader into a fairy-tale atmosphere.

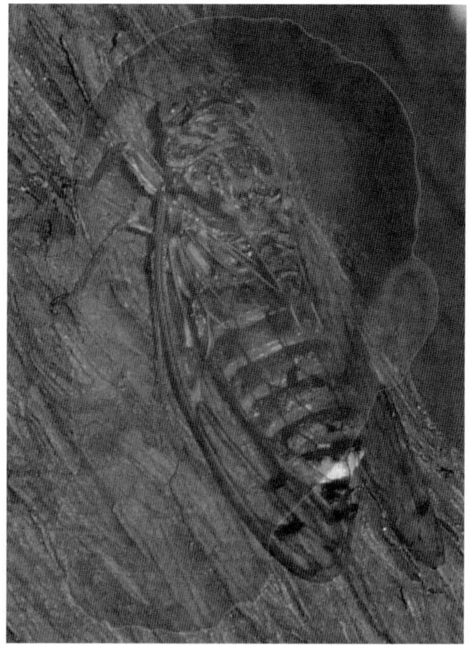

Figure 1.2 *Galileo and the cicada* by Nicholas Wade. A photograph of a cicada taken on Monte Pisano (a place familiar to Galileo) is combined with Galileo's attentive features. The portrait of Galileo is based upon a painting by Filippo Furini, also known as Pippo Sciamerone (see Tongiorgi Tomasi, 2005).

he chanced to hear a delicate sound, and, being unable to imagine what it could be except some small bird, he set out to capture it.

Arriving at the road, he found a shepherd boy who was blowing into a kind of hollow stick and moving his fingers about on the wood, thus drawing from it a variety of notes similar to those of a bird, though by quite a different method. Astonished, and led on by his natural curiosity, he gave the boy a calf in exchange for his whistle [*zufolo*][5] and retired to solitude. Realizing that if he had not chanced to meet the boy he would never have learned of the existence of two methods for forming musical notes and very sweet songs, he tried traveling far from his home in the hope of meeting with some new adventure. The very next day he happened to pass near a small hut, and, hearing a similar tone within, he went inside to find out whether it was a whistle or a blackbird. There he found a boy holding a bow in his right hand and sawing upon some fibres[6] stretched upon a concave piece of wood. The fingers of the left hand (which supported the instrument) were moving, and without blowing the boy was drawing from it various notes, and most sweet ones too. Now, you who are participating in this man's intelligence and sharing in his curiosity, judge his astonishment![7] Finding himself to have two unexpected

5 Notice the economic disproportion in the exchange between the shepherd boy and the man interested in the sounds of birds. This is also a way for Galileo to show how scientific endeavour is not primarily intended to acquire richness and material advantages.

6 *Nervi* (nerves) in the original.

7 These words addressed directly by the narrator to his listeners serve also to qualify the readership to which the *Saggiatore* is addressed, one made of people rich in curiosity and intelligence (*ingegno* in the original, meaning intelligence, ingenuity, and similar).

> new ways of forming tones and melodies, he began to believe that still others might exist in nature. His wonder increased when upon entering a certain temple he glanced behind the gates to learn what it was that had sounded, and perceived that the noise had emanated from the hinges and fastenings as he had opened the gate. Again, impelled by curiosity, he entered an inn expecting to see someone lightly bowing the strings of a violin, and instead saw a man rubbing the tip of his finger round the rim of a goblet and drawing forth from it a very sweet sound. And later he observed that wasps, mosquitoes, and flies did not form separate notes from their breaths, as did his original birds, but made steady tones by the swift beating of their wings. In proportion as his amazement grew, his belief diminished that he knew how sounds were created; nor could all his previous experience have sufficed to make him understand or even believe that crickets, which do not fly, could draw their sweet and sonorous shrilling not from breath but from a scraping of wings. And when he had almost come to believe that there could be no further ways of forming notes-after having observed in addition to what has been recounted numerous organs, trumpets, fifes, stringed instruments of various sorts, and even that little iron tongue which when placed between the teeth makes strange use of the buccal cavity as a sounding box and of the breath as a vehicle of sound-when,[8] I say, he believed that he had seen everything, he found himself more than ever wrapped in ignorance and bafflement upon capturing in his hand a cicada, for neither by closing its mouth nor by stopping its wings could he diminish its intensely strident sound, and yet he could not see it move either its scales or any other parts.[9] At length, lifting up the armor of its chest and seeing beneath this some thin, hard ligaments, he believed that the sound was coming from a shaking of these, and he resolved to break them in order to silence it. But everything failed until, driving the needle too deep, he transfixed the creature and took away its life with its voice, so that even then he could not make sure whether the song had originated in those ligaments. Thereupon he was reduced to such diffidence on his understanding that when asked how sounds are generated he used to reply tolerantly that although he knew some of the ways, he was certain that many more existed which were unknown and unimaginable. (SAGGIATORE, pp. 94–96; transl. pp. 234–236 slightly revised)

1.3 **Reflections on a fable**

For people reading *Saggiatore*, the surprise encounter with the characters and rhythm of a fairy tale (intermixed as we know within the argumentative pages of polemics on comets) is accompanied by other elements that would not be expected by Galileo's readers, particularly modern ones. For many, the reference to Galileo and to his science evokes the scientific revolution of the seventeenth century, and the idea of a science which arrives (through experiments and logical reasoning) at crystal-clear and indubitable knowledge. It calls to mind the picture of a universe regulated by well-defined rules and knowledge for anybody provided with adequate investigation tools, according to the metaphor of the world as an open book, which is presented in its best known version in *Saggiatore*. When speaking about philosophy (a word meaning science and knowledge in a wide sense) Galileo writes:

> Philosophy is written in this grand book, I mean the universe, which stands continually open to our gaze. But it cannot be understood unless one first learns to comprehend the language and comprehend the characters in which it is written. It is written in the language of mathematics, and its characters are triangles, circles, and other geometric figures, without which it is humanly impossible to understand a single word of it; without these one is wandering about in a dark labyrinth. (SAGGIATORE, p. 25; transl. pp. 183–184)

---

[8] The instrument corresponds in this case to the Jew's harp.

[9] In Galileo's epoch the mechanism of sound production in a variety of insects was sufficiently known due to the great interest in the matter of anatomists and natural philosophers. For a modern vision of the subject—and particularly for the song production in cicadas—see Haskell (1960) and Young and Bennet-Clark (1995).

The allusion to the 'language of mathematics' (*lingua matematica*), to the 'characters' that correspond to 'geometric figures', strengthens the idea of Galileo as the scientist of certainties, ready to hypostasize scientific knowledge to mathematical certainty (with its character of logical absoluteness, according to the modern acceptance of the word 'mathematics'). This scientific paradigm has long been exalted as that to which all sectors of knowledge should eventually conform. As such, Galilean science has been considered as a science of the past, rigid and incapable of confronting new forms of knowledge. Four centuries after Galileo we discover in physics (a territory traditionally considered as Galilean) and in other fields as well (biology, meteorology, geology, and various social sciences) phenomena that cannot be referred to physically determined mechanisms which are knowledgeable in an absolute way (and thus to the paradigms considered as typical of Galileo's science).

With relation to this rather simplistic way of considering Galileo and his science, this 'fable of sounds' creates many difficulties and raise many questions, and its apparently sceptical conclusion might seem founded on the presupposition of unknowability with respect to reality.

A conclusion like this based on the apparently literal sense of this text, of Galileo as a sceptical thinker, would lead to an opposite error which is as misleading as that of Galileo as the scientist of certainty. As already mentioned, he did not have the opportunity of accurately observing the comets which appeared in the second half of 1618, and he was therefore not in a position to provide a satisfactory theory capable of accounting for the nature of these celestial bodies. This interpretation is supported by a marginal annotation written by Galileo in his personal copy of Grassi's *Libra* (and also inserted in *Saggiatore* as a comment to the fable). With reference to a popular saying, Galileo wrote ironically: 'I tell you that I have the cicada in my hand, and I don't know how she sings; but I can well speak about the comet'. The fable of sounds could simply be a literary *divertissement* (on a theme suggested by a popular saying), due to the condition of justified uncertainty, directed against somebody who pretends to be speaking about distant and difficult matters, when, in the evidence of facts, he is incapable of grasping the meaning of matters just in front of him. That said, the narration seems to communicate, in the allegorical language of a fable, some of the fundamental aspects of the way in which Galileo conceives the scientific enterprise and, more generally, the voyage leading humans to knowledge.

It is indeed a voyage. It is not by chance that the protagonist decides to leave his home, when, as a consequence of the encounter with the shepherd boy, he realizes that if he remained in his 'very solitary place' he would not learn the various ways in which sounds are produced in nature. Besides the 'very suave songs' of his birds, there are other sounds intentionally produced by artificial instruments of different construction and mechanism, and even those unintentionally emanating 'from the hinges and fastenings' of the temple gate. And also those produced by other animals, in a way very different from that of his beloved birds.

As happens on all voyages, the path to knowledge is open to adventures and unexpected discoveries, sometimes beyond the limits of established categories and predefined mental schemes. It can thus induce wonder and amazement, but nevertheless it might not prevent us from discovering what we are looking for in a simple and direct way. It is an open path, and those who advance through it discover the richness and variety, but also the complexity, of the ways in which nature operates. As they progress further in knowledge, they become progressively aware of the much that remains to be discovered. It also takes them to the Socratic awareness that they know nothing. On the other hand, those who do not feel the need to begin their voyage of knowledge will try vainly to subjugate the variety of natural phenomena to their a priori schemes.[10]

Not even in the works of his maturity does Galileo pretend to have found a new system of knowledge and therefore he does not attempt to present new truths in a developmental way. His intention is to open a new path towards the knowledge of reality. On the one hand he reassures us, through the metaphor of the 'book of universe', that nature can be known. On the other hand, he warns us that, in addition to wonders and surprises we can meet with difficulties and failures. This contributes to explaining Galileo's choice of the literary form of the dialogue, which is explicit in his two main works (the *Dialogue* of 1632 and the *Discorsi e dimostrazioni matematiche intorno a due nuove scienze* of 1638),[11] but appears also more or less implicitly in some earlier works.

In the *Dialogue*, knowledge emerges and develops from encounters between different and somewhat contrasting propositions, and sometimes the 'discourse' does not yield absolute certainties. Instead, it highlights new ways of investigation and research. In a somewhat analogous way (as well as in the fable of sounds) the voyage of knowledge begins after the chance encounter with someone; in this case, the researcher cannot arrive at knowledge if he remains confined in his home—'a very solitary place'.

The distinguishing characters of the protagonist of the new path of knowledge are indicated from the beginning: 'a very perspicacious mind and an extraordinary curiosity'. These features differentiate the inquisitive spirit of the new science with respect to traditional culture. Curiosity, an attribute generally considered as a reproachable vice in the philosophical and theological tradition of the Middle Ages, becomes for Galileo one of the emblems of the new science. The superlative *perspicacissimo* ('very perspicacious' from the Latin *perspicere*—to see through, to see beyond) refers to a visual metaphor. It contrasts the doubtful reliability of visual appearances in traditional culture; this is particularly the case with telescopic observations where visual perceptions cannot be confirmed by tactile sensations.

At the same time *perspicacissimo* evokes the telescope indicated as '*perspicillum*' in *Sidereus nuncius*, Galileo's first astronomical work,[12] published in 1610. In addition to being driven by curiosity, the figure of the fable is moved by *meraviglia* (wonder, marvel: a term that we found again in the fable together with other words belonging to the same semantic area as *stupefatto*—astonished, amazed—and *stupore*, amazement). For Galileo, discovery and knowledge are indeed characterized by a strong emotional dimension; in addition to wonder and amazement, we find in his work

[10] This theme appears in other works by Galileo and is particularly vibrant in the conclusion of the 'first day' of the *Dialogue*. Here Sagredo, the Venetian aristocrat who is one of the debaters, says: 'It always seems to me extreme rashness on the part of some when they want to make human abilities the measure of what nature can do and knows how to do. On the contrary, there is not a single effect in nature, even the least that exists, such that the most ingenious theorists [*i più specolativi ingegni*] can arrive at a complete understanding of it. This vain presumption of understanding everything can have no other basis than never understanding anything. For anyone who had experienced just once the perfect understanding of one single thing, and had truly tasted how knowledge is accomplished, would recognize that of the infinity of other truths he understands nothing' (DIALOGO, p. 94; transl. p. 101).

[11] 'Discourses and mathematical demonstrations relating to two new sciences...' from now on simply *Discourses*.

[12] As we shall see in Chapter 2, Galileo had already published two astronomical pamphlets, respectively in 1605 and 1606a, but in a pseudonymous form.

other expressions of a veritable pathos of knowledge: a new instrument can be 'admirable', 'human inventions' are 'to be admired' (*ammirande*), the conclusions of a mathematical demonstration can be 'full of marvel and delight', an observation can be *bellissima* (very beautiful), a phenomenon can be *meraviglioso* (marvellous), a thought *bellissimo*, properties of natural motions are *bellissime passioni* (very beautiful qualities), and the body of the moon appearing to the inquisitive gaze of a telescope is '*pulcherrimum atque visu iucundissimum*' ('very beautiful and extremely delightful to be seen').

Another feature of the protagonist of the fable is the delight he derives from his contacts with nature. This is also a distinguishing characteristic of the Galilean attitude to knowledge. He 'raised many birds as an amusement—*trastullo*—much enjoying their songs' which is a characteristic that insinuates a clear element of leisure in the endeavour of new science. Together with pleasure and delight, we find taste (*gusto*), which can be 'great' or even 'very great', to characterize repeatedly the phases of knowledge in many passages of the *Dialogue* and *Discourses*; this occurs particularly in the sayings of Sagredo, one of the three discussants. In the encounter between the man of the fable and the shepherd boy another attitude typical of the new scientific spirit emerges: the capability of deconstructing a newly encountered phenomenon and separating it into its various constitutive elements ('blowing into a kind of hollow stick and moving his fingers about on the wood, thus drawing from it a variety of notes'). This represent a new perceptive and inquisitive attitude, characteristic of scientific analysis, different from that typical of common observation, which allows us to look at things as if we were seeing them for the first time.

The final episode with the cicada raises a series of questions and leaves the reader somewhat puzzled: the insect dies after 'the armour of its chest' is pierced in an attempt to discover the mechanism of sound production. This alludes to the potentially destructive nature of scientific experiments. Certainly a very profound transformation has occurred in the experience of the 'very perspicacious' man since the time that he had been raising birds for his amusement and enjoyed listening to their songs. In contrast to the very melodic character of the initial bird songs, the cry emitted by the cicada is perceived as 'an intensely strident sound', a noise (*altissimo stridore, strepito*), that is no longer associated with the elements of melody and delight typical of bird songs. From a playful activity, the scientific enterprise changes its character becoming a complex investigation, with uncertain results, needing an active and potentially destructive intervention, in order to broaden the vision of reality. From the field of observation one is obliged to move towards the more engaging and promising path of knowledge which embraces the uncertainties of experiments.

There are other allegorical features of this fable. For example, the awareness that sound production in the animal kingdom is based upon mechanisms similar to those operating in the physical world (Figure 1.3). On the one hand, with the tools he is able to contrive, the man can imitate the known sounds produced by animals (in the whistle the sound is produced through a breathing process similar to that operating in birds). On the other hand, after noting that sounds could be produced in a variety of ways (by 'sawing upon some fibres stretched upon a concave piece of wood', by the movement of 'the hinges and fastenings' of a moving gate, or by 'rubbing the tip of his finger round the rim of a goblet') he is able to formulate a hypothesis of sound production in the animals that he has encountered and even in the animals he will encounter later.[13]

[13] As we shall see, this attitude will be a source of inspiration for the iatromechanical theory adopted by the 'modern scientists' (*novatores*) of the second half of the seventeenth century, such as Giovanni Alfonso Borelli and Marcello Malpighi.

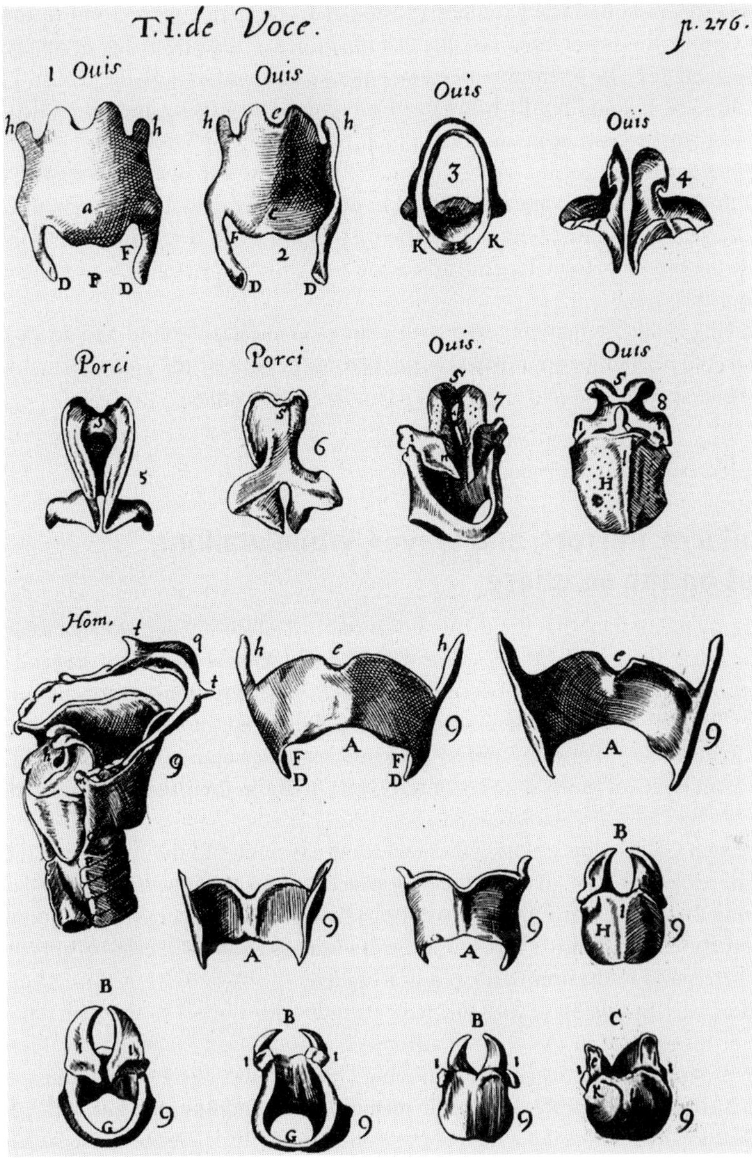

Figure 1.3 The cartilages of larynx from *De visione, voce, auditu* (1600) by Fabricius ab Aquapendente. Fabricius, one of the greatest anatomists of Padua University, is particularly known for his embryological work and for the discovery of valves in veins, a discovery that opened the way for William Harvey's works on blood circulation. The anatomical tables painted in colour, by artists of the Venetian school (*Tabulae Pictae*), are among the most beautiful anatomical illustrations of all time. Forgotten for centuries, they were rediscovered in 1909 by the Italian anatomist Giuseppe Sterzi in the archives of the Marciana library of Venice and recently restored (and exhibited in the same library: Rippa Bonati and Pardo-Tomás 2004). They serve as illustrations for a monumental work of human and animal anatomy, the *Theatrum totius animalis fabrica* (Theatre of the whole animal structure) which was never published. Compared to the images of Casseri (Figure 1.2), the images illustrating the printed works of Fabricius are more essential and modern. Fabricius was an important physician and surgeon, and Galileo was among his patients.

The possibility exists that the hypothesis formulated might not correspond to the reality of nature. For Galileo, this is not, however, due to a fundamental unknowability of nature. As in any path of human enquiry, no scientific enterprise emerges at its outset with the certainty of success. If this was the case, it could hardly bring us to achieve the surprising and unpredictable results which characterize the genuine discoveries in their most elevated phases.

Galileo's message is that nature can be known. It might, however, operate in ways that are quite different to those to which we are accustomed in our ordinary daily life. This should encourage true researchers to be cautious about the knowledge they acquire. Alternatively, it will induce them to appreciate the vast and fascinating territories towards which they could direct their unbounded spirit of inquisitiveness.

Before leaving Galileo's man endowed with a very perspicacious mind and an extraordinary curiosity, it would perhaps be appropriate to quote some famous words from the final scene of the first Act of Shakespeare's *Hamlet*, inspired by a similar open attitude:

> There are more things in heaven and earth, Horatio,
> Than are dreamt of in your philosophy.

1.4 Simulacra, mirrors, and waves, while walking at sunset on the seashore

We have already mentioned that the theory advanced by Galileo in *Saggiatore* to account for the nature of comets is flawed. The Pisan scientist denied that comets are real bodies and accounted for their visibility on the basis of optical effects similar to those responsible for the aurora borealis, rainbows, and other more or less comparable luminous appearances seen in the sky under particular circumstances. For him, comets were nothing other than images due to the reflection of sunlight from layers of moist vapours of terrestrial origin in their ascension towards the vault of heavens.[14]

To some extent Galileo's optical hypothesis of comets is similar to the conception (also flawed) that he had developed about two decades earlier to account for the appearance of a strong light in the sky, having the characteristics of an exceptionally brilliant new star. Another common motif in the two situations was Galileo's incorporation of vision as a source of celestial appearances that might not correspond to the immediate physical reality.

We will deal later in this book with Galileo's attitude with respect to the new star within the framework of his interest in the sensory aspects of astronomical investigations. Here we limit ourselves to a passage from *Saggiatore* signifying Galileo's interest in visual appearances. This highlights his ability to illustrate a scientific phenomenon (and one that has both physical and perceptual features) with prose of a high literary standard. With reference to the fable of sounds, we could say that, in addressing his proposals to Cesarini, Galileo invites us to walk along the seashore (*marina*) at sunset and observe the variable appearances of sunlight reflected from the surface of the sea.

What Galileo portrays is a kind of 'natural' visual experiment concerning a phenomenon which, in the context of *Saggiatore*, serves to account for the appearance of comets. As we shall see later (particularly in Chapters 8, 11, and 12), in the *Dialogue* a similar explanation would be of great

---

[14] Despite Galileo's erroneous explanation of comets, it must be recognized that their most striking visual appearance, namely their long luminous tail, is the consequence of optical phenomena due to the encounters of sunrays with the long trail of vapours emanating from the ice core of their heads.

importance to account for the appearance of the brightness of the moon, and thus to deal a final blow to ancient cosmology.

As often happens with Galileo, in both *Saggiatore* and *Dialogue* great science is married to great literature.

> The better to explain a point which is of the utmost importance and which may perhaps give someone (I shall not say Sarsi) a new idea, let your Excellency[15] fancy himself at the seashore at a time when the water is quite tranquil and the sun is already declining toward the west. You will see a very bright reflection of the sun in the surface of the sea near the vertical line passing through the solar disc.[16] This will not spread over a large area;[17] indeed, if the water is very peaceful as I said, you will see a pure image of the solar disc bounded as in a mirror. Next let a light breeze spring up and ruffle the surface of the water, and simultaneously your Excellency will see the sun's image[18] begin to break into many parts and spread and extend into a larger space. If you were close by, you might be able to distinguish the broken pieces of the image from one another, but from a greater distance you would not see this separation because of the narrowness of the intervals between the pieces, or because by their great brilliance the shining parts would mix together and behave as do several fires close together which from afar appear to be one. Now let the ruffling proceed into greater waves, and that multitude of mirrors from which the image of the sun will be reflected to the eye according to the various slopes of the waves will extend into wider and wider intervals. Next, withdraw to a greater distance and climb a hill or some other prominence in order to see the water better, and the lighted field will appear one and continuous. From a very high mountain about sixty miles from the Bay of Leghorn, on a clear but windy day about an hour before sunset, I have seen a very bright strip spreading to right and left of the sun and occupying a length of tens and perhaps hundreds of miles which was the same kind of reflection of sunlight as those just mentioned. Now let Sarsi imagine most of the sea on both sides to be removed so that there remains only a breadth of two or three miles (p. 101) at the middle, pointing toward the sun. This surely would all be illuminated, and it would not be movable with every motion of the observer to one side or the other—unless perhaps he were to move several miles, for then he would begin to lose the left side of the image (if he moved toward the right) and the bright image would become constricted until it was made very thin and even vanished entirely. But it is not in this way that the image would actually move with the motion of the observer; rather, we should continue to see it entire, though all of it would move so that its center would always correspond with the direction of the sun, which for other people observing it at the same time would correspond with various other points on the horizon. Here I wish to tell your Excellency something that has occurred to me as the solution of a maritime problem. Experienced sailors sometimes recognize that a wind will come to them from a certain part of the sea before long, and they say that a sure sign of this is to see the air in that direction more bright than it would ordinarily be. Consider, your Excellency, whether this might not arise from a wind disturbing the waves over there already. From such waves, as from many mirrors

[15] Virginio Cesarini, to whom *Saggiatore* is dedicated.

[16] The 'vertical line' here is the celestial meridian passing through the observer, that is the great circle going from the North to the South of the globe and intersecting the observer.

[17] The reflection of the image of the sun seen in this situation will be just a little larger than the image seen directly on the sky.

[18] In the original, image is here *simulacro* (*simulacrum*). This is a word reminiscent of *De rerum natura* of Lucretius, and was largely used in a similar context by Leonardo, as we shall see in Chapter 11. The Latin poet used the term *simulacra* to translate the Greek expression 'eidola', meaning the elements that, according to the atomistic theory of vision, were emitted by external objects and making vision possible by penetrating inside the eye. As we shall see, atomism provided a reference for various aspects of Galileo's science, including his theory of sensations.

spread over a wide area, there would originate a much brighter reflection of the sun than would exist if the sea were calm. Then that part of the vapor-laden air may be made brighter by this new light and by the diffusion of that reflection. This air, being high, sends also some reflection of light to the eyes of the sailors, while they, being low and far off, would not be able to receive the primary reflection from that part of the sea which is already being ruffled by the wind twenty or thirty miles away. And that is how they perceive and predict a wind from afar. But pursuing our original idea, I say that the solar rays do not impress the image of the sun with the same size in all materials, or I should say upon all surfaces. In some, namely those which are plane and smooth like a mirror, the solar disc is shown to us as bounded and as equal (p. 102) to the actual sun; in smooth convex surfaces it appears smaller to us, and in concave ones it appears sometimes smaller and sometimes larger and sometimes even the same, in accordance with the different distances between the mirror, the object, and the eye. If the surface is not even but is wavy and full of elevations and depressions (composed, as we might say, of a great multitude of little mirrors placed at varying tilts and exposed to the eye in thousands of ways), then this same image of the sun, divided into thousands of pieces, will meet our eye as thousands of parts spread over a large space. Thus it will impress us as a collection of many little bright patches [*piazzette*, i.e. properly 'small piazzas']. The number of these will make it appear from a distance as a single continuous luminous field, stronger and more vivid in the center than toward the edges. At the edges the light becomes languid, and finally it vanishes mistily when the obliquity of the eye to this surface no longer causes the visual rays to find any waves to reflect them toward the sun. This large image is also capable of moving with a movement of the eye, provided the surface where the reflection takes place continues beyond the limits of the image. If the material occupies a small space (smaller than that of the whole image), it will continue to appear bright until the eye arrives at that boundary beyond which the obliquity of incident rays upon the material causes the reflections to be no longer directed toward the sun, when the light vanishes and is lost. (SAGGIATORE, pp. 100–102; transl. pp. 240–242)

1.5 Reflections on sunlight along the seashore

Here Galileo enunciates the principle of so-called 'diffuse reflection'. It is a common phenomenon that occurs in the visibility of objects with no intrinsic luminance and with more or less irregular surfaces; it is different to the reflection from mirrors, polished glasses, and static liquids. He makes this connection with reference to the reflection of sunlight at dusk for two main reasons. The first is because it has direct relevance to the optical hypothesis of comets that he has been developing. The second is that the variations in the sea's surface at sunset offer him the possibility of a 'spontaneous' experiment. The phases of this experiment are marked by three moments which develop in an apparently natural sequence, with minimal intervention of the observer-experimenter. The person walking along the seashore (Cesarini, but also the reader) is implicated in the experiment simply through a kind of impersonal invitation. First, he is asked to imagine to be 'at the seashore at a time when the water is quite tranquil and the sun is already declining towards the west'; secondly, to wait while 'a light breeze springs up and ruffles the surface of the water'; and thirdly, that 'the ruffling proceeds into greater waves'. Only at the end, the invitation requires a less spontaneous and obvious action, because it implies that the reader 'withdraw to a greater distance and climb a hill or some other prominence' and finally go on 'a very high mountain about sixty miles from the bay of Leghorn', following Galileo who seems to be there just by chance.

As mentioned earlier, in the *Dialogue* the physical principles underlying diffuse reflection will be enunciated within the context of the explanation of lunar brightness. In this situation Galileo makes recourse to a true experiment, carried on by the three debaters, Salviati, Sagredo and Simplicius. It is the famous experiment of the mirror on the white wall which is performed through a rapid sequence and efficacious movements of the protagonists directed by Salviati, Galileo's alter ego.[19]

In the case of *Saggiatore* we become aware of a potentially revolutionary perceptive process through the suggestions evoked by an apparently leisurely and pleasant situation. Is it not charming to watch the sunset while walking along the seashore waiting for a light breeze to disturb the surface of the water? Is it not similarly pleasant to climb a hill or a high mountain 'on a clear but windy day' and to gaze from afar at the quivering surface of the sea?

In addition to providing an aesthetic dimension, *Saggiatore* invites us to be involved in the scientific adventure. Then we discover what might be hidden beneath the surface of the sea as the wind increases in intensity. In the beginning, when 'the water is very peaceful' we would 'see a pure image of the solar disc bounded as in a mirror'. As the wind freshens, this perfectly bounded image progressively fragments and spreads over increasingly wider regions. Galileo tells us that this happens because the surface, initially similar to a horizontal mirror, becomes divided into a multiplicity of small surfaces, as in a 'multitude of mirrors', with different inclinations, each one reflecting a more or less partial image in different directions. Eventually (and with relation also to the observation distance), these multiple images would fuse together, producing a diffuse brightness, where the image of the sun is no longer discerned.

In his writings Galileo makes a clear distinction between 'diffuse' and 'mirror-like reflection'. The diffuse type is that underlying the vision of most common objects in our visual world (like the surface of a wall or table, or the page of a book), and in particular of almost all non-light-emitting objects that we see because they reflect the light from a source like the sun. The peculiarities of this type of reflection explain why objects appear to be luminous even when it is unlikely that a true reflection (i.e. a mirror type one) could occur. This happens because the surfaces of most natural objects are made up of many minute mirrors oriented according to various inclinations capable of reflecting

[19] In chapters 11 and 12 we will return to the mechanism of diffuse reflection, and particularly on its use by Galileo in the context of his cosmological observation and his consideration on vision process. As we shall see, about the time of Galileo, the phenomenon had been considered by Paolo Sarpi, a friar of the order of Servites, who was an expert on optics and probably played an important role in Galileo's development of telescope. After Galileo, Isaac Newton would utilize the concept of diffuse reflection in his experiments on colours, following the elaboration of the Tuscan scientist. On the basis of this concept, the English scholar explains why a paper, which is perceived as white under natural illumination, would still appear so if illuminated indirectly through the light reflected by a paper painted with multiple colours. This would happen if the coloured paper source is kept at a certain distance from the other one (Newton, 1671/1672). This is so because the paper surface is made up of a myriad of minute reflecting surfaces oriented in different directions. By reflecting, according to their orientations, the rays of various colours, these surfaces would mix these rays and, by consequence, would lead to the white appearance of the other paper receiving the mixture of their lights and, in turn, reflecting the rays in various directions. If a polished metal is substituted for the 'white' paper, its surface will, on the contrary, show the multi-coloured aspect of the coloured paper, due to a mirror-like reflection mechanism. As, however, the metallic surface is made progressively more irregular by scraping, again the surface would recover its white appearance. In the *Philosophical Transactions* article in which he describes this experiment, Newton presents another suggestive version. The surface of a white wall (i.e. of a wall appearing white under ordinary illumination), would continue to appear white, even if illuminated by the light coming from a distant window, whose panes are made of glasses of various colours. This happens even if an observer placed near the white wall would perceive the different colours of the window panes. Newton uses this experiment to show that, contrary to the objections of Hooke, the rays of different colours maintain their individuality even when, by combining together, they produce the appearance of white (see Newton, 1671/1672).

minute fragmented images of the light source ('a collection of little bright patches') that will be eventually reach the eye. It is because of the diverse inclination of these multiple reflecting small surfaces that reflection occurs under the various angles between the observer, light sources, and macroscopic surface of the object.

Towards the end of the passage Galileo alludes to the mechanism of diffuse illumination in order to account for a phenomenon that occurs in everyday life, and is known to 'experienced sailors'. They become aware that wind is approaching from some point on the horizon when they 'see the air in that direction more bright than it would ordinarily be'.

Galileo frequently intertwines scientific theories and observations from everyday life. The correspondence with ordinary events serves to support the value of the theory and, moreover, to provide evidence of the usefulness and applicability of scientific knowledge.

This attitude is typical of the new science advocated by Galileo but it was not so obvious until the first phase of the Renaissance, when knowledge tended to be considered mainly as a means to elevate humans above the most ordinary and prosaic aspects of life. Its possible practical implications were relatively neglected, as if they were not suitable for the superior minds of philosophers. Galileo's attitude represents an instance of developing a connection between the knowledge derived from real life—especially due to the practice of craftsmen and technicians-and the science which leaves the ivory towers of academic culture, the courts of princes, and the cells of monks and humanists (places where learning with practical implications was generally considered mean and vulgar).

In Galileo's writing we find a link between the inquisitive attitude of the man of science who looks at the sun declining towards the sea ('a man endowed by nature with a very perspicacious mind and an extraordinary curiosity') and the 'experienced sailors' who watch the horizon in order to understand the direction of winds. This represents a crucial moment in the progress of humankind—a moment in which two forms of learning merge together. On the one hand, an ancient learning based on the experience derived from probing nature's clues; this was crucial for the primitive hunters (who identified footprints to distinguish the animals to be pursued and chased from those to be avoided), and for fishermen (interested in knowing the direction of winds in order to avoid thunderstorms and shipwrecks). On the other hand, a more modern and more efficacious knowledge, based on experiments and logical interpretations; this does not disregard the other form of knowledge but, by investigating its bases and foundations, succeeds in extending its scope and capability of prediction.

We will return later in this book to Galileo's elaboration of the reciprocal 'diffuse' reflection between the earth and the moon and on its importance for the renewal of cosmology. What is important to note here is that he discovered that the moon shines in the nocturnal sky without exploring sidereal space with a spacecraft, but by simply remaining still, on the earth's surface.[20]

Perhaps not entirely still. This is because the intellectual journey leading him to assume that the moon shines as it does because of the irregularity of its surface (and also the earth—because of the irregularity of its own surface—shines and therefore does illuminate the moon) in some way begins with a voyage. Or better simply with a walk at sunset along the seashore. As a matter

[20] At the time when Galileo was writing his *Dialogue*, someone had ventured virtually on a voyage to the moon. Indeed Johannes Kepler, the other great protagonist of modern scientific revolution had written his *Somnium, seu De Astronomia lunari*, a book based on an imaginary voyage to the moon. Although the great astronomer had conceived this work since his youthful years, the volume was only published in 1634, four years after his death, due to the vicissitudes of his mother, Katharina Guldenmann. Katharina had been accused of being a witch and had undergone a long trial from which she was eventually acquitted. In the *Somnium*, considered as one of the first science fiction novels, Kepler envisions a spacecraft journey to

of fact, the principle accounting for the moon's brilliance is the same as that responsible for the changing appearance of the sun's reflection on the sea surface as this becomes more turbulent under the action of the wind.

As the fable of sounds reminds us, we must always be aware of the limits of enquiry, like the man who was reduced to great 'diffidence in his understanding'. Moreover, we cannot but be amazed by the power of science in widening the frontiers of human knowledge.[21]

At the beginning of the third millennium we can still be amazed in thinking that the explanatory principle capable of accounting for the lunar splendour can be derived from the observation of the changing aspect of the sun's reflections from the sea's surface. It is perhaps more difficult to realize how revolutionary the consequences of Galileo's achievement were in his day. This is because it was then totally unexpected that one could account for a celestial phenomenon on the basis of an experiment performed on earth. There was indeed a fundamental contrast with the principles of classical physics and cosmology; these stipulated that the sublunary and the superlunary worlds had different properties (the first was corruptible, mutable, and subject to death whereas the second was incorruptible, immutable, and perennial) and obeyed essentially different physical laws, not to mention being made of different components. More on this will be said later in the book.

1.6 Galileo's artistic eye

One could perhaps say that the ancient Aristotelian-Ptolemaic cosmos, which had remained static for millennia (with the earth at the centre, and the celestial bodies revolving around it in their crystalline orbs)-started to be undermined on the basis of the speculations of a man walking along the seashore.

Those who are not inclined to feel the emotion intrinsic to scientific adventure (and present in Galileo's pages) could object that, by widening the limits of human knowledge, science was dissolving the poetic enchantment aroused for centuries by contemplation of the universe. Or that the increased knowledge contributed to making the world in which we happen to live more prosaic. Everyone is entitled to their own opinions. Many believe that there is an irreconcilable opposition between a scientific mindset and an artistic attitude. To those people we would like to point out that one of the reasons why Galileo succeeded in accounting for the mutual reflection of earth and moon was related to his interest (and talent) in the artistic field, and particularly in painting. As a matter of fact, he derived the explanation of the phenomenon largely from the consideration of the 'secondary lumen' developed by Italian painters since the time of Leonardo. These considerations explained why an illuminated body, even one with a rough surface, could become a source of illumination for surrounding places not directly struck by the (primary) light source. Galileo was well aware of pictorial techniques, and particularly of the problem of shadows

---

the moon and, besides considering the specific conditions of life on the planet, he discusses in detail the appearance of the sky seen from the point of view of the lunar residents. By proposing a 'lunar astronomy', he aimed mainly at demonstrating the inconsistency of the objections against the Copernican system based on the centrality of an earthly viewpoint. Kepler was obliged to postpone the publication of this book because of the possible negative consequence on his mother's trial. As a matter of fact, in the book the mother of the narrator is presented with some of the features of a witch. The *Somnium* is a great literary text, although the literary charm of Kepler's prose is completely different from that of Galileo.

21 In this context, it is perhaps appropriate to mention that, on the basis of his telescopic observations, Galileo succeeded in calculating the height of lunar mountains with an error of only about twenty per cent, while in his era the height of the highest peaks in the Alps were estimated to be two thousand metres. We will discuss this point in Chapter 9.

and chiaroscuro so important in the representation of external world on the surface of a painting. In his youth he had attended drawing courses at the Accademia Fiorentina (Florentine Academy) and followed the lectures on drawing and perspective delivered by Ostilio Ricci, mathematician to the Medicean Court. Galileo was, moreover, acquainted with many painters, and particularly with Ludovico Cigoli, the author of a treatise on perspective. Galileo wrote a famous letter to Cigoli in 1612 on the relation between painting and sculpture (Panofsky, 1954; see Chapters 6 and 14).

Galileo's familiarity with painting techniques also allowed him to represent graphically the moon as seen in his first telescopic observations in the period 1609 to 1610 (Bredekamp, 2009; Bredekamp et al., 2011). His own representations are shown in Figure 1.4. Moreover, and most importantly, it allowed him to interpret these images correctly as he understood that dark or bright spots visible on the moon's surface were due to the presence of craters and mountains, and not due to intrinsic variations of luminosity or transparency, as was traditionally held to be the case. Galileo's eye that viewed the moon through his telescope was that of a scientist as well as an artist.

1.7 The globe of jasper and the small orange of China

To those who are still of the opinion that science deprives the world of its poetic charm, we would like to present a passage from the *Dialogue*. It is the place in which Sagredo argues against those who wish to endow the celestial bodies with attributes of immutability and incorruptibility because they believe that without these attributes they would be degraded to the level of earth, the site of mutability and of imperfection.

From the *Dialogue*:

SAGREDO. I cannot without great astonishment—I might say without great insult to my intelligence—hear it attributed as a prime perfection and nobility of the natural and integral bodies of the universe that they are invariant, immutable, inalterable, etc., while on the other hand it is called a great imperfection to be alterable, generable, mutable, etc. For my part I consider the earth very noble and admirable precisely because of the diverse alterations, changes, generations, etc. that occur in it incessantly. If, not being subject to any changes, it were a vast desert of sand or a mountain of jasper,[22] or if at the time of the flood the waters which covered it had frozen, and it had remained an enormous globe of ice where nothing was ever born or ever altered or changed, I should deem it a useless lump in the universe, devoid of activity and, in a word, superfluous and essentially nonexistent. This is exactly the difference between a living animal and a dead one; and I say the same of the moon, of Jupiter, and of all other world globes. The deeper I go in considering the vanities of popular reasoning, the lighter and more foolish I find them. What greater stupidity can be imagined than that of calling jewels, silver, and gold 'precious,' and earth and soil 'base'? People who do this ought to remember that if there were as great a scarcity of soil as of jewels or precious metals, there would not be a prince who would not spend a bushel of diamonds and rubies and a cartload of gold just to have enough earth to plant a jasmine in a little pot, or to sow the seed of a small China orange and watch it sprout, grow, and produce its handsome leaves, its fragrant flowers, and fine fruit. It is scarcity and plenty that make the vulgar take things to be precious or worthless; they call a diamond very beautiful because it is like pure water, and then would not exchange one for ten barrels of water.[23] Those who so greatly exalt incorruptibility, inalterability, etc. are reduced to talking this way, I believe, by their great desire to go on living, and by the terror they have of death. They do not reflect that if men were

[22] A variety of quartz, although here it indicates mainly a generic crystal-like, reflecting matter.

[23] Sagredo alludes here to the 'paradox of value' of economic theories. This stipulates that the value of goods does not depend on their intrinsic utility, but on their relative scarcity or abundance. This paradox had been dealt with in Italy long before Galileo's time (see, for instance, the *Lezione delle monete*—'Lecture on

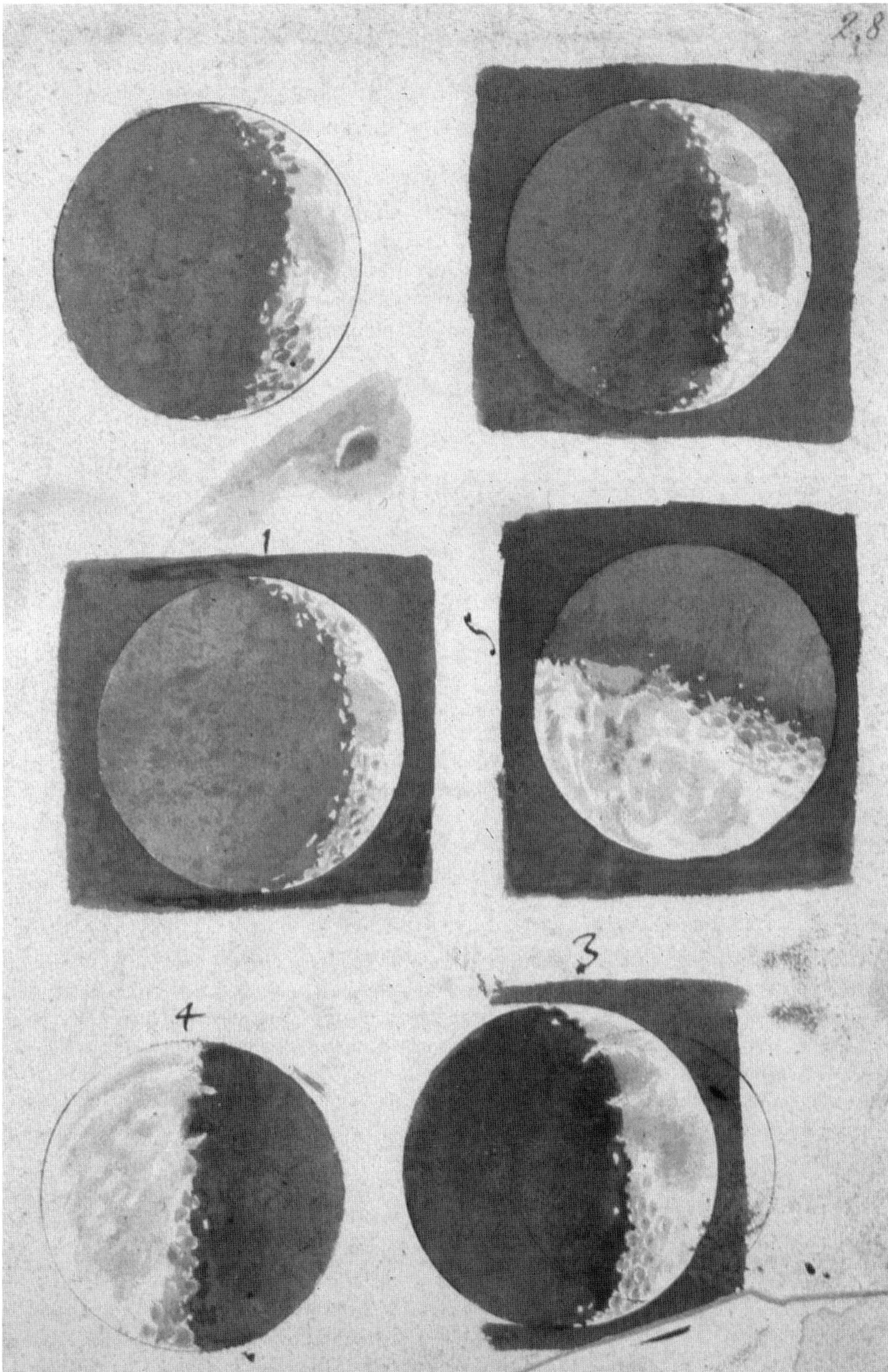

Figure 1.4 Phases of the moon drawn by Galileo (BNF GAL 48, F28r; © Biblioteca Nazionale of Florence, Italy).

immortal, they themselves would never have come into the world. Such men really deserve to encounter a Medusa's head which would transmute them into statues of jasper or of diamond, and thus make them more perfect than they are.

SALVIATI. Maybe such a metamorphosis would not be entirely to their disadvantage, for I think it would be better for them not to argue than to argue on the wrong side. (DIALOGO, pp. 50–51; transl. pp. 58–59)[24]

When reading the passage concerning 'jasmine' and 'China orange' it is difficult not to share the opinion of Italo Calvino, who considered Galileo as the greatest writer of Italian literature. At the same time, it is difficult to think that the charm of science, and of Galilean science in particular, is necessarily 'cold' and devoid of the emotional enchantment that only poetry and art can offer.

On the literary side, it is worth noting that after the expression of 'lyrical pathos' pronounced by Sagredo as an exaltation of mutation against the incorruptibility (a genuine 'praise of life'), the emotional register of the prose descends towards the ironic accents of Salviati's words, according to a decrescendo rhythm, somewhat similar to the octaves of *Orlando Furioso* by Galileo's favourite poet, Ludovico Ariosto.

1.8 **A Barbary horse, one hundred Friesian horses, and the eggs of Babylonia**

With reference to this rather gentle irony, we would like to conclude with another passage from *Saggiatore*. These pages are marked by wit and polemic force, two main aspects of this text, based on a more than lively controversy. Here Galileo addresses some of the main tenets of the old culture. On one side, its insistent reference to the authority of the 'ancient authors'. On the other side, its endorsement of the testimony and opinion of the multitudes, which are valued more than the direct and personal observation of natural phenomena:

I cannot help wondering that Sarsi[25] still wishes to persist in proving to me by means of witnesses that which I can see at any time by means of experiment. Witnesses are examined in doubtful matters which are past and impermanent, not in those which are factual and permanent. Thus it is necessary for a judge to seek by means of witnesses to determine whether it is true that Peter injured John last night, but not whether John is injured, for this he is able to see and to make the *visu reperto*.[26] Furthermore, I say that

money'—by Bernardo Davanzati, a Florentin humanist and merchant, written in 1558). In less ancient times, and in a somewhat different context, Michael Faraday expressed a vision somewhat similar to that of Sagredo, by comparing, in his famous *Natural history of a candle*, the beauty of a flame with that of diamonds and other precious objects: 'You have the glittering beauty of gold and silver, and the still higher lustre of jewels like the ruby and diamond; but none of these rival the brilliancy and beauty of flame. What diamond can shine like flame? It owes its lustre at nighttime to the very flame shining upon it. The flame shines in darkness, but the light which the diamond has is as nothing until the flame shines upon it, when it is brilliant again. The candle alone shines by itself and for itself' (Faraday, 1861, p. 29).

24 The theme of the conflicting relation between a supposed perfection in shape and matter of the celestial bodies versus the possibility of life, dealt with by Sagredo in this passage, is present, somehow with similar words, in a letter addressed on 16 July 1611 to Gallanzone Gallanzoni, secretary of the French Cardinal François de la Joyeuse (OG XI, pp. 148–149).

25 Lothario Sarsi, was, as already mentioned, the pseudonym used by the Jesuit Orazio Grassi in signing his *Libra astronomica*.

26 The phrase used in forensic pathology to indicate the forensic test, which was largely based on anatomo-clinical inspection.

even in conclusions of which one may attain a knowledge only by reasoning,[27] the testimony of many men is worth little more than that of few, it being certain that the number of those who reason well in difficult matters is much smaller than the number of those who reason badly. If reasoning were like carrying burdens, where several horses will carry more sacks of grain than one alone, I should agree that several reasoners would avail more than a single one; but reasoning is like running and not like carrying, and one Barb horse[28] will outrun a hundred Friesian horses.[29] So when Sarsi brings in such a multitude of authors, it does not seem to me that he strengthens his conclusion, but that he ennobles Sig. Mario's[30] cause and mine by showing that we have reasoned better than many men of great reputation. If Sarsi wants me to believe from Suidas[31] that the Babylonians cooked eggs by whirling them rapidly in slings, I shall do so; but I must say that the cause of this effect is very far from that which he attributes to it. To discover the truth I shall reason thus: 'If we do not achieve an effect which others formerly achieved, it must be that in our operations we lack something which was the cause of this effect succeeding, and if we lack but one single thing, then this alone can be the cause. Now we do not lack eggs, or slings, or sturdy fellows to whirl them; and still they do not cook, but rather they cool down faster if hot. And since nothing is lacking to us except being Babylonians, then being Babylonians is the cause of the eggs hardening.' And this is what I wished to determine. Is it possible that Sarsi in riding past has not observed the coolness brought to his face by the continual change of air? And if he has indeed felt this, can he prefer to believe things which happened two thousand years ago in Babylon, as related by others, rather than present things which he himself experiences?[32] (SAGGIATORE, p. 187; transl. pp. 302–303)

---

[27] In the original the word used here is *discorso*, a term full of meaning in Galileo's prose, referring to the verbal form *discorrere* in footnote 2.

[28] An Arab horse, very fast in running, so called because they originate from Barbary, the westward region of Morocco (largely corresponding to present-day Maghreb). In Galileo's times the Barb horses were well known in Tuscany, because they were used in the horse races of the popular tournament of Siena, the *Palio*.

[29] Horses originating from Friesland, employed particularly as draught and working horses because of their strength and endurance. As highlighted particularly by Italo Calvino in his *Lezioni americane* ('American lectures', first published in 1988) Galileo plays here on the linguistic proximity of the original words for reasoning (*discorso*) and for running (*corsa*). On another issue, we could remark that Galileo's attitude in this particular context seems different from that of another great protagonist of the modern scientific revolution, Francis Bacon. In chapter 26 of his *Sapienza veterum*, Bacon remarks that in the *lampadedromia* (the torch relay race dedicated to Prometheus), success was not determined by the fast running of single athlete, but by an ensemble of runners capable of achieving an appropriate fit between the speed and the requirement that the torch flame does not extinguish, as could happen with extremely fast runners (Bacon, 1609). In this way Bacon remarked on the collaborative character of research in the new science, in opposition to the work of few great minds, as was more the case in Galileo's writings.

[30] Galileo alludes here to Mario Guiducci (1585–1646), one of his former students, who in 1619 had signed the *Discorso sulle comete* ('Discourse on comets'), a work largely due to Galileo himself. Grassi directed his *Libra astronomica* against this *Discourse*.

[31] Suida or Suidas is the title of a Byzantine encyclopaedic compilation. It was popular in the Renaissance and was usually referred to as an author rather than a book.

[32] Notice that Galileo's argument about the relation between movement and heat is largely flawed. As he knew well, movement produced heat through the effect of friction, and, therefore, it is in principle possible that Babylonians succeeded in cooking eggs by whirling. The cooling sensation on the face caused by riding fast is an indirect consequence of the evaporation of the transpired liquid at the skin surface, and also of the removal of warm air layers surrounding the face. This error of Galileo's does not undermine the polemic efficacy of his attacks on Grassi.

Chapter 2

Subtleties of vision and of the scientific revolution

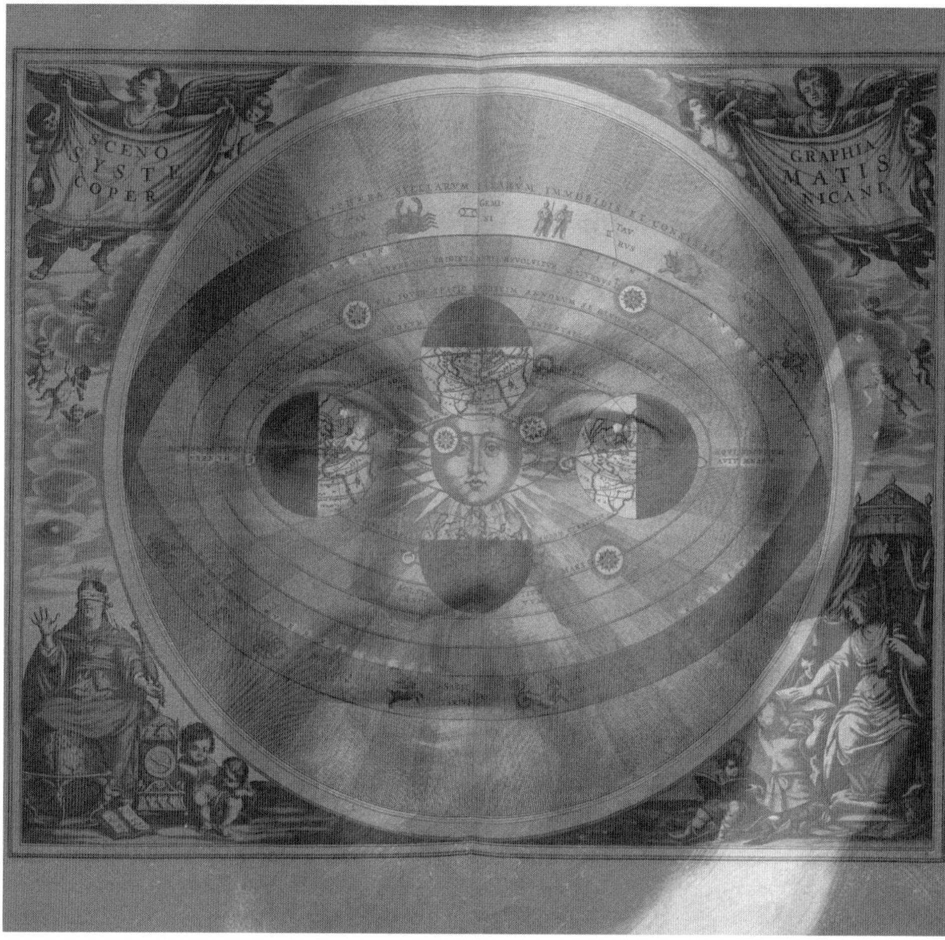

Figure II *Galileo's world view* by Nicholas Wade. The portrait of Galileo (derived from a painting by Passignano) is combined with a representation of the cosmic system according to Copernicus (reproduced from Cellarius, A. *Harmonia macrocosmica seu Atlas universalis et novis*, 1601, Amstelodami, apud Joannem Janssonium). Galileo's eyes are in the hemispheres of earth illuminated by the central sun.

Credit: The Copernican system of the sun, from the 'Harmonia Macrocosmica', published in Amsterdam, 1660 (engraving), Cellarius, Andreas (c.1596–1665) / Bibliotheque Nationale, Paris, France / The Bridgeman Art Library.

Upon a hillside will the woolly flocks
Be cropping their goodly food and creeping about
Whither the summons of the grass, begemmed
With the fresh dew, is calling, and the lambs
Well filled, are frisking, locking horns in sport:
Yet all for us seem blurred and blent afar—
A glint of white at rest on a green hill.
Again, when mighty legions, marching round,
Fill all the quarters of the plains below,
Rousing a mimic warfare, there the sheen
Shoots up the sky, and all the fields about
Glitter with brass, and from beneath, a sound
Goes forth from feet of stalwart soldiery,
And mountain walls, smote by the shouting, send
The voices onward to the stars of heaven,
And hither and thither darts the cavalry,
And of a sudden down the midmost fields
Charges with onset stout enough to rock
The solid earth: and yet some post there is
Up the high mountains, viewed from which they seem
To stand—a gleam at rest along the plains.[1]

These two images are apparently very different. Indeed, what can be more unlike the tranquil flocks of sheep on a hillside than the restless wandering of horses and warriors in the tumult of battle? Still, both views are used by the great Latin poet Lucretius (in the second book of his *De rerum natura*) to reject a possible objection to his conception of the universe based on the more or less casual encounters between minute elements in rapid motion. These are the *semina* (seeds) or *primordia rerum* (origins—primeval elements—of things), i.e. the 'elementary particles' or 'atoms' of present-day terminology. The objection faced by Lucretius is that based on the impossibility of perceiving through the senses the continuous stirring of these minute particles that, by their encounters, produce material bodies.

The difficulty of perceiving the consequences of invisible interactions due to the small size of the elements in motion is compared by the poet to the difficulty of seeing the motion of things located at great distances. An important point in the comparison is that distant images, besides appearing small, might appear still, even if they are in motion. This is a consideration based on a relatively common visual experience, even more common now than in the Roman era because of air travel. Looking down from an aircraft cabin window we might be surprised to see the waves as still, despite the motion of the sea. Conversely, looking upward from the ground towards a distant airplane that moves at great speed, we might have the same impression of an immobile object. After sunset, because of this apparent immobility, we might be prone to another perceptual error: we could assume that a brilliant spot against the dark sky might be a bright star although it could be due to the reflection of sunlight from the metallic surface of the airplane.

2.1 The old cosmos: a world of senses

The same illusion holds for the nocturnal sky: we see multitudes of immobile stars embedded in a similarly immobile vault of the heavens. Despite their apparent immobility, stars are undergoing

1 The translation of the Latin from Lucretius, 2004, pp. 38–39.

various forms of motion. One is due to our own movement, as we are rapidly transported both by the diurnal rotation of our planet around its axis and by the annual revolution of the earth around the sun. We make a tour of the world in just one day, while the orbital movement around the sun transport us at an average speed which is more than 50 times faster. The celestial bodies are also moving with respect to one another (with relation to a reference point usually assumed by astronomers to be the centre of the solar system). These movements can occur at extremely high velocities and yet they still evade our perception and usually require sophisticated astronomical techniques to be detected. Moreover, they can be resolved only for stars located relatively close to our position as observers.

For millennia the apparent immobility of stars resulted in them being referred to as 'fixed stars'. This phrase denoted their perceptual rather than objective immobility, and it served to distinguish them from 'wandering stars', i.e. planets. This was the case even though planets also appeared to be stationary in the nocturnal sky. However, their motion had been appreciated since the very dawn of civilization; it was inferred rather than perceived because planets also look perceptually still and their changing positions could be established after comparison with those of nearby 'fixed stars' at different periods of the year. Thus, the conception of wandering planets is not based on an immediate perceptual experience but is the outcome of complex reasoning and calculation. Apart from some very peculiar and rare phenomena like shooting stars and meteors, everything in the nocturnal sky appears immobile despite the various motions of the stars and planets.

These celestial observations have resulted in one of the most ancient beliefs: the existence of constellations which are so deeply rooted in our mythological and astrological imagery. In three-dimensional cosmic space, the stars of a given constellation are not particularly close to one another; moreover, they are characterized by reciprocal movements, their distances being subject to continuous changes. On physical grounds the constellations do not therefore possess the attributes of coherent and stable ensembles usually associated with the idea of visual objects. Nevertheless, they are perceived as the images of definite celestial entities (although different people, depending on their mythology, folklore, and science, identify different ensembles and assign different features to them).

In sum, the apparent immobility of the fixed stars, and the relative immobility of the stars in a constellation, are due to a perceptual phenomenon analogous to that alluded to by Lucretius with his metaphor of distant flocks, and of horses and battling warriors.

2.2 The vault of heavens

It was not only the apparent immobility of stars but also the idea of a vault of the heavens that was based on visual perception. Besides appearing immobile and vague, all distant objects seem to be at the same distance. In three-dimensional space, the locus of the points situated at the same distance from the observer is a near spherical surface with the observer at its centre, and this accounts for the vault-like aspect of the sky above us.

These considerations apply not only to the luminous points in the starry sky. They also concern the weak and diffuse luminosity of the diurnal sky leading to its appearance as a blue vault. The blue sky is due to the scattering of sunlight by air particles. In the nineteenth century, Lord Rayleigh (John Strutt) demonstrated that scattering is much more intense for the short-wavelength rays (i.e. the blue region of the visible spectrum) than for the long-wavelength rays (corresponding to the red region). This results in the bluish appearance of light reaching us indirectly and also, particularly at sunset, in the yellowish appearance of direct sun rays, which correspond to the fraction of sunlight reaching our eyes after being deprived of the scattered component.

The vaulted blue sky above us thus depends on the presence around the earth of a gaseous atmosphere.[2] Its spherical appearance is, however, in no way due to the fact that the gases of the atmosphere surrounding the earth's surface wrap our planet like a spherical shell. It results from a perceptual phenomenon similar to that responsible for the vaulted appearance of the starry nocturnal sky. Perceptual measurements of the apparent distance of the vault during the day (as well as during the night) show that we see it located surprisingly close to us. The perceptual distance of the vault of the sky is indeed of the order of only hundreds of metres rather than of kilometres (or light years as it should be if we would consider the starred dome of nocturnal sky).

We will deal with the problem of the perceptual distance of the sky in some detail later when treating Galileo's interpretation of the moon (or sun) illusion. The important point to make here is that one of the main foundations of the world view in classical Greek science, the idea of a spherical and closed cosmos, is based on visual perception.

This is the *machina mundi* (machine of the world), the extremely complex system consisting of a variable number of spheres (or orbs or skies), rotating at different speeds around the centre of the universe—earth. Already present in pre-Socratic philosophy, and developed afterwards in different forms, particularly by Eudoxus, Aristotle, and later by Ptolemy (Figure 2.1), this conception dominated the Western and Arabic traditions for centuries. In a simple version it consisted of the seven orbs of planets (from moon to Saturn, all supposed to be planets of Earth), surrounded by the eighth orb, that of the fixed stars. Outside, there was a ninth orb of the 'prime mover', usually considered as the source of the movement of all orbs below (Figure 2.2). In the Middle Ages this model was endowed with deep religious significance, becoming an essential aspect of the conception of the world. Specific angels have been associated with each orb, sometimes assuming the role of governing its movement (from below upwards: angels, archangels, principalities, powers, virtues, dominions, thrones, cherubims, seraphims). The outermost sky of the religious cosmos was supposed to be immaterial and timeless, the perfect Empyrean, a residence fit for Almighty God (Figure 2.2). This conception represents the physical, philosophical, and theological framework of one of the greatest poems of the Middle Ages, the *Divina Commedia* by Dante Alighieri.

With the improvement of astronomical measurements, new complexities were added to the model of the world in order to 'save the appearances', i.e. to make the observed movements of celestial bodies correspond to the predictions of the model. Eventually the system became so complex and so physically implausible that novel conceptions emerged. Among them was the model developed by Nicolaus Copernicus, based on the unmoving and central sun (Figure 2.3). Although his eye was located on earth, his world system rotated around the sun. The Copernican system would be at the very heart of the scientific revolution of the seventeenth century, a fundamental phase of development of Western civilization of which Galileo would be one of the main players.

A point already alluded to in Chapter 1 should be noted here. A fundamental aspect of the traditional cosmological conception, already present in Aristotle, was the idea of an essential physical difference between the lower, terrestrial world (i.e., the earth and the various zones immediately surrounding it: the sphere of water, air, and fire up to the orb of the moon) and the upper or celestial world, from the orb of the moon up to the fixed stars and beyond. According to classical science, the terrestrial or sublunary world is the place of mutability and corruptibility (also implying

[2] In the absence of a light-scattering atmosphere (as happens, for instance, around the moon) there would be no blue vault of heavens, although an observer on the moon would still perceive around him a sphere of fixed stars.

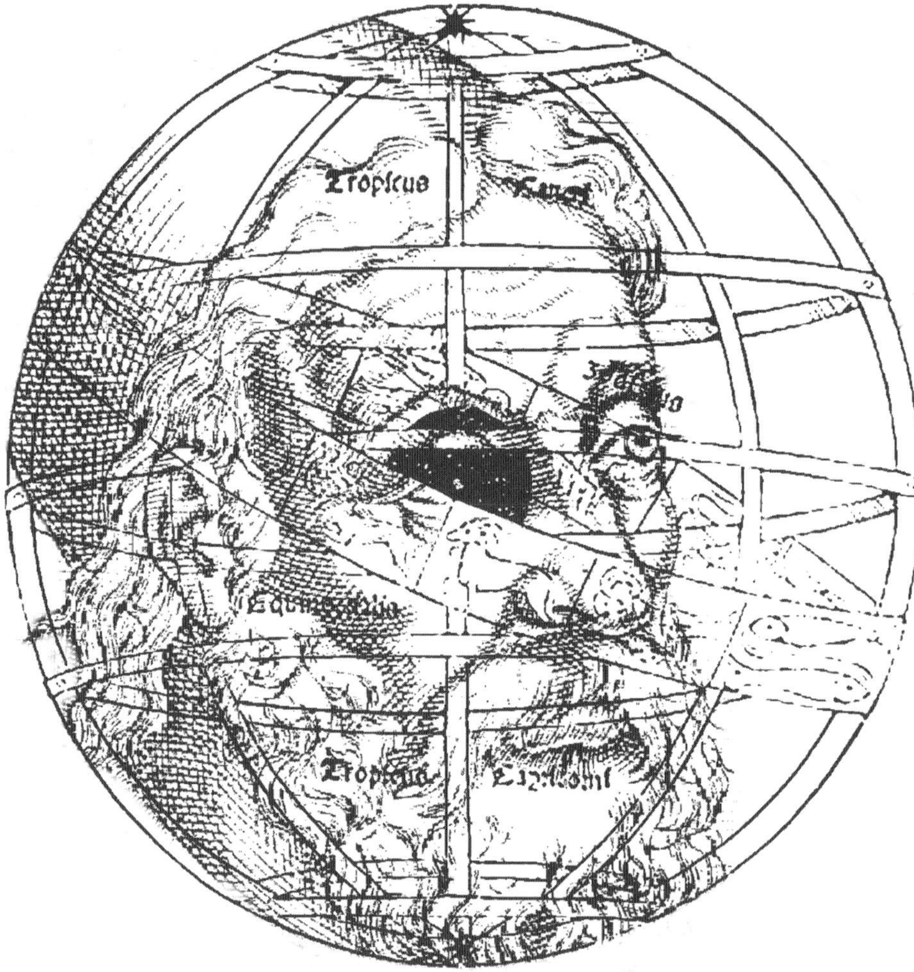

Figure 2.1 *Ptolemy's world* by Nicholas Wade. Ptolemy provided a mathematical description of the rotations of the stars in his book now called the *Almagest*. His was a theory in which the earth was the centre of the universe and all the planets rotated around it in circles. Ptolemy's geocentric model was based not only on astronomical observations but also on some basic aspects of perception. If the earth was moving would it not be felt as such? However, we are not sensible to any such motions and so it was a reasonable inference that the earth-bound observer was stationary and that Ptolemy's eye was at the centre of the universe.

the interplay of life and death), due to continuous interaction of the four elements of classical physics (earth, water, air, and fire). By contrast, the celestial or superlunary world consists of a single crystal-like material, characterized by immutability, incorruptibility, and intangibility: the ether or 'quintessence'. In the terrestrial world various forms of violent motion are possible; these are due to accidental causes in addition to natural motions. The latter result from the tendency of any of the elements to reach their own natural sphere (the element of earth towards the centre of the universe, and the other elements towards the spheres of water, air, and fire, respectively).

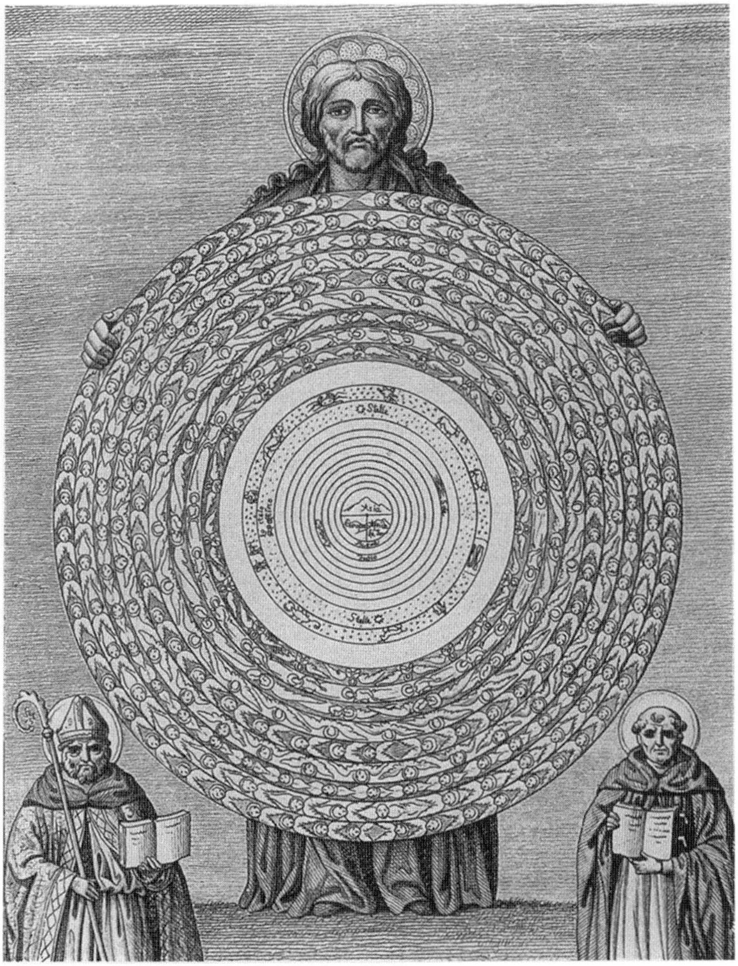

Figure 2.2 A representation of the cosmos in an engraving derived from a medieval fresco in the monumental Camposanto of Pisa.

In the celestial world the only possible motion is circular. This is because of the geometrical perfection as well as the periodicity of circular motion.

There were many reasons why the philosophers and astronomers of antiquity adopted the intricacies of this complex *machina mundi*. One was most probably based on vision: the spherical appearance of the vault of the heavens led to the supposition of the spherical conformation of the cosmos itself. This is also attested by the Greek word used to describe the sky, *koílos*, meaning 'concave' (from which arose the Latin *caelum* and the various similar forms of neo-Latin languages, including the English 'celestial').[3] Borrowing a beautiful phrase from Alexandre Koiré (and also used by Erwin Panofsky) in a Galilean and cosmological context, we could say that the conception of a spherical cosmos is produced, at least partially, by a *hantise de la circularité* deeply rooted in our visual mechanisms (Koyré, 1939; Panofsky, 1954).

[3] The English words 'cavity' and 'cave' have a similar origin.

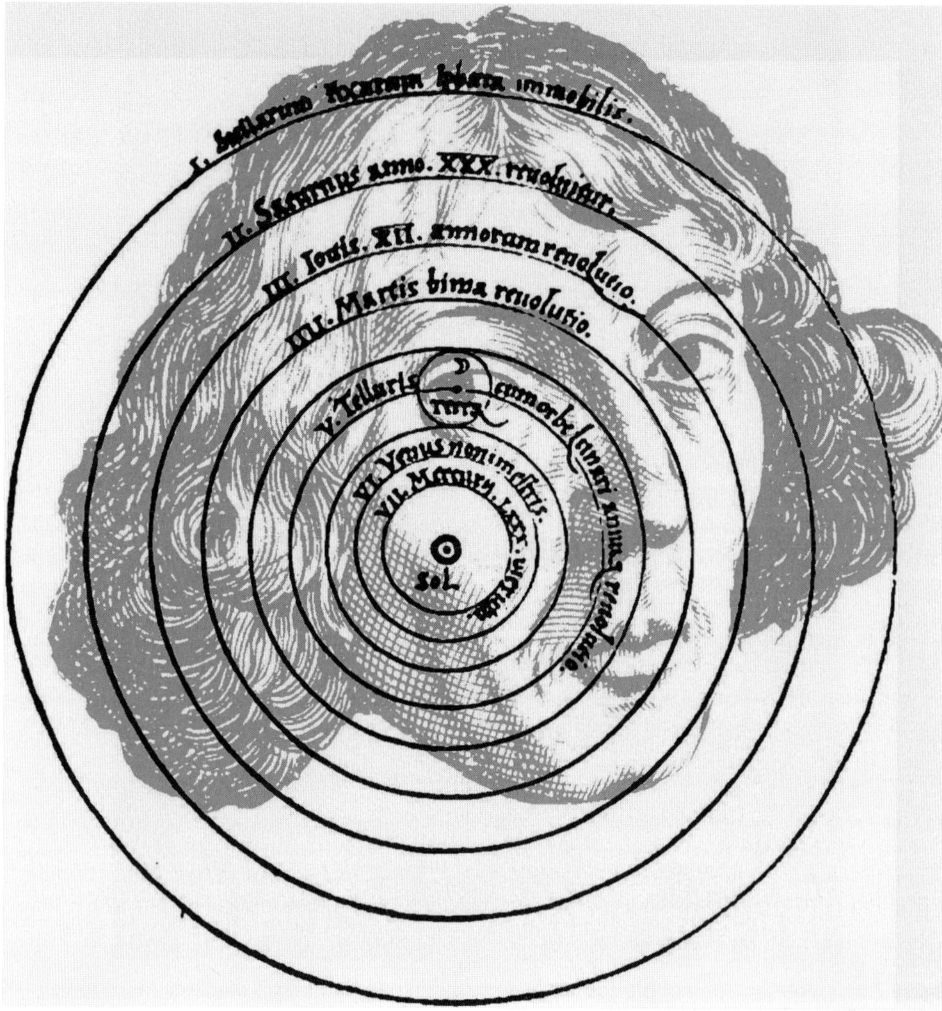

Figure 2.3 *The world of Copernicus* by Nicholas Wade. Nicolaus Copernicus disturbed Ptolemy's harmony of the spheres by proposing that the sun rather than earth was the centre of the universe. That is, although the eye of the observer is located on earth it does not lie at the centre of the world. In the illustration the eye of Copernicus is based on earth but the sun is at the centre; he was able to see beyond the confines of earth. In the model, Copernicus placed the earth and moon together, with Mercury and Venus closer to the sun and Mars, Jupiter and Saturn more distant. The planets have notes of the durations of their revolutions. The outermost circle is 'the immovable sphere of fixed stars'.

2.3 **Galileo and the sensory deconstruction of cosmic appearances**

The problem of mutability of the skies became a hotly debated issue from the second half of the sixteenth century, when the classical Aristotelian-Ptolemaic cosmology was in crisis. This was exacerbated by the appearance of prominent new stars (and of various comets) which attracted the interest of many astronomers and philosophers.

In Padua, Galileo observed a particularly bright new star in mid-October 1604. It was actually a supernova, afterwards called SN 1604, and also designated as Kepler's Supernova because it was studied in detail by the German astronomer, who published the results of his observations two years later in *De stella nova in pede Serpentarii* (Kepler, 1606). This new star represented Galileo's first opportunity to engage in a public debate on astronomical matters. It would also lead to his first works in print on these themes (two small polemical volumes) published in 1605 and 1606; their character anticipates some of his works published after his first telescopic observations. Both volumes appeared under pseudonyms, and were possibly both written by Galileo in collaboration with some friend or colleague. The immutability and incorruptibility of the sky is addressed from various points of view in both of these works, and the second (*Considerazioni d'Alimberto Mauri sopra alcuni luoghi del discorso di Ludovico delle Colombe intorno alla stella apparita 1604*[4]) involves annotation of a sensory character which would recur in later works. One is based on the possibility of seeing movements and changes in distant objects.

Ludovico delle Colombe was a Florentine philosopher and astrologer who invokes some classical Aristotelian arguments for the incorruptibility of the celestial world. Moreover, he explicitly says that the mutation and corruption normally occurring 'in the inferior things' because of their elemental composition 'cannot indeed be seen to occur in the celestial matter'. Galileo answers with piercing irony:

> Here is an argument for the incorruptibility of the sky drawn from the difference of elemental and celestial matter; behold:
>
> On earth beans are seen to dry, cucumber to blossom, cabbages to appear, and at the same time many animals decay. None of these effects are perceived in the sky. Therefore the matter of the sky is different from that of the earth below. Therefore, if the latter is corruptible and changeable, it follows that celestial [matter] is completely alien to these properties.
>
> But I hear someone whispering in my ear, 'Oh, but if the Author [i.e. Colombe] will have it that stars of the first magnitude, which are more than 107 times as large as earth, cannot be seen without spectacles, how will he ever know whether up above, even 100 miles away from us, things that small are created or destroyed? For even a distance of twenty miles loses mountains from our view, to say nothing of oaks and beeches'.—An objection that indeed will lose the Author some little reputation among the learned, unless I remind them that he is a supernatural Astrologer, and hence able quite well to divine whether or not those bagatelles of corruption exist here. (MAURI, fol. 4/transl. p. 85 revised)

A similar defence of those who pretend to see in the celestial bodies mutations analogous to those occurring on the earth was present in Galileo's other pseudonymous work on the new star published one year earlier. This was a text written in the dialect of Padua, *Dialogo de Cecco di Ronchitti da Bruzene in perpuosito de la stella nuova*,[5] with the aim of pitilessly ridiculing the fancy lucubrations on the new star expounded in the same year by another peripatetic philosopher, Antonio Lorenzini.

Many years later, Galileo will play the same tune again, although with a more graceful irony (and with some additional arguments), in a discussion between Salviati and Simplicio, two of the discussants in his masterpiece, the 1632 *Dialogue*. Like Colombe and Lorenzini, Simplicio is in this dialogue the defender of traditional doctrines and supports incorruptibility of the sky.

---

4 'Considerations of Alimberto Mauri on some places of the discourse of Ludovico delle Colombe about the star appeared in 1604.' From now it will generally referred simply as MAURI.

5 'Dialogue concerning the new star, by Cecco di Rochitti from Brugine.'

SALVIATI. As to the first, for whose force you appeal to experience, I wish you would tell me precisely what these alterations are that you see on the earth and not in the heavens, and on account of which you call the earth alterable and the heavens not.

SIMPLICIO. On earth I continually see herbs, plants, animals generating and decaying; winds, rains, tempests, storms arising; in a word, the appearance of the earth undergoing perpetual change. None of these changes are to be discerned in celestial bodies, whose positions and configurations correspond exactly with everything men remember, without the generation of anything new there or the corruption of anything old.

SALVIATI. But if you have to content yourself with these visible, or rather these seen experiences, you must consider China and America celestial bodies, since you surely have never seen in them these alterations which you see in Italy. Therefore, in your sense, they must be inalterable.

SIMPLICIO. Even if I have never seen such alterations in those places with my own senses, there are reliable accounts of them; besides which, *cum eadem sit ratio totius et partium*,[6] those counties being a pan of the earth like ours, they must be alterable like this.

SALVIATI. But why have you not observed this, instead of reducing yourself to having to believe the tales of others? Why not see it with your own eyes?

SIMPLICIO. Because those countries are far from being exposed to view; they are so distant that our sight could not discover such alterations in them.

SALVIATI. Now see for yourself how you have inadvertently revealed the fallacy of your argument. You say that alterations which may be seen near at hand on earth cannot be seen in America because of the great distance. Well, so much the less could they be seen in the moon, which is many hundreds of times more distant. And if you believe in alterations in Mexico on the basis of news from there, what reports do you have from the moon to convince you that there are no alterations there? From your not seeing alterations in heaven (where if any occurred you would not be able to see them by reason of the distance, and from whence no news is to be had), you cannot deduce that there are none, in the same way as from seeing and recognizing them on earth you correctly deduce that they do exist here. (DIALOGO, pp. 39–40; transl. pp. 47–48)

In addition to mutability (and motion), there were other perceptual phenomena of great importance in Galileo's endeavour which aimed at deconstructing the astronomical appearances (both the direct ones and those provided by the telescope) and providing support for the new conception formulated by Copernicus. In Chapter 1 we alluded to the problem of reflection, which was considered a distinguishing feature of the superlunary bodies with respect to the terrestrial world in the old cosmology. Galileo's elaboration on visual contrast and contour phenomena was of particular relevance in this context. As we shall see in Chapter 3, these phenomena imply that the brightness of a visual object is not a simple function of its physical luminance, but depends on that of the background or of nearby objects; similarly, the perceived contour of a visual feature depends on the luminance of the adjacent areas.

The vision of distant objects (like astronomical bodies) imposed a new critical reflection on visual appearances and their correspondence (or lack of it) with physical reality. This is because, in the case of distant objects, we cannot support the visual data with those from other sensory systems, and especially that provided by touch. Moreover, as distance increases the information provided by a change of viewpoint relative to the position of the observed object becomes less and less relevant. In general, distant objects are less amenable to the various forms of experimental manipulations by which the impression based on direct visual appearance can be confirmed (or falsified).

6 Since the rationale should be the same for the whole or the part.

2.4 Looking at the sky from the top of a Caucasian mountain

Because of its importance in the interpretation of astronomical appearances, Galileo's attention to the senses and their possible fallacies would become particularly vibrant in the period of his first astronomical observations and it would be one of the themes of *Sidereus nuncius*. However, his sensory interests certainly antedate the discussion of the new star of 1604. This is evident from a letter in 1597 addressed to Jacopo Mazzoni, a former teacher of Galileo in Pisa. Mazzoni had just published a book comparing the philosophies of Plato and Aristotle. Although private in character, this letter probably circulated amongst Galileo's friends. It is of interest here because Mazzoni raised an objection to the Copernican system which was addressed by Galileo who developed an argument based on considerations of geometrical optics. This anticipates some of his future methodological attitudes in interpreting telescopic images.

According to Mazzoni, if the sun was at the centre of the universe and the earth relatively peripheral, during the night we would see a much smaller portion of the vault of the heavens than during the day. This would be because in the night we would be farther from the centre of the universe (which—according to the Copernican system—corresponds to the centre of the vault and of the sun), and therefore the line of our sight would bisect the cosmic globe in an asymmetrical way. To support his view, Mazzoni invoked the Aristotelian consideration that compared to a person staying on the plain, an observer on the top of a Caucasian mountain would start seeing the sun much earlier at sunrise and much later at sunset. Galileo countered this argument on geometrical and perspective grounds (and with the help of two illustrations—Figure 2.4). For the purpose of seeing more or less of the sphere of the heavens what matters is the elevation of the observer with respect to the earth's surface, rather than their absolute displacement from a (putative) centre of the universe. On the basis of the contemporary cosmological assumptions concerning the dimensions and distances of the universe (and particularly the diameter of the sphere of the heavens and the distance between the earth and the sun), Galileo was able to show that variations of viewpoint on earth were miniscule relative to the cosmic distances involved.

The rebuttal of Mazzoni's argument against the Copernican system represents Galileo's implicit support of the new vision of the world elaborated by the Polish astronomer. In his letter to Mazzoni there is indeed an explicit pronouncement about Copernicus, whose opinion Galileo considers 'more probable than that of Aristotle and Ptolemy'. It is likely that, despite the fact that he was teaching astronomy according to the classical geocentric tradition, Galileo had been adhering to the Copernican system from a much earlier stage. This comes out particularly from a letter written in the same year and addressed to Johannes Kepler, where he informs his correspondent that he 'had come toward Copernicus' opinion since many years' (OG X, p. 68). Galileo also wrote (in the letter to Kepler) that by taking into account Copernicus's views he had been able to account for phenomena that were difficult to explain by other theories. Nevertheless he refrained from siding publicly with the Copernican opinion because of its general discredit among learned people which was causing 'hilarity and repulsion'. With these words, he was probably alluding to the fact that ironic comments would be cast on those people who adhered to the Copernican system but lacked good arguments against a series of objections generally raised against the theory. The most important of these objections (and the most repeated, since the publication, in 1543, of *De revolutionis orbium coelestiusm*) were those connected to the impossibility of perceiving the consequences of the earth's movement. It was argued that if the earth were to move, we should be aware of its in various ways: flying birds or clouds would be lagging westward as a consequence of the rapid eastward motion of the earth; in an analogous way, a stone dropped from the top of

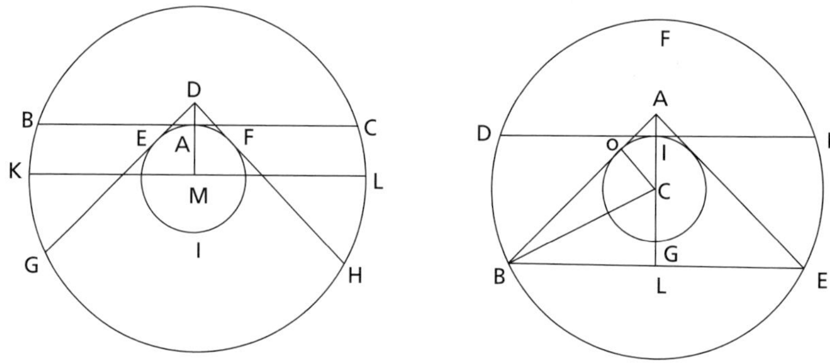

Figure 2.4 Galileo's schemes to answer the objection developed by Jacopo Mazzoni against the Copernican system on the basis of the supposed different visibility of the vault of the sky between night and day. The figure on the left allows Galileo to show that, as far as the visibility of different portions of the sky is concerned, a modest elevation of the observer (D) relative to the earth's surface has greater consequences than a larger displacement from the centre of the world (assuming that the observer remains on the surface of the earth). The observer is first supposed to be at the centre of the globe (M); afterwards on the earth's surface (B), and, finally, at an elevation D with respect to the earth's surface. The figure on the right allows Galileo to make quantitative measurements of the supposed effects on the basis of geometrical procedures. The fact that the vault of the heavens (or sphere of the fixed stars) does not exist physically does not diminish the strength of Galileo's argument against Mazzoni (and thus implicitly in favour of the Copernican system: from OG II, pp. 199–200[8]).

a tower would fall down in a westerly direction (as also would happen for an arrow shot vertically upward); finally because of the centrifugal consequences of the motion, objects would tend to leave the ground and rise up towards the sky with ruinous effects for animals, buildings, and towns.[7]

Starting from the letter to Mazzoni, in the large majority of his writings dealing with astronomical matters Galileo would attempt to provide arguments to support the Copernican system. This would often occur in an indirect or implicit way, due to the strong resistance of many civil and religious institutions of the age, and particularly the Catholic Church, against the new astronomy of Copernicus and his followers, which resulted eventually in the prohibition of Copernicus's work by the Holy Office in 1616. In order to achieve his goals, in some of his writings Galileo would play on the theme of ambiguity, and would use a technique referred to as 'honest dissimulation', a strategy that allowed people to express their opinions without the fear of incurring the wrath of the censors, but making the messages intelligible to expert readers.

In the case of the letter to Mazzoni, Galileo's visual argument dealt mainly with geometrical considerations, and such arguments would be used later in several circumstances (such as

[7] These were just some of the objections that in the works of his mature age, and particularly in the *Dialogue conceming the two chief systems of the world*, Galileo would show totally inconsistent and well accountable for by his inertial theory of motion.

[8] As indicated in the Bibliographic Abbreviations at the beginning of our book, the notation OG followed by the volume number refers to the National Edition of Galileo works, cited as Galilei, G. (1890–1909) in the References at the end of the book.

discussing the localization of sunspots with relation to the sun's surface, and in the calculation of the altitude of lunar mountains). Geometrical considerations were common in classical astronomy although they did not necessarily imply a physical correspondence with reality.

As we shall see starting from Chapter 3, in other circumstances Galileo's interest in visual phenomena had different and more sensory dimensions that we could qualify as psychophysical in modern terminology. This was particularly the case when he invoked contrast phenomena in order to reveal the possible fallacies of the immediate visual appearance as an indication of the physical brilliancy of celestial objects, or when he discussed the problem of the correspondence between the visual and physical dimensions of celestial objects.

Chapter 3

Casting light on Galileo's contrasts

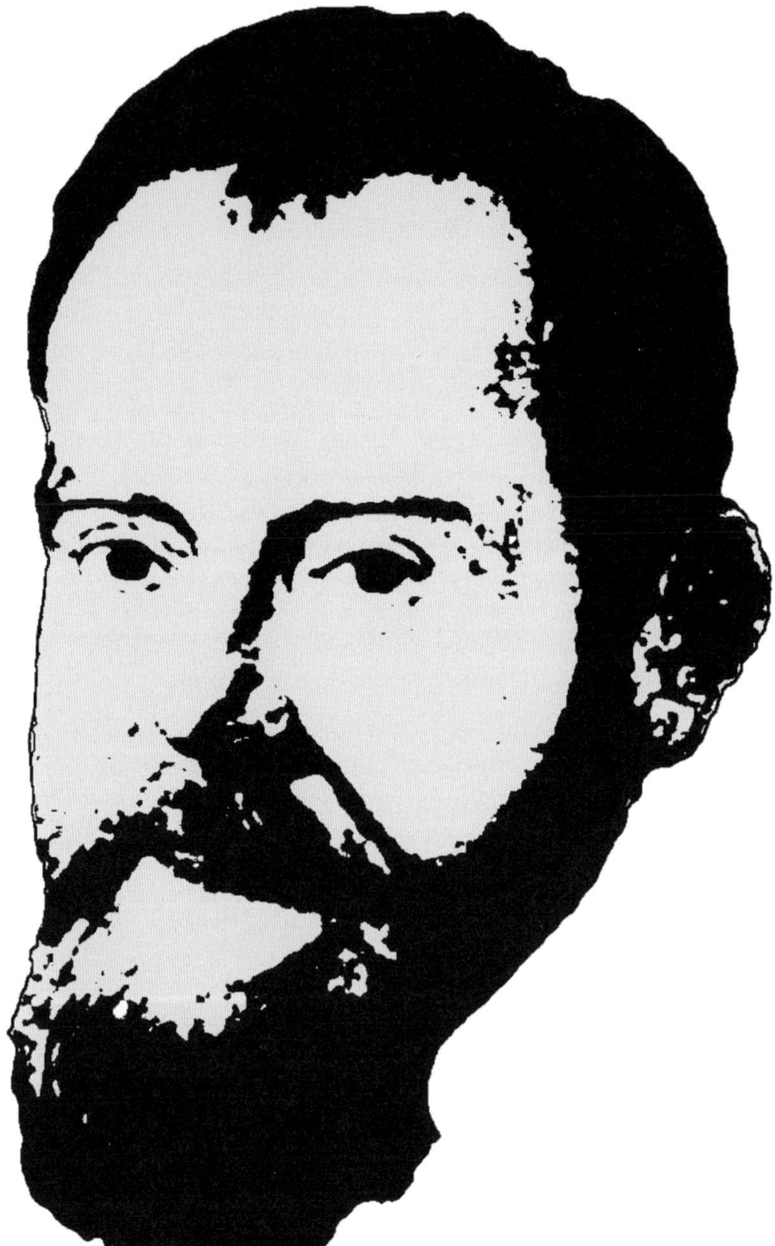

Figure III *Galileo in contrast* by Nicholas Wade. Galileo's bold features are rendered in black-and-white after a painting by an unknown artist, possibly Filippo Furini also known as Pippo Sciamerone (see Tongiorgi Tomasi, 2005). Despite the high contrast and loss of detail, Galileo can still be readily recognized.

3.1 Contrasting views

Naïve realism—the belief that perception provides a faithful copy of the external world—is questioned by a range of common experiences amongst which are constancy and contrast phenomena. They are so common, and we are so accustomed to seeing them, that we are usually unaware of their continuous occurrence. For example, the words printed on this page appear black, and much darker than the white background; they continue to appear so even when the intensity of the light falling onto the page is increased so that the light reflected from the printed characters is greater than the background was in the previous dimmer illumination. In other words, from very weak illumination to dazzling light the background will appear white and the written characters black. Indeed, with a light meter which can measure luminance, it can be shown that the intensity of the black letters on a bright summer's day is much greater that of the white background indoors under ordinary illumination.

To give another example, a piece of coal will appear black and a sheet of white paper will appear white, even when the intensity of the light they reflect is changed over a wide range. Even more strikingly, if the paper is in shadow, it may reflect less light than the coal, but the coal will still appear darker than the paper. Again, this is dependent on being able to perceive the intensity of the ambient illumination. If the paper and the coal are placed side by side and the coal is illuminated by a hidden spotlight, it can be made to appear whiter than the paper. These constancies are also influenced by perception of the three-dimensional space in which illuminated objects are placed. The phenomenon is called lightness constancy (Gilchrist, 2006), and without it survival would be virtually impossible.

The same considerations apply to most of the objects we observe as a consequence of reflections of light from them. Without lightness constancy we could no longer recognize the things around us, like the face of a familiar person, or respond appropriately to potentially dangerous objects. It would also be somewhat embarrassing if we could only read the written words on the page of a book under particular ambient illumination. Lightness constancy results in recognition under variable conditions of illumination whereas brightness contrast renders small differences in lightness easier to discriminate. They are usually referred to as simultaneous contrast phenomena. They generally refer to the apparent brightness or colour of one region in a pattern when it is surrounded by another having a different brightness or colour. For example, in Figure 3.1 the central grey circles all reflect the same amount of light, i.e. they have the same physical luminance, but there is a difference in their perceived brightness. This difference in brightness (a perceptual dimension) where there is no difference in luminance (a physical dimension) is due to the surrounding regions in each case. When the surround is lighter than the central grey circle the latter appears darker than when surrounded by a darker region. If the surrounds were

Figure 3.1 Simultaneous brightness contrast. The central circles are all the same luminance, but their brightnesses are influenced by the areas surrounding them. If the surround is darker then the grey circle looks brighter, and vice versa.

coloured then the central grey areas would also appear slightly coloured, but in the complementary colour to that of the surround. For instance, if the surround was red then the physically grey centre would appear greenish; if it was blue then the centre would appear yellowish.

These effects have been manipulated systematically by artists for centuries. They were well known to the scholars of the classic Greek and Roman period. Chinese artists of the Sung dynasty (960–1279) used them in a highly refined way to strengthen the perception of brightness. In the Western world, Leonardo in his *Trattato della pittura* described the effects of placing darker and whiter pigments next to one another. Many subsequent painters made recourse to contrast phenomena in order to enhance the perceptual brightness (or darkness) of a detail in their pictorial compositions, and this is particularly evident in the attempt to represent luminous objects, especially sources of light. Good examples can be found in the paintings of Caravaggio, Rembrandt, Georges de La Tour, and Seurat.

In Galileo's time, painters were familiar with techniques for alluding to solid objects on a flat canvas, like contrast and other perceptual phenomena. These were described in a variety of treatises and manuals for artists together with directions on the use of chiaroscuro, illumination and reflection phenomena, dark-and-shadow effects, and linear perspective. Galileo was well versed in painting (see Chapter 1) and he used his knowledge as an aid to interpret the visual experiences connected to his telescopic and cosmological research.

3.2 On dark and light contrasts and on the sun and moon

The interpretation of local contrasts was significant in Galileo's disputes with the German Jesuit, Christoph Scheiner (Figure 3.2). This took place a few years after the publication of *Sidereus nuncius* in 1610. The debate concerned the discovery and interpretation of the spots on the surface of the sun that were visible with the newly invented telescope. According to traditional cosmology (strongly supported by Jesuits) the sun, being a perfect sphere, could not have imperfections on its surface like these spots. Also embarrassing to traditional astronomy was the fact that the spots observed by both Scheiner and Galileo were not fixed and seemed to move over the sun's surface and eventually disappear. These phenomena added another problem for the traditional view which maintained that the superlunary world was unchanging and unchangeable. In order to undermine the potentially revolutionary relevance of the sunspots and provide support for classical cosmology, Scheiner assumed that the spots were not actually on the surface of the sun. He argued that they resulted from the momentary congregation of a cluster of small satellites rotating around the sun. Because of their small size, these satellites would not normally be visible unless they happened to concentrate in front of the sun. This could result in them intercepting sunlight and appearing as dark spots on its surface. In this way, Scheiner could rescue the doctrine of celestial immutability without denying the reality of his own observations and also those by other astronomers.

Scheiner's theory of sunspots was expounded in 1611 in his *Tres Epistolae de Maculis solaribus scriptae ad Marcum Welserum* ('Three letters on sunspots written to Mark Welser'), which were published in the following year by Welser's private press (Scheiner, 1612a); he was an important banker and public councillor in Augsburg and was closely connected to the Society of Jesus. Welser spoke Italian because he had lived in Italy and studied in Padua; he was acquainted with Galileo and his circle and became a fellow member of the Accademia dei Lincei. Accordingly he sought Galileo's advice on Scheiner's observations. The three letters did not appear under Scheiner's name but bore the signature of *Apelles latens post tabulam* ('Apelles hidden behind the painting', a pseudonym already adopted on previous occasions and derived from an anecdote narrated by Plinius the Elder in relation to the famous Greek painter, Apelles of Kos).

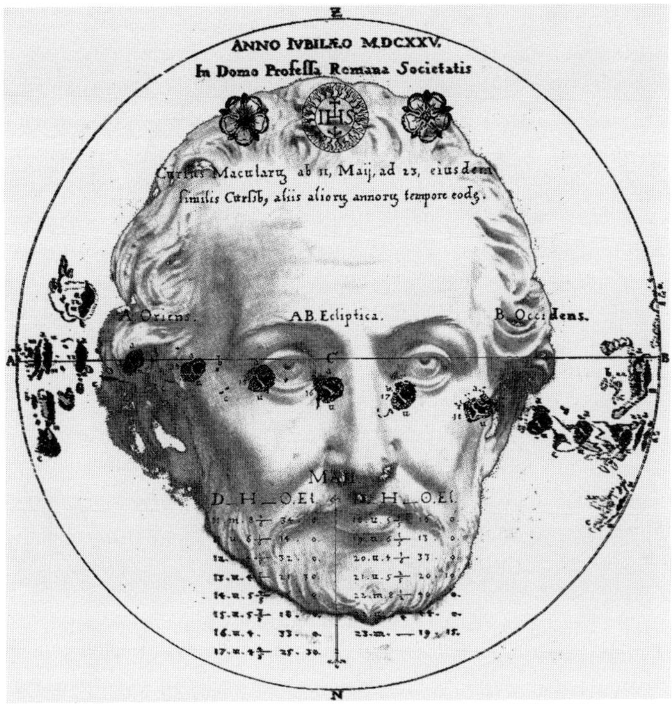

Figure 3.2 *Scheiner's sunspots* by Nicholas Wade. Christoph Scheiner's representation of sunspots seen during May 1625 (from *Rosa Ursina*, 1630) encloses his portrait which is derived from a nineteenth-century bust illustrated in Daxecker (2004).

The first letter described the 'rather blackish spots like dark specks' against the surface of the sun, noting that these spots could not be due to objects present in the terrestrial atmosphere. Scheiner did not consider it likely that the spots were located on the surface of the sun:

> It has always seemed to me unfitting and, in fact, unlikely, that on the most lucid body of the Sun there would be spots, and that these would be far darker than any ever observed on the Moon, except for one very small one.[1] (MACULIS, F2 r; transl. p. 62)

Galileo's (Figure 3.3) response to Scheiner was also written in the form of three letters also addressed to Welser. It was published in 1613 by the Accademia dei Lincei under the title *Istoria e dimostrazioni intorno alle macchie solari e loro accidenti* ('History and demonstrations concerning sunspots and their accidents'). In the letters Galileo refuted almost all the assertions and interpretations contained in Scheiner's *Tres Epistolae*. He based his refutations on a series of

[1] '*In Sole, corpore lucidissimo, statuere maculas, easque nigriores multo quam sint in Luna unquam visae (praeter unicam parvulam), mihi inconveniens semper est visum, et vero necdum fit probabile*'.
The dark small spot on the moon surface alluded to by Scheiner is likely the Grimaldi basin, located near the border of the moon, slightly on the south (lunar coordinates: longitude 68.6° W, latitude 5.2° S) which is considered the darkest zone of the moon's surface.

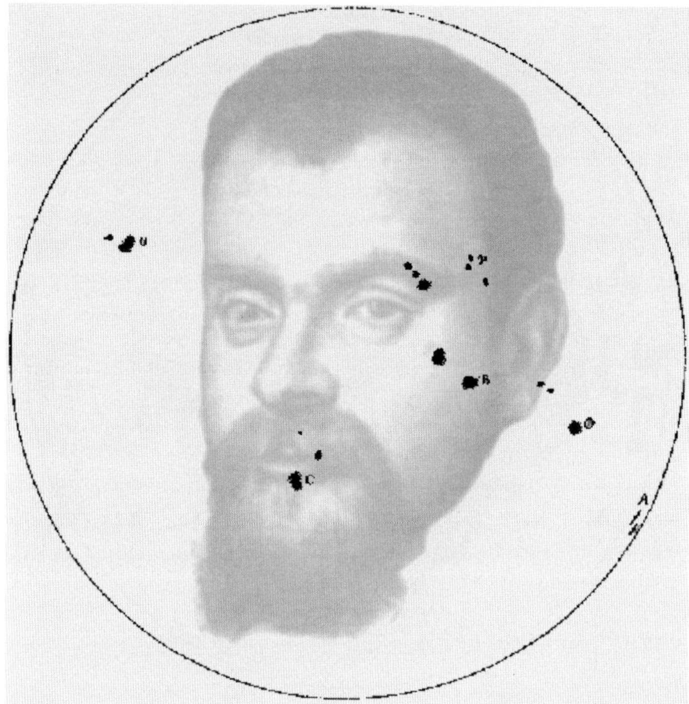

Figure 3.3 *Galileo's sunspots* by Nicholas Wade. Galileo's illustration of sunspots (from *Istoria e dimostrazioni intorno alle macchie solari*, 1613) encloses his face derived from a portrait of him, painted by Domenico Tintoretto when Galileo was 42 years old (see Fahie, 1929).

arguments, relying on his own observations of the phenomena, and particularly on geometrical 'demonstrations' about the location of the sunspots relative to the surface of the sun. The *Istoria* is one of the most important of Galileo's works and the first printed work expounding general arguments of an epistemological character. It can be considered as a kind of elaborate treatise on how immediate visual appearances might be surprisingly different from expectations regarding the physical reality, particularly relating to observations of distant objects. It also indicated how, despite such deceptions, important knowledge concerning reality could be extracted.

3.4 Very brilliant, dark spots and impossible comparisons in the sky

Let us first consider how Galileo deals with Scheiner's assertion that sunspots 'would be far darker than any spot ever observed on the Moon' (with the unimportant exception of 'a very small one' on the lunar surface). In a way which seems paradoxical, Galileo develops a series of arguments which would conclude that these apparently dark sunspots are physically very brilliant, and much more so not only than the dark zone of the moon, but even than the (apparently) intensely luminous regions of the moon's face. In his first letter Galileo develops his argument in this way:

> What Apelles said in that passage, namely, that the spots appearing on the Sun are much darker than any ever observed on the Moon, I believe to be absolutely false. On the contrary, I believe that the spots one sees on the Sun are not only less dark than the dark spots one sees on the Moon, but [also] that they

are no less bright than the most luminous parts of the Moon even when it is most directly illuminated by the Sun. And my reasoning is as follows. Even though at its evening rising Venus is filled with such great splendour, it is not visible until it is many degrees from the Sun, especially when both are high above the Orient. This is because those regions of the ether, surrounding the Sun, are no less bright than Venus itself, and from this it can be argued that if we could put the Moon, shining with the same light that it has when full beside the Sun, it would in fact remain invisible, as it would do when located in a field no less shining and bright than its own face. Now consider [the fact that] when we gaze at the very bright solar disc with the telescope—that is, with the spyglass—how much brighter it appears than the surrounding field, and when we then compare the blackness of the solar spots both with the light of the Sun itself and with the darkness of the adjacent setting, we will find from the one and the other comparison that the spots of the Sun are not darker than the surrounding field. If therefore, the darkness of the solar spots is not greater than that of the field that surround the Sun, and also if the splendour of the Moon would remain imperceptible in the brightness of the same surroundings, then it follows as a necessary consequence that the solar spots are by no means less bright than the brightest parts of the Moon, even though against the most dazzling background of the solar disc they manifest themselves as dark and black. And if these spots yield nothing in brightness to the most luminous parts of the Moon, how bright will they be in comparison with the dark spots of the Moon, especially if we were referring to those caused by the projected shadows of the lunar mountains, which—compared to the illuminated parts—are no less black than the ink compared to this paper? And I intend this not so much to contradict Apelles as to show that it is not necessary to suppose that the material of the spots is very opaque and dense, as one must reasonably assume the matter of the Moon and the other planets to be, for density and opacity similar to that of a cloud interposed between the Sun and us is sufficient to cause such a darkness and blackness. (ISTORIA, pp. 12–14; transl. pp. 91–92)

Galileo articulates the comparison between the brightness of sunspots with those of the moon under similar background illumination through a series of logical steps. We will try to identify and separate these steps with the twofold aim of facilitating the reader's comprehension and of unveiling how the Pisan scientist succeeds in making a visual comparison which is impossible to perform in reality. To succeed in his purpose Galileo first invokes Venus, the brightest planet in the night sky, as having an intermediate brightness so facilitating comparison of the sun and moon under similar conditions. The physical impossibility of the experiment is that it would require seeing the moon in its full phase near the sun; this would allow the comparison of the dark and light zones of the two celestial bodies under the same background illumination. This is astronomically impossible because of the astronomical relationship between sun, earth, and moon and because the luminosity of the moon is due to reflection of sunlight: when the moon is visually close to the sun (astronomically, in 'conjunction' with it) it would become invisible being in the phase of a new moon.

In the first step of his demonstration Galileo says that, despite its apparent brightness (superior to that of the moon), Venus becomes invisible when it is near the sun, an effect accountable for by the fact that it is not as bright as the halo surrounding the sun. The second step assumes that the full moon, being less brilliant than Venus, would also become invisible if it could be seen near the sun. With Venus as an intermediate element, Galileo has thus succeeded in making the luminous region surrounding the sun the common background for the comparison between the moon and the sun. He is now ready for the third logical step of his thought experiment. With the help of the telescopic observation he goes on to establish a comparison between the brightness (or darkness) of the solar spots with both the ordinary regions of the sun's surface and the sky's surface immediately surrounding the sun.

This darkness of the circumsolar area seems to be in contrast with the previous annotations pointing to its brightness. As, for instance, when Galileo wrote that 'those regions of the ether, surrounding the Sun, are no less bright than Venus itself', or when he spoke of the moon 'which would in fact remain invisible, as would it do when located in a field no less shining and bright than its own face'. This happens because—as he is well aware—the brightness of a visual object depends on the background against which it is observed. To be able to withstand the extremely great clarity of the sun body one needs to filter or attenuate sunlight in some way and this results in a dark appearance of the halo surrounding the sun.

Galileo now arrives at his conclusion (step 4) that the sun spots, even though 'they manifest themselves as dark and black', are indeed brighter than 'the most luminous parts of the Moon', a conclusion which appears paradoxical, but is so only for a naïve realist who is ready to accept sensory experiences as veridical indications of physical reality.

3.5 **The sadness of seeing the earth dark**

Galileo's third letter on sunspots was written after Scheiner had published another tract on the same matter, also composed of a series of letters addressed to Welser (*De Maculis solaribus et stellis circa Iouem errantibus, Accuratior disquisitio*—'On sunspots and on the stars wandering around Jupiter, a more accurate enquiry': Scheiner, 1612b). One of the themes dealt with in Galileo's third letter is that of the brightness of the moon. We have already mentioned in Chapter 1 (in connection with sunlight reflected from the sea) that Galileo attributed the brightness of the moon to diffuse reflections, similar to those from any irregular surface illuminated by an external source. Invoking this process meant that the surface of the moon is irregular; this corresponded with Galileo's telescopic observations of the moon with its craters, mountains, and various other inequalities (see Chapters 5 and 6). This was not a minor aspect of the cosmological discussion of the age, inasmuch it represented—in Galileo's hands—an important argument against the traditional cosmology of Aristotle and Ptolemy. In classical science, the moon shines under the action of the sun's rays because it is a sphere with a perfectly polished surface, being made of extremely pure crystal-like matter (the quintessence, a faultless and immutable substance, profoundly different from the four elements forming the sublunary world). Its brightness was thus produced by reflection comparable to that of a mirror.

These characteristics of the moon (in common with other superlunary bodies) were in contrast with those of earth, a place of irregularity and mutation. Moreover, earth was considered as an opaque body incapable of reflecting the sun's rays because of its 'elementary'[2] composition and the roughness of its surface. Galileo shows that the moon can shine brilliantly in the sky just because its surface is as irregular as that of the earth. Paradoxically, it shines because it seems unsuited to reflection, at least according to the common sense view of the matter.

As mentioned previously, in the case of sunspots, Scheiner had developed an ad hoc explanation, based on the variable aggregation of the swarm of minute satellites, in order to face the revolutionary implication of the presence of irregularities and variations on the surface of 'the most lucid body of the Sun'. In a similar way, he tried to face the upsetting consequences of an irregular lunar surface for traditional cosmology; this would make the moon similar to the earth, thus undermining the essential distinction between the earthly and celestial worlds. Scheiner supposed that the apparent irregularities visible on the moon's surface were due to the partial penetration of rays from the sun on a lunar body made of a translucent material. This hypothesis was already current among the scholars adhering to traditional cosmology (see Chapter 11). They had been

---

[2] In the language of peripatetic science 'elementary' meant to be made of the four elements of the sublunar world (earth, water, air, and fire).

obliged to find an explanation for the apparent lack of homogeneity of the lunar surface that had been visible long before the invention of the telescope. They did not wish to assume that lunar surface is in fact irregular.[3]

In the third letter on sunspots, Galileo develops his attacks on Scheiner by trying to understand the psychological and historical reasons for adhering to the traditional view. He addresses this question not only to 'the common people'—*il popolo*—but also to philosophers and scientists—'the Aristotles and Ptolemys'.

Galileo writes:

> But because Apelles is so unwilling to concede that such a powerful reflection of light comes from the terrestrial globe, and so ready to admit that the lunar body is transparent and can be penetrated by the rays of the Sun, as he argues here and even more openly toward the end of these discussions, I want to adduce one or two of the many reasons that persuade me that the former conclusion is true and the latter false. If these were by some chance resolved in Apelles' favour, they would be able to change my opinion. In the meantime, I will not be silent about the fact that I strongly suspect that this common notion—that the earth, as dark opaque, and rough as it is, is incapable of reflecting the light of the sun, while, on the contrary, the Moon and the other planets reflect it well—is prevalent among the masses because we never have occasion to see it from some dim and remote place while it is illuminated by the Sun. By contrast we often see the Moon when it is in the dark field of the sky, and we are encumbered by nocturnal gloom. And here it happens that when we lower our eyes to the Earth, after having fixed them on the wondrous splendour of the Moon and of the stars, we are in some fashion saddened by its darkness, and we form a dread of it as a thing repugnant by its nature to all radiance. We fail to consider that the density, darkness, and roughness of the material, in no way prevent it from receiving and reflecting the light of the Sun, and that illumination is a gift and a quality of the Sun, and requires no excellence at all in the bodies that are to be illuminated by it. On the contrary, it is rather necessary to deprive them of certain more noble features such as transparency of substance and smoothness of surface, rendering the matter opaque and its exterior rough and rugged. And I am very certain, in contrast to popular opinion, that if the Moon were polished and smooth like a mirror, not only would it not reflect the light of the Sun to us as it does, but it would also be absolutely invisible, as if it were not there. And in its proper place I will make this manifest with clear demonstrations. (ISTORIA, pp. 133–134; transl. pp. 283–284)

Galileo presents his account of the reluctance to accept the possibility that the Earth could shine like the moon (and that the moon shines, not despite of, but because of the unevenness of its surface) in a lively and emotional way. He makes reference to the hypothetical sadness of someone who would look down to the darkness of the earth after having contemplated the fascinating splendour of the moon.

Galileo develops another of his thought experiments in order to undermine this attitude which, he believes, is largely based on the impossibility of seeing the earth illuminated by the sun against the dark, nocturnal sky. The purpose of this experiment is to create virtual conditions in which the comparison between the earth and the sun could be made in somewhat similar situations. The problem is that, at least in his time, it was impossible for people to look at the earth illuminated by

[3] In the *Dialogue*, with reference to the hypothesis of a moon perfectly regular in its surface, but appearing irregular because of its unevenly transparent parts, Sagredo made the comparison of the lunar body with the 'mother of pearl', which 'even when brought to an extreme polish, it appears to the eye so pitted and raised in various places that even touching it can hardly make us to believe to its smoothness' (Galileo, 1632, p. 79). The theme of moon surface irregularities will be dealt with in various chapters of this book and particularly in Chapters 6 and 7.

the sun against the nocturnal sky. The ideal condition for the observer was to view 'full earth' from the moon. This would correspond to the situation of astronomical opposition between the earth and moon with respect to the sun, and would imply the absence of the sun's direct illumination of the lunar surface. A voyage to the moon was then possible only in the imagination of poets (for instance, his favourite Ariosto who would let Astolfo fly to the moon with his hippogriff in search of Roland's sense).[4]

Galileo's strategy consists of creating a different comparison, bringing the moon against the background of the diurnal sky and placing it in direct relation with terrestrial objects, like clouds or the top of a tower or a wall illuminated by the sky:

> But not to stray from the matter at hand, I say that I find it easy to believe that if we had never happened to see the Moon by night, but only during the day, we would have formed the same impression of it as we have of the Earth. For, if we consider the Moon during the day, when on occasion it is more than a quarter illuminated and it happens to be in the wisps of some white clouds, or perhaps near the peak of a tower or a wall whose colour is of a middling brightness, when these bodies are directly illuminated by the Sun such that one might compare their lustre with the light of the Moon, their splendour will surely be found to be no less than that of the Moon. Therefore, if they were able to remain illuminated in this fashion even in the darkness of the night, they would appear to us no less luminous than the Moon. Nor would they illuminate the places around them less than it does, up to that distance from which their apparent size would be no smaller than the lunar size. But these clouds and walls, stripped of the rays of the Sun, remain at night not less dark and black than the Earth. (ISTORIA, pp. 134–135; transl. p. 294)

As Galileo remarks, from a comparison of this type, it would emerge that the splendour of the terrestrial object 'will surely be found to be no less than that of the Moon'. The common conviction that the moon is much more luminous than the Earth was due to the fact that terrestrial objects cannot be seen as illuminated by the sun at night.

3.6 Galileo's artistic reflections

In continuing his argument, Galileo confirms that the earth reflects sunlight like the moon, and further compares the moon with terrestrial objects. This is again a thought experiment which draws on Galileo's favourite theme of diffuse reflection (see Chapter 1 and also Chapter 12). More specifically it is inspired by the discussion amongst Italian painters of the so-called 'secondary lumen'. This is based on the observation of light passing through a hole into a dark room illuminating a wall opposite. If the diameter of the hole is such that it would subtend a visual angle no larger than that of the moon, then the light reflected from the wall would be intense enough to illuminate a second room communicating with the first one. The secondary illumination would be sufficient to read a book more easily than with direct moonlight:

> We should, moreover, derive great certainty about the Earth's ability to reflect light from seeing how much it spreads in a room deprived of all other illumination and lit only by the reflection from a wall facing it that happens to be struck by the Sun, even if that reflection passes through a hole so small that from the place in the room where it strikes its diameter does not appear to subtend an angle greater than that of the visual diameter of the Moon. Nevertheless, this secondary light is so powerful that when it has struck and passed from a first room into a second it will still be no less luminous than the first reflection of the moon [*che non punto cederà alla prima reflessione della Luna*]. A clear and

[4] As mentioned in Chapter 1, Kepler imagined a voyage to the moon in his *Somnium, seu De Astronomia lunari*, mainly in order to undermine astronomers' objections to the Copernican system.

> available proof of this is that we will read a book more comfortably by the second reflection from the wall than we would by the primary reflection from the Moon. (ISTORIA, p. 135; transl. p. 284)

The use of reading as an estimate of luminance is an indication of Galileo's awareness of the unreliability of the immediate perception as a clue to the physical reality of the visual world and of the importance of contrast phenomena. Galileo goes further in providing other indications of the similarity between moon and earth reflection, again making a thought experiment based on an apparently impossible comparison between celestial and terrestrial objects under comparable conditions. First the comparison between 'a flame on a distant mountain at night' and 'a star grazing the horizon'; a comparison from which he concludes that the light from the star might be indistinguishable from that from the flame. Then a second comparison is based on the supposition of 'the Earth burning and wholly inflamed'. If a flame could appear like a star then under these conditions the earth would appear like a brilliant star if observed from a dark and distant place (for instance, from the moon during the lunar night). The third step is to compare the brightness of a flame with that of 'a stone or a piece of wood directly struck by a beam of sunlight' (a comparison that does not require a thought experiment). The fact that a flame in full sunlight viewed from some distance would become invisible means that it irradiates less light that that reflected by the stone or the wood illuminated by the sun.

All this amounts to saying that the earth, struck by the sun's light, would in principle shine towards the moon as the moon shines towards the earth (and, because of their different sizes, much more terrestrial light would reach the moon, than lunar light reaching earth). In sum, Galileo has succeeded in transporting his ideal observer (and with him the readers of his book) into space to let them contemplate the brightness of the earth illuminated against the darkness of the nocturnal sky. This achievement would require a spacecraft journeying to the moon; or simply the acute mental elaborations of 'a man endowed by nature with a very perspicacious mind and an extraordinary curiosity', as Galileo undoubtedly was. But let us conclude this chapter in Galileo's own words from the *Istoria* describing this last impossible comparison:

> Finally, I add that there will be few who, observing a flame on a distant mountain at night, might not have wondered whether they were seeing a fire or a star grazing the horizon, the latter's light appearing no greater than that of a flame. From this, one would suppose not only that were the Earth burning and wholly enflamed, it would appear no less bright than a star if seen from the dark part of the Moon, but also that every rock and every clod of dirt struck by sunlight is considerably brighter than if it were on fire. This will easily be observed if a lighted candle is brought near a stone or a piece of wood directly struck by a beam of sunlight, for the flame is by comparison invisible. And thus the Earth, struck by the Sun and seen from the dark part of the Moon will appear as bright as all other stars, and as much more light will be reflected to the Moon [from the Earth] as the Earth exceeds the Moon in size, the surface area of our globe being, that is, about twelve times as large as the lunar body appear to be to us. Besides, at New Moon, the Earth is closer to the Sun than is the Moon when it is full, and therefore the one is more strongly illuminated, that is, from nearer by; the light from the Earth will therefore reflect more forcefully to the Moon than will that from the Moon to the Earth. For these and many other reasons and experiences that for the sake of brevity I will omit, the reflection of the Earth should, in my opinion, be considered sufficient to explain the secondary light of the Moon. There is no need to bring up any transparency, least of all the degree of transparency attributed to it by Apelles, in which I seem to see certain inexplicable contradictions. (ISTORIA, pp. 135–136; transl. pp. 284–285)

Chapter 4

The lunar candour and the litheosphorus

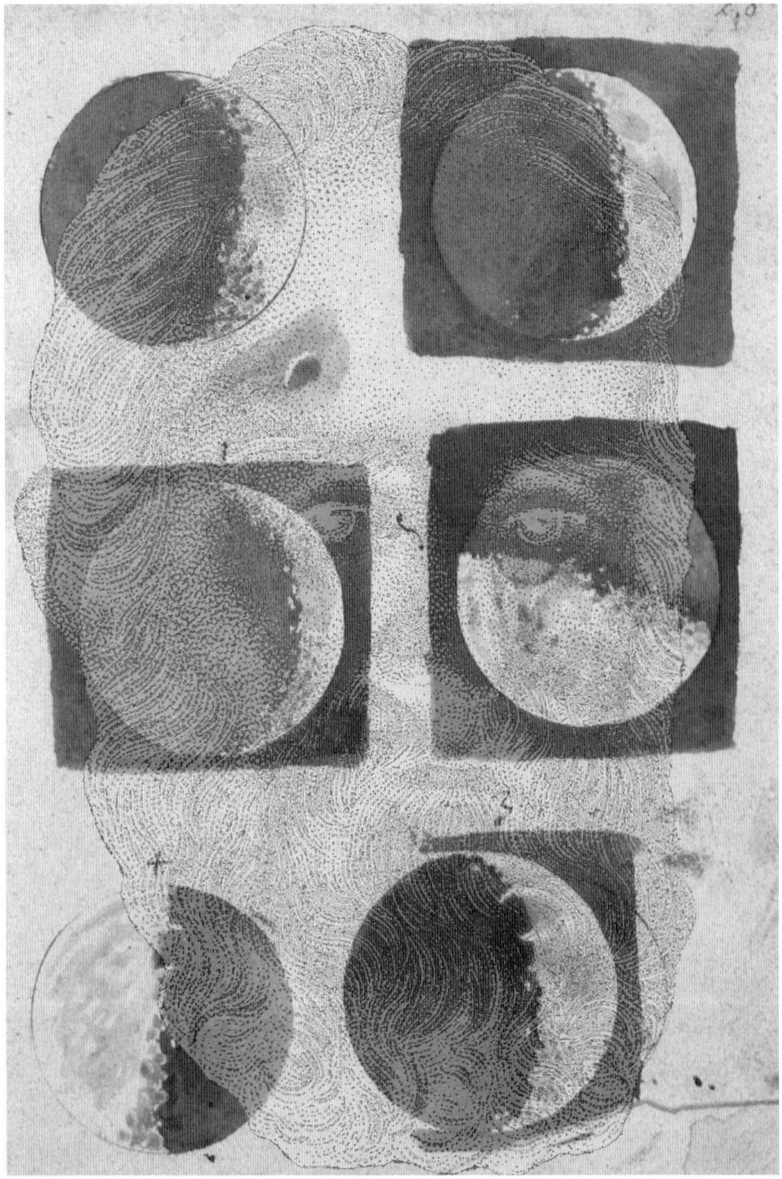

Figure IV *Galileo's lunar candour* by Nicholas Wade. Galileo's painting of phases of the moon (courtesy of the Biblioteca Nazionale, Florence) is combined with a low-contrast portrait of Galileo derived from an engraving (in Knight, 1834) based on a painting by Alan Ramsay.

4.1 What was already known about moon and clouds

The theme of the luminance of the moon indicated Galileo's deep concern with the topic of light reflection. It is one of the most important aspects of his interpretations of sensory appearances and he returns to it repeatedly in his work. It also represents a fundamental feature of his arguments against traditional cosmology. This was because it pointed to the applicability of the same physical laws to the supralunar and terrestrial world, thus undermining the essential separation between the sky and earth, which was an essential tenet of traditional cosmology. The relevance of Galileo's conclusion in this context justifies the way Bertolt Brecht introduces the third scene of the first act in his *Life of Galileo*. This scene portrays the first telescopic observation of the moon, together with Galileo's consideration of the similar physical properties of the earth regarding their similar capacity of reflecting sun light:

> *January ten, sixteen ten:*
> *Galileo Galilei abolishes heaven.*[1]

The strong reactions to Galileo's astronomical and cosmological conclusions, particularly by the Catholic Church, more than justify the acute way the great German dramatist reflected on this important aspect of Galileo's work.

The luminance of the moon is one of the most important themes on the 'First Day' of Galileo's *Dialogue*. Galileo's alter ego, Salviati, directs the scene addressing Sagredo, a Venetian aristocrat fully open to the new science, and Simplicio, the defender of traditional cosmology. Simplicio is strongly anchored in the ideas and conceptions of 'old authors' and principally Aristotle and his followers, the peripatetics. He is reluctant to admit that 'the earth can reflect light from the sun no less strongly than the moon can'. Challenging him, Salviati says that he knows from the outset, better than Simplicius himself, the reasons of his difficulties. This attitude reflects an important aspect of the *Dialogue* (also present in other Galileo's works and—for instance—in the *Istoria*). This is the effort made by Galileo to penetrate and make clear the reasons for the resistance encountered by both common people and philosophers in accepting the new science, and the tendency to adhere tenaciously to the old knowledge, even in the presence of strong contrary evidence.

Salviati refers initially to the comparison, already present in the third letter on sunspots, between the luminance of the moon during daylight and that of 'a little cloud' (*una nugoletta*) illuminated by the sun:

SIMPLICIO. Whether I reason well or badly, you might indeed know better than I do; but whether I reason well or badly I shall never believe that you can see into my reasoning better than I.

SALVIATI. Even that I shall make you believe in due course. Tell me, when the moon is nearly full, so that it can be seen by day and also in the middle of the night, does it appear more brilliant in the daytime or at night?

SIMPLICIO. Incomparably more at night. It seems to me that the moon resembles those pillars of cloud and fire which guided the children of Israel; for in the presence of the sun it shows itself like a little cloud, but then at night it is most splendid. (DIALOGO, pp. 80–81; transl. p. 87)

Afterwards, Salviati remarks that the particular brightness of the moon at night does not correspond to physical reality but is the consequence of a psychophysiological effect:

SALVIATI. So that if you had never happened to see the moon except by day, you would not have judged it brighter than one of those little clouds?

---

[1] Brecht, 1955, p. 22; transl. 1967, p. 35.

SIMPLICIO. I do believe you are right.

SALVIATI. Now tell me, do you believe that the moon is really brighter at night than by day, or just that by some accident it looks that way?

SIMPLICIO. I believe that it shines intrinsically as much by day as by night, but that its light looks greater at night because we see it in the dark field of the sky. In the daytime, because everything around it is very bright, by its small addition of light it appears much less bright.

Salviati induces Simplicio to conclude that the brightness of the moon at night does not necessarily imply an essential difference of the lunar matter with respect to the matter of the earth:

SALVIATI. Now tell me, have you ever seen the terrestrial globe lit up by the sun in the middle of the night?

SIMPLICIO. That seems to me to be a question that is not asked except in sport, or only of some person notorious for his lack of wit.

SALVIATI. No, no; I take you for a very sensible man, and ask the question in earnest. So answer just the same, and then if that I am talking nonsense, I shall be taken for the brainless one; for he is a greater fool who asks a silly question than he to whom the question is put.

SIMPLICIO. Then if you do not take me for a complete simpleton, pretend that I have answered you by saying that it is impossible for anyone who is on earth, as we are, to see by night that part of the earth where it is day; that is to say, the part which is struck by the sun.

SALVIATI. So you have never chanced to see the earth illuminated except by day, but you see the moon shining in the sky on the darkest night as well. And that, Simplicio, is the reason for your believing that the earth does not shine like the moon; for if you could see the earth illuminated while you were in a place as dark as night, it would look to you more splendid than the moon. Now if you want to proceed properly with the comparison, we must draw our parallel between the earth's light and that of the moon as seen in daytime; not the nocturnal moon, because there is no chance of our seeing the earth illuminated except by day. Is that satisfactory?

SIMPLICIO. So it must be.

SALVIATI. Now you yourself have already admitted having seen the moon by day among little whitish clouds, and similar in appearance to one of them. This amounts to granting at the outset that these little clouds, though made of elemental matter, are just as fit to receive light as the moon is. More so, if you will recall in memory having seen some very large clouds at times, white as snow. It cannot be doubted that if such a one could remain equally luminous on the darkest night, it would light up the surrounding regions more than a hundred moons. If we were sure, then, that the earth is as much lighted by the sun as one of these clouds, no question would remain about its being no less brilliant than the moon. Now all doubt upon this point ceases when we see those same clouds, in the absence of the sun, remaining as dark as the earth all night long. And what is more, there is not one of us who has not seen such a cloud low and far off, and wondered whether it was a cloud or a mountain; a clear indication that mountains are no less luminous than those clouds. (pp. 81–82/pp. 88–89)

Soon afterwards Galileo returns to the argument that light from the sun when reflected from a wall illuminates a dark room more intensely than the rays coming directly from the moon. In contrast to the *Istoria*, he does this by recourse to a true experiment portrayed by Sagredo, the other debater. As in the previous text, among the arguments invoked by Sagredo in support of his (and Salviati's) views is that of the readability of a book under different conditions of illumination.

SAGREDO. But why any more arguments? Yonder is the moon, more than half full, and over there is a high wall. Come this way so that the moon is seen beside the wall. Now look; which appears the brighter to you? Do you not see that if there is any advantage it belongs to the wall? The sun hits that wall, and from there it is reflected to the walls of this room; thence it is reflected into that chamber, so that it arrives there on its third reflection; and I am absolutely certain that there is more light there than if the light were arriving directly from the moon.

SIMPLICIO. Oh, I do not think so, for the light which the moon gives, especially at the full, is very great.

SAGREDO. It seems great from the darkness of the shadowy surroundings, but it is not much absolutely; less than that of the twilight a half hour after sunset.This is obvious, because earlier than that you do not see enough to distinguish upon the ground the shadows of things illuminated by the moon. You could tell whether this third reflection in that chamber gives more light than the moon by going in there and reading a book, and then testing whether it is easier to read by moonlight. I believe it would be harder.

By addressing himself to Simplicio, Salviati can thus conclude his discourse with these words:

SALVIATI. If you are satisfied now, Simplicio, you can see how you yourself really knew that the earth shone no less than the moon, and that not my instruction but merely the recollection of certain things already known *to you* have made you sure of it. For I have not shown you that the moon shines more brilliantly by night than by day; you already knew it, as you also knew that a little cloud is brighter than the moon. Likewise you knew that the illumination of the earth is not seen at night, and in short you knew everything in question without being aware that you knew it. Hence there should be no reason that it should be hard for you to grant that reflection from the earth can illuminate the dark part of the moon with no less a light than that with which the moon lights up the darkness of the night. More, because the earth is forty times the size of the Moon. (p. 83/pp. 89–90)

4.2 **The secondary lumen of the moon and the recent booklet by an 'old' author**

The reference here is to the possibility that sunlight reflected from the earth towards the dark zone of the moon might be responsible for the faint glimmer visible on the lunar region not directly illuminated by the sun. This is referred to as the 'secondary lumen' of the moon. First Salviati considers the weak visibility of our satellite during eclipses in the nocturnal sky. This is different from the faint luminosity of the dark part that is visible mainly in the days near the thin crescent phase. To support his contention, Salviati develops psychophysiological considerations of the effects of visual contrast:

SIMPLICIO. I really thought that the secondary light of the moon was its own.

SALVIATI. Well, you knew about that, too, and did not perceive that you knew it. Tell me, did you not know yourself that the moon shows itself brighter by night than by day with respect to the darkness of the surroundings? And from that did you not know in general every bright body looks brighter when the surrounding are darker?

SIMPLICIO. I knew that perfectly well.

SALVIATI. When the moon is crescent and the secondary light looks bright to you, is it not always close to the sun and is it not consequently seen in twilight?

SIMPLICIO. So it is, and many times I have wished that the sky would darken so that I could see that light more clearly, but the moon has set before the night grew dark.

SALVIATI. Oh, then you knew perfectly well that this light would have appeared greater in the dark of night?

SIMPLICIO. Yes indeed, and still greater if the bright light of the horns lit up by the sun could be removed, the presence of which much obscures the lesser light.

SALVIATI. Does it not happen sometimes that one can see the whole disc of the moon in blackest night, without its being illuminated by the sun at all?

SIMPLICIO. I do not know that this ever happens except in a total eclipse of the moon.

SALVIATI. Well then, at that time its light ought to look most vivid, being in a very dark field and not obscured by light from the luminous horns. How bright has it looked to you in that state?

SIMPLICIO. Sometimes I have seen it copper-colored and a little whitish [*albicante*], but other times it remained quite dark so that I have lost sight of it.

SALVIATI. If what you could see so clearly in the twilight despite the obstacle of the adjacent splendor of the horns were the moon's own light, how could all other light be removed from it in the darkest night, and its own light fail to appear? (pp. 83–84/pp. 90–91)

Simplicio tries to respond to Salviati's pressing arguments by referring to a 'recent booklet' (*Disquisitiones mathematicæ de controuersiis et nouitatibus astronomicis*—'Mathematical investigations on astronomical controversies and novelties') published in 1614 by Galileo's adversary Scheiner (Figure 4.1). This time there is overt declaration of authorship although Scheiner appears only as the mentor of his student Georg Locher. In this work, in line with his general conception about the constitution of the moon as a partially transparent body ('as a cloud or a crystal'), the German Jesuit attributed the 'secondary light' of the moon to the penetration of sunlight after being diffused from the zone directly illuminated by the sun (Scheiner & Locher, 1614, p. 61):[2]

SIMPLICIUS. Wait a moment, please, for I have just remembered reading in a recent booklet of theses, which is full of novelties, that 'This secondary light is not caused by the stars nor by the moon's own light, and still less is it communicated from the earth; it derives from the illumination of the sun itself, which penetrates its whole body because the substance of the lunar globe is somewhat transparent. But this more vividly illuminates the surface of the hemisphere which is exposed to the sun's rays, and the interior, drinking in and soaking up this light so to speak, like a cloud or crystal, transmits it and makes...' This, if I remember correctly, he proves by authority, experience, and reason, adducing Cleomedes, Vitellio, Macrobius, and some other author, a modern; adding that experience shows this light to look rather bright in daytime when the moon is near is near conjunction (that is, when it is crescent), and shines most brightly along its limb. Moreover, he writes that in solar eclipses, when the moon is under the sun's disc, it is seen to be translucent, especially around the extreme edges. (p. 85; pp. 91–92)

Through Salviati, Galileo replies and offers a proof of his singular capacity for critical analysis of visual appearances. At the same time he gives his old adversary another lecture on the theme of the fallacy of senses. Namely, what Scheiner had supposed to be a physical consequence of sunlight on the translucent lunar body is largely due to the effect of visual contrast. Galileo is referring to the apparently more intense brightness of the obscure part in the periphery of the moon's surface, farther from the directly illuminated part.

Salviati/Galileo initially remarks that Scheiner does not even have the privilege of being 'the first author to hold such an opinion' and that, contrary to the old authors who could not rely on the new evidence, he has persisted in an error that was against the results of 'thousands of experiments'.[3] Afterwards, he develops his 'sensory' criticism to Scheiner's opinions by suggesting a simple experiment to get rid of the effects of visual contrast and arrive at a better appreciation of the physical intensity of seen objects:

SALVIATI. But let us get back to showing Simplicio the futility of the arguments of his modern author, in which there are falsehoods and fallacies and contradictions. First, it is false that this secondary light

[2] In Chapter 8 we will discuss in some depth the arguments developed by Scheiner and Locher in their *Disquisitiones*. Many pages of the *Dialogue* are dedicated to the rebuttal of the anti-Copernican arguments elaborated by Scheiner in his attempt to defend the traditional cosmology strongly advocated by the Catholic Church.

[3] The idea of a variable transparency of the moon's body has indeed a very long history, going back to classical Greek science, and had been a matter of particularly intense discussions through the Middle Ages (see Chapter 11).

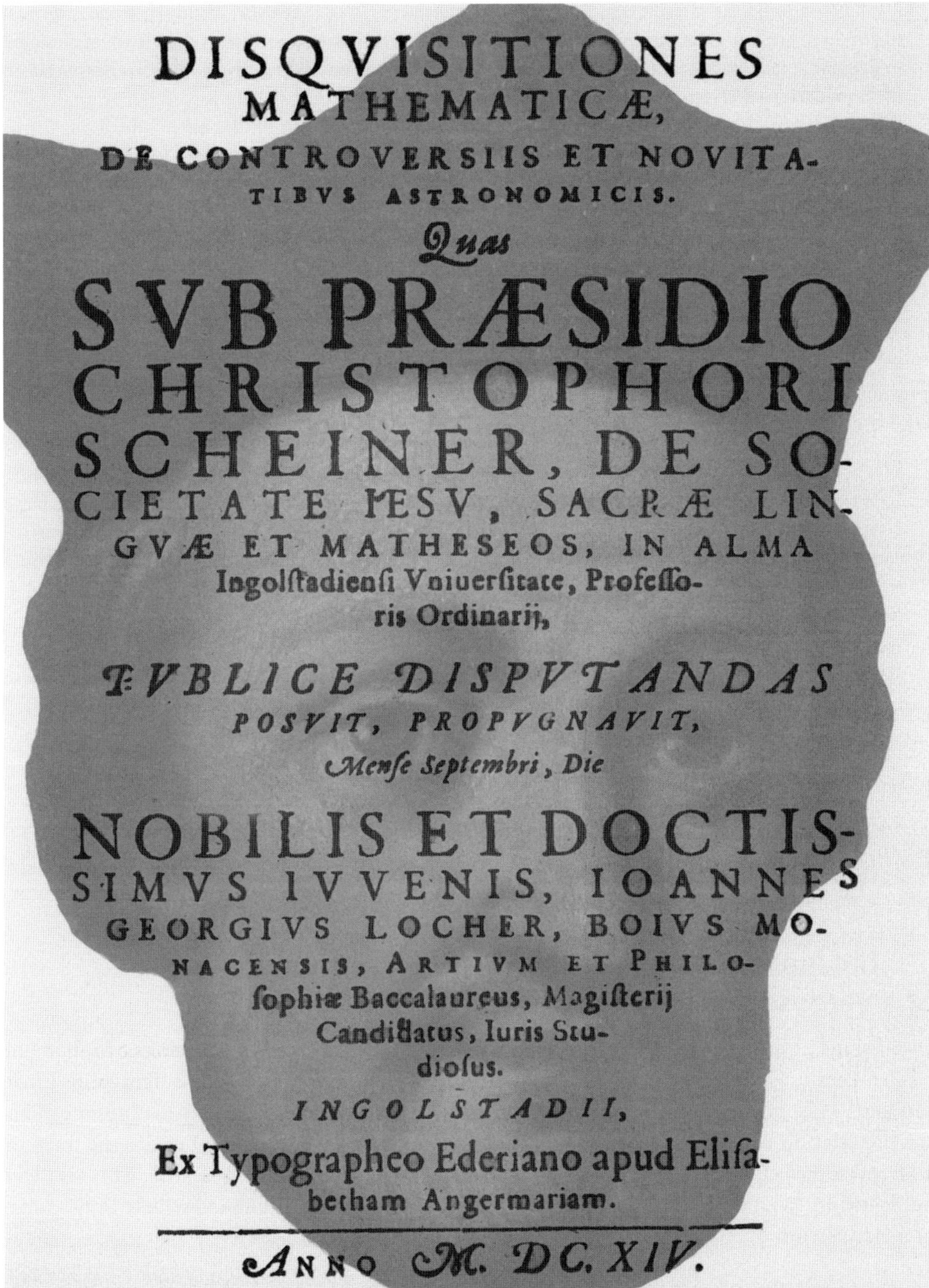
DISQVISITIONES
MATHEMATICÆ,
DE CONTROVERSIIS ET NOVITA-
TIBVS ASTRONOMICIS.
Quas
SVB PRÆSIDIO
CHRISTOPHORI
SCHEINER, DE SO-
CIETATE IESV, SACRÆ LIN-
GVÆ ET MATHESEOS, IN ALMA
Ingolſtadienſi Vniuerſitate, Profeſſo-
ris Ordinarij,
PVBLICE DISPVTANDAS
POSVIT, PROPVGNAVIT,
Menſe Septembri, Die
NOBILIS ET DOCTIS-
SIMVS IVVENIS, IOANNES
GEORGIVS LOCHER, BOIVS MO-
NACENSIS, ARTIVM ET PHILO-
ſophiæ Baccalaureus, Magiſterij
Candidatus, Iuris Stu-
dioſus.
INGOLSTADII,
Ex Typographeo Ederiano apud Eliſa-
betham Angermariam.
ANNO M. DC. XIV.

Figure 4.1 *Scheiner's Disquisitiones* by Nicholas Wade. Scheiner's portrait is derived from a photograph of a painting in the Stadtmuseum Ingolstadt. It is combined with the title page of his *Disquisitiones*.

> is brighter around the extreme margin than in the central parts, so that a sort of ring or circle is formed that is more brilliant than the rest of the field. It is true that the moon shows such a circle when observed in twilight at its first appearance after new moon, but that originates deceptively in differences between the boundaries which terminate the lunar disc over which this secondary light is spread. For on the side toward the sun, the light is bounded by the bright horn of the moon; on the other side, it has for its boundary the dark field of the twilight, in relation to which it appears lighter than the whiteness of the lunar disc-which on the other side is obscured by the greater brilliance of the horns. If only this modern author had tried placing between his eye and the primary brilliance some screen such as the roof of a house or some other partition, so that only the part of the moon outside the horn remained visible, he would have seen it all equally luminous. (pp. 86–87/pp. 93–94)[4]

Salviati's words, with the reference to the trick of the occultation of the 'primary brilliance' by means of an interposed object (with the aim of attenuating the effects of visual contrast)[5] are reminders of those from *Sidereus Nuncius* where Galileo discussed the phenomenon of the 'faint brightness' in the dark unilluminated part of the moon:

> When, both before and after conjunction, the Moon is found not far from the Sun, she offers to our sight not only that part of her globe that is adorned with shining horns, but also a certain thin, faint periphery that is seen to outline the circle of the dark part (that is, the part turned away from the Sun) and to separate it from the darker field of the ether itself. But if we examine the matter more closely, we will see not only the extreme edge of the dark part shining with a somewhat uncertain brightness (*incerta quadam claritate*), but the entire face of the Moon-that part, namely, that does not yet feel the brightness of the Sun-made white by some not inconsiderable light. At first glance, however, only a slender shining circumference appears on account of the darker parts of the sky bordering it, while, on the contrary, the rest of the surface appears darker because the nearness of the shining horns makes our sight dark. But if one chooses a place for oneself so that those bright horns are concealed by a roof or a chimney or another obstacle between one's sight and the Moon (but positioned far away from the eye), the remaining part of the lunar globe is left exposed to one's view, and then one will discover that this region of the Moon, although deprived of sunlight, also shines with a considerable light, and especially when the chill of the night has already increased through the absence of the Sun. For in a darker field the same light appears brighter. (SIDEREUS, p. 14; transl. p. 53, slightly modified)

4.3 The lunar candour and the luminous stone of a verbose philosopher

Discussions of the secondary lumen (or secondary light) of the moon are present in many of Galileo's texts. He refers to the phenomenon under several names like 'ash light' and 'lunar candour'. It is, however, particularly developed in the last work printed in his lifetime. This is a dissertation wholly dedicated to the phenomenon and written in 1640 under the form of a *Lettera al Principe Leopoldo di Toscana* (Letter to Prince Leopold of Tuscany). This text was published in 1642, the year of Galileo's death, after having been circulated widely in the form of a manuscript.

---

4 Among the arguments invoked by Galileo in the *Dialogue* to undermine the idea that the secondary light of the moon depended on a transparency of the moon's body was the fact that, if this were the case, we would see it exclusively during the eclipses of the sun.

5 This expedient is already present in the manuscript of Leonardo, some of which were probably a source of inspiration, direct or indirect, for Galileo, as we shall see in Chapter 11.

It is remarkable that the *Lettera* was written by Galileo when he had become almost completely blind (see Chapter 14). It is largely concerned with fallacies of visual impressions. By that time he was confined to his house in Arcetri, as a consequence of the condemnation inflicted on him by the Church. Despite his restricted vision of the external world, his passion and his intellectual vivacity were in no way tamed.[6]

For Galileo, the reason for this letter on the lunar candour had been the publication of the *Litheosphorus, sive de lapide Bononiensi* ('Litheosphorus, that is on the Bologna stone', Figure 4.2). It was concerned with the causes of the phosphorescence of the so-called 'Bologna stone' (a mineral named by the author of the book with the more imposing term of litheosphorus). The book was a long and verbose treatise, full of erudition but lacking genuine scientific ideas, written in the typical style of late peripatetic works by Fortunio Liceti, an Aristotelian philosopher then professor at the University of Bologna.[7]

The stone dealt with in the book was a mineral (baryte as we now know), discovered at the beginning of the century by an amateur alchemist of Bologna, Vincenzo Casciarolo, on Monte Paderno, a mountain just outside the town. It was called by a variety of sometimes fanciful names, like 'Luciferin stone', 'moon-' or 'sun-stone', 'sponge of light', and 'shining stone'; the last alluded to its property of becoming bright in the presence of a light source and retaining this for a certain time in the darkness.

The readers of Galileo's works know about the episode narrated by Giulio Cesare Lagalla (another Aristotelian philosopher and professor in Rome) of the Pisan scientist giving a demonstration of the properties of the stone in 1611, during his first visit to Rome. Galileo's performance was made in the presence of a number of Roman prelates and scholars and was considered by him as evidence of the corpuscular nature of light. As already mentioned (see Chapter 2), the Pisan scientist adhered to a conception of the structure of matter largely based on atomism. Within this framework Galileo assumed that the phosphorescence of the stone was due to its capacity of capturing the corpuscles of light and releasing them slowly in the absence of external light sources, thus producing a faint glimmer. This explanation was in contrast with the non-corpuscular Aristotelian conception of the nature of light.

In *Litheosphorus* the discussion on the singular stone was developed by Liceti in order to provide an explanation of the faint light seen in the dark zone of the moon. It was an alternative interpretation to Galileo's, which was based on the reflection of sunlight from the earth towards the lunar surface. Liceti assumed that the moon had properties similar to that of the Bologna stone and that its phosphorescence, once excited by the sunlight, could be maintained long enough to account for the dim lunar light. As we shall see in Chapter 11, a similar hypothesis had been discussed by medieval scholars within the framework of a theory of the impregnation or imbibition of the moon's body by the light of the sun.

---

6 Indeed, in the initial part of the letter on lunar candour, Galileo remarks on his difficulty, by saying that in preparing his manuscript he was obliged to 'make recourse to the help of the eyes and pen of others', and this makes a difference similar to that which, in a game of chess would be 'to play with the open eyes, or with the eyes bandaged or closed'. This might refer simply to the activity of preparing the manuscript, or could perhaps imply that Galileo also asked some of his assistants to perform for him some sensory experiments on the visibility of the lunar candour or on terrestrial objects irradiated by the moon. No doubt in doing this Galileo was guided by the memory of the observations he had made in the previous years. In the final chapter of this book we will return to Galileo's astronomical endeavours in the period of his declining sight.

7 Before moving to Bologna Liceti had taught at the Universities of Pisa and Padua.

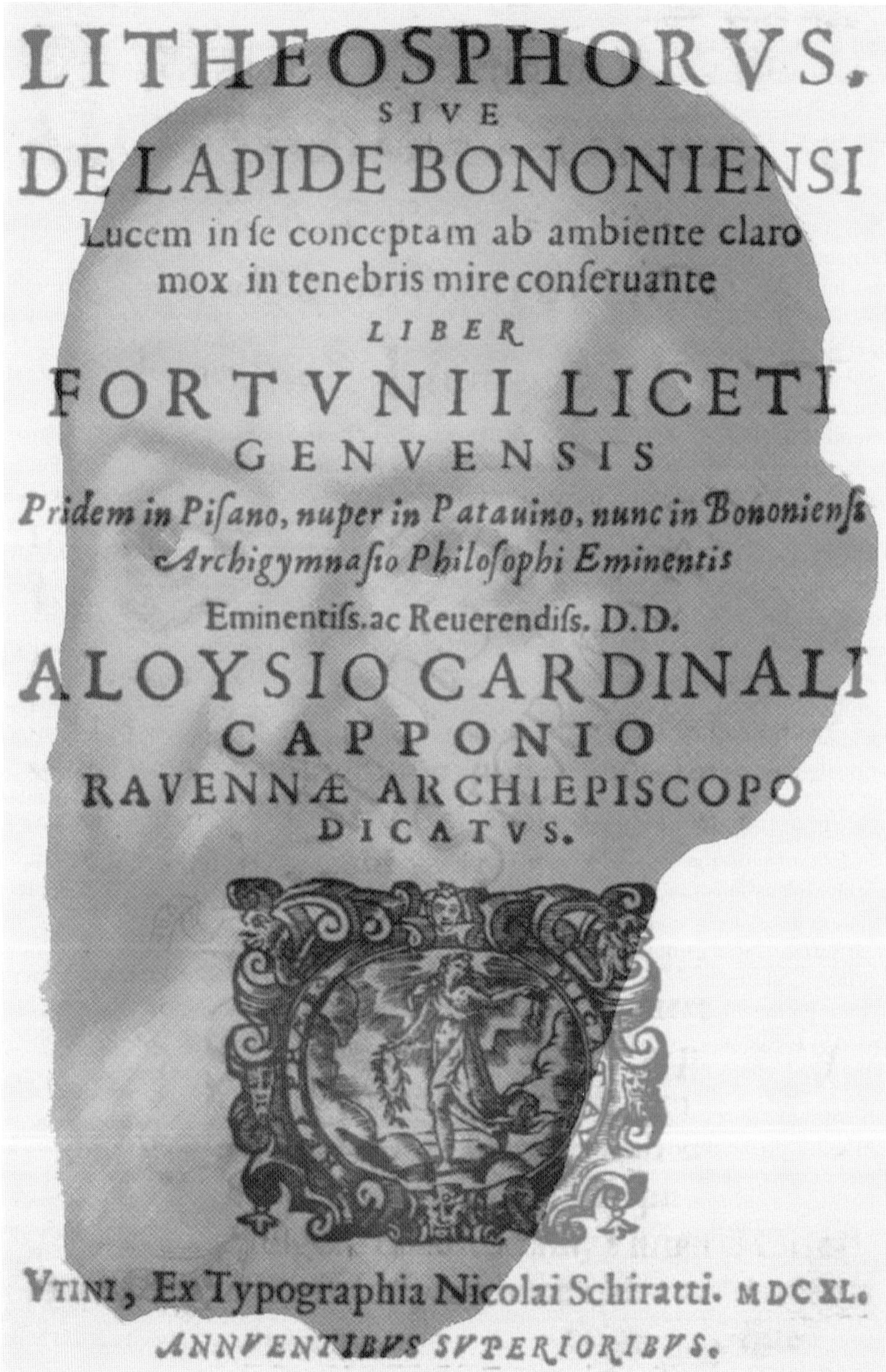

Figure 4.2 *Galileo's Bologna stone* by Nicholas Wade. Galileo's portrait is derived from a detail of a portrait by Sustermans and placed in the title page of Fortunio Liceti's *Litheosphorus*.

Liceti was ready to admit the absence of an intrinsic self-luminosity of the matter of the moon. This had been entertained by some theologians on the consideration that the moon, being the symbol of the Virgin, should shine as a luminous pearl (see Reeves, 1997).

These are the words whereby Liceti invoked the moon-litheosphorus analogy:

> If, on the other hand, the Moon is totally obscure and opaque, as believed by the very illustrious personage [i.e. Galileo], on the other hand do I believe that it has a great and noble analogy with the Bologna stone; such as, in the absence of the Sun, and in the shadow of both the earth (when it sets), but of itself (that is in the conjunction with the Sun), in the part not struck by the solar rays, the Moon would keep for a certain period the light absorbed from the sun rays. (Liceti, 1640, pp. 247–248)

Taking advantage of the discussion with a prolix and largely out-dated philosopher, strongly anchored to the traditional doctrines and incapable of reflecting deeply on the physical facts, Galileo develops in his *Lettera* an important discussion on the scientific method largely based on the critical evaluation of sensory data and on the elaboration on the errors of knowledge.

We will not enter in detail into the various arguments developed by him in order to support his hypothesis of the lunar candour and to undermine the objections and the theories of his adversary. We will limit ourselves to considering some points which highlight Galileo's interest in visual appearances. His arguments are analogous to the discussion present in the *Istoria* on the reasons leading people to maintain old views and to resist the modern explanation about the luminosity of the moon (and of the earth).

Galileo writes:

> I wish to interpose here a thought of mine, whatever it could be, in order to find out the reason why speculative minds have missed this, in my opinion, true and rather conclusive reason of the origin of lunar candour from the reflection of sunrays by the Earth surface. While the Sun is above the horizon, and illuminates our terrestrial hemisphere, in whatever position the Moon is situated, its candour does not appear visible to us. This is why nobody in this particular time would be inclined to believe that the lumen of our Earth might have the strength to illuminate the part of the lunar surface not struck by the sun. Even much less therefore one would happen to think that the surface of the Earth, devoid of splendour, would be strong enough to whiten [*incandire*] the Moon. I mean powerful, while it is dark, to bring the light there where it did not bring [the light] while it was luminous. This is why, after the sunset, when the Earth has got dark, at the moment we see the lunar candour manifesting itself, popular judgement could invoke any other cause except the Earth. Therefore men, being persuaded by this first and simple apprehension, either did not reflect on the matter, or tried to find out the reason in any other thing, excepts the terrestrial splendour (OG VIII, pp. 504–505).

Galileo develops a series of arguments to demonstrate the inconsistency of one hypothesis put forward by Liceti in order to account for the lunar candour, based on the presence of an atmosphere around the moon that could return the light of the sun onto the dark zone of the lunar surface.[8] He then examines the assertion that the lunar candour was fainter than the illumination

[8] It is worth recalling here that Galileo himself had initially supposed, in order to account for some of the appearances of the lunar surface when seen through the telescope, the presence 'just as around the Earth, there is around the lunar body a certain orb of denser substance than the rest of the ether, able to receive and reflect a ray of the Sun, although not endowed with so much opacity that it can inhibit the passage of vision (especially when it is not illuminated)' (SIDEREUS, p. 12; transl. pp. 49–50). The idea of a lunar atmosphere had a long history, going at least up to the epoch of Plutarch, as we will mention in Chapters 6 and 11.

received from the earth on nights of the full moon. Galileo's discourse developed on this point is of significance for the general theme of this book, because it reveals his great attention for the possible fallacies of the senses (and also his enjoyment in making them manifest).

Galileo declares from the outset the possible deception of vision 'at the first apprehension', and the need 'in order that vision could occur with certainty and without the deception of the sense', to make recourse to 'a correction to be made through the help of the right rational discourse' (OG VIII, p. 511). Afterwards, with a reasoning partially corresponding to that on the apparent blackness of the sunspots, he considers how it could it be that what is darker appears brighter, and vice versa. The problem, he says, is that if we remain on earth we cannot establish a reliable, direct comparison between the light that the earth receives from the sun, and the lunar candour caused by the rays reflected from the earth onto the moon. The reason is that we normally observe the earth from very near ('not more than three or four cubits'), a distance 'incomparably less than that of the whitening moon situated in the conjunction,[9] which exceeds by far the three hundred millions of cubits' (p. 512).

4.4 The moon, the earth, and twilight

In order to establish a reliable comparison of the true physical illumination that the two bodies of the solar system receive from each other, it would be necessary for the observer to fly to the moon, and from its surface observe the zone of the earth not struck directly by the sunrays.

But let us leave the words to Galileo, who takes into consideration, on the one hand, the illumination of the earth by the full moon, and on the other, the candour of the moon caused by the earth when this exposes to the moon its face totally illuminated by the sun. This would correspond to a condition of 'full earth' that, for a lunar observer happens in the astronomical condition of 'conjunction'. For the terrestrial observer this would result in the moon appearing thinly falcate:

> Most excellent Signor Liceti, in order to judge of the present argument without fallacy, it would be necessary that, first, you should note apart what appears to your sight while, being on the Earth, you look at the Lumen on the earth, and compare it to the candour of the Moon when it is situated in conjunction. Afterwards, you should note, again apart, what would appear to your sight when you would be settled on the moon whitened [*incandita*] by the terrestrial Lumen, and thence you could see the Earth, very far from you, illuminated from the Moon. If in the one and the other experience you would happen to find that the Earth appears more white [*candida*] that the whitened [*incandita*] Moon situated under your feet, you would have well rightly concluded. But I think that the second experience would make you change mind, and to judge wholly the contrary of what that the first sight persuaded you about this. Let thus stop in this case the faith that the intellect should credit to the sense. Let us, moreover, add that, in the case of two visible objects, of a different size, the smaller would encumber less the eye with light than the bigger, even though they had the same specific splendour [*splendore in specie*]. Now let one notice that the lunar disc is comprised under a very acute angle, since its base does not subtend more than half a degree; but the angle that from the widest divarication is constitute in the eye, being more than right, subtend more than ninety whole degrees. This angle is totally encumbered from the luminous area and place of the Earth, when we look at it from near. Since the amplitude of this big angle is more than two hundred times of the other, acute, one that comprises the lunar disc, we have no wonder in taking for good the apparent majority of light in gazing at the Earth, than at the whitened [*incandita*] moon. Nothing I tell of the difference of the two mentioned angles that is much less than the difference of the two solid angles originating from them: indeed the angles formed by the

[9] The conjunction is, in this case, the astronomical situation leading to the new moon, with the illuminated part of the moon being invisible from the earth.

> visual rays are solid. Of these, the one which has for its bases the terrestrial surface exposed to the eye, despite its very small size, is more than forty thousand times larger than the other, the one based on the lunar disc. (OG VIII, pp. 512–513)

The impossible experiment, needing an improbable journey to the moon, is carried out by Galileo in a virtual way with the force of his intellectual imagination. It is again a thought experiment, aimed in this case at comparing, under similar conditions of observation, the brightness of the dark part of the moon illuminated by the earth (the lunar candour) with the brightness of the earth illuminated by the moon. Also in this case Galileo makes recourse to an intermediate term in order to carry out his apparently impossible comparison. In this case it is the mediocre brightness of twilight (*crepuscolo*).

Let us listen to his own words:

> Since we cannot put one against the other side by side [*a petto a petto*], the candour of the Moon and the lumen of the Moon on the Earth, it seems to me that we could judge between them with enough assurance if we make comparison of both of them with a third illuminated body; since, if it were that the splendour of this third body would exceed the lumen of the Moon, but would in turn be won by the candour of the Moon, we could then assert without doubt that the candour of the moon exceeds the lumen of the Moon on the Earth. An appropriate middle term for this comparison appears to me to be the splendour of twilight, if we establish a comparison between it and the other two. Once the Sun has set, one would see for a good space of time the Earth surface to be more clear because of the twilight than when it is illuminated by the full moon. We can be ascertained of that from seeing any minuteness whatsoever on the Earth in a much more distinct way in the sunset light than what we can see, after the twilight has passed over, in the presence of moon light. This effect can be, moreover, confirmed in a manifest way: if indeed we would have on the Earth some obscure body, as for instance a column, or even our own body, the light of the full Moon would not produce in the Earth a shadow of the tenebrous body until the twilight has so decreased that the lumen of the Moon might prevail on it. This is a clear indication that the lumen of the Moon is for a long time, after the beginning of the sunset, much less than the twilight. Let us then add another experience, also useful to confirm that the illumination of the twilight is much stronger than that of the full moon. Let us look from far to some large building situated on some eminent place, distant from us, say, three or four miles. Certainly, we could keep seeing it well for a long time at the sunset, and we would lose its view only after a notable diminution of the twilight. However, after twilight when the illumination of the full Moon would appear, it could easily happen that we could no longer see that same building. Less is therefore the lumen of the Moon on the earth compared to the lumen of twilight; on the other hand, we need not wait until the twilight has greatly weakened in order to see the candour of the Moon, since we could see it whitening in the same lumen of the twilight; but, on the contrary, a rather long time is required before the Moon would be able to produce shadows. Less is therefore the lumen of the Moon on the Earth compared to the candour of the Moon surface. (OG VIII, pp. 513–514)

It is perhaps useful to summarize Galileo's reasons for concluding that the earth illuminates the dark part of the moon more than the moon illuminates the earth:

(1) For some time after sunset, twilight is more intense than the light the earth receives from the full moon. To ascertain this important point he went beyond immediate appearances, and made recourse to three more reliable criteria, namely (a) in twilight we could see more minute details of terrestrial objects than those visible in full moonlight (evidence already invoked in the *Istoria* in a similar context), (b) it requires a long time after sunset for the moonlight to produce an evident shadow, and (c) if we keep sight of a distant building in twilight it remains visible for a long time after sunset, whereas it would hardly be visible by moonlight.

(2) The light on the dark part of the moon is faintly visible soon after sunset, which means that it is comparable to the twilight in the first period after the setting of the sun.

(3) It is thus logical to conclude that the light reflected from the earth to the moon's surface is more intense than the light of the sun reflected from the moon onto the earth.[10]

This conclusion allows Galileo to reassert the importance of the correct logico-mathematical discourse in order to amend the data of sense, which 'in some circumstances, in its first apprehension, might be deceiving and needing correction', and to point to 'the difference which exists between the discourse of the mathematicians and of the pure natural philosophers'.

There are many other themes that Galileo discusses in the letter on lunar candour that we cannot deal with here. Some of them recur in his writings, as we shall see in Chapter 5 for the case of the 'diffuse reflection' already alluded to in Chapter 1. We do not consider the way Galileo undermines Liceti's assumption of the partial transparency of the lunar body, an essential element of his hypothesis of the moon shining in a similar way to the Bologna stone after having absorbed sunlight.

We prefer to conclude this chapter with the passage in which Galileo criticizes one of his adversary's theories—implying the reverberation of sunlight by a dense atmosphere surrounding the moon (an 'ambient ether surrounding the Moon') in the phenomenon of lunar candour. As we have noted earlier, Galileo had considered such a possibility in the period of his first astronomical observations but had afterwards abandoned it. In the *Lettera*, he provides evidence against Liceti's supposition from a careful examination of the telescopic appearances of the moon, and particularly from the sight of the peak of a lunar mountain illuminated by the light of the sun:

> I can with clear evidence make it manifest that the ambient ether of the Moon is much less dense than the part of vaporous air surrounding the earth. The vapours around the Earth are dense in such manner that the Sun, when is near to the horizon, illuminates a wall, or any other opaque body facing it, very weakly compared to the lumen it offered when it was for many degrees elevated above the horizon. This notable difference can only proceed, in my opinion, from the need that, near the setting, the sunrays have to traverse for a very long space the vapours surrounding the Earth; whereas the rays of the sun, when it is very elevated, must traverse for a smaller space the vapours between the Sun and the interposed opaque object. If there were no vapours, and the air were very thin, the illumination from the Sun would be always of the same vigour, so much from elevated places as from lower ones, provided that they would be received with the same angles in the illuminated surfaces. Let us suppose that we could make a comparison of two places on the Moon, one receiving the sunrays after passing very obliquely through the dense ether of the Moon, and the other receiving them directly (that is to say proceeding for a short path through the ambient ether). From which it would follow, in the case we would see the illumination of the two places to be equal, the ambient ether surrounding the moon to be very little more dense that the remaining most pure ether. But we can see frequently these two places. As a matter of fact, when the Moon in the quadrature with the Sun, if we consider the border separating the part of the moon illuminated by the sunrays from the other dark, we see in this last one, some peaks of mountains rather apart and far from the said border: these peaks, at the moment that they illuminated by the sun, before the lower parts, despite the obliquity of the sunrays receiving them, nevertheless they shine with the same splendour and lumen as any other part of at the centre of the illuminated part. This happens despite that at the separated peak the sunrays arrive by intersecting obliquely the ambient ether, whereas they arrive directly or less obliquely to the noted places. This is a manifest sign that it is very small the impediment caused by the ambient ether to the penetration of sunrays, and, by consequence, very faint the lumen that the dark part of the Moon can receive from it. (OG VIII, pp. 524–525)

[10] Unlike Galileo, Paolo Sarpi (of whom much will be said in Chapter 12, particularly with reference to the moon's secondary light) held the opinion that the dark light of the moon was less intense than twilight (see Sarpi's *Pensieri*, p. 66—*pensiero 53*).

Chapter 5

Sensory surprises

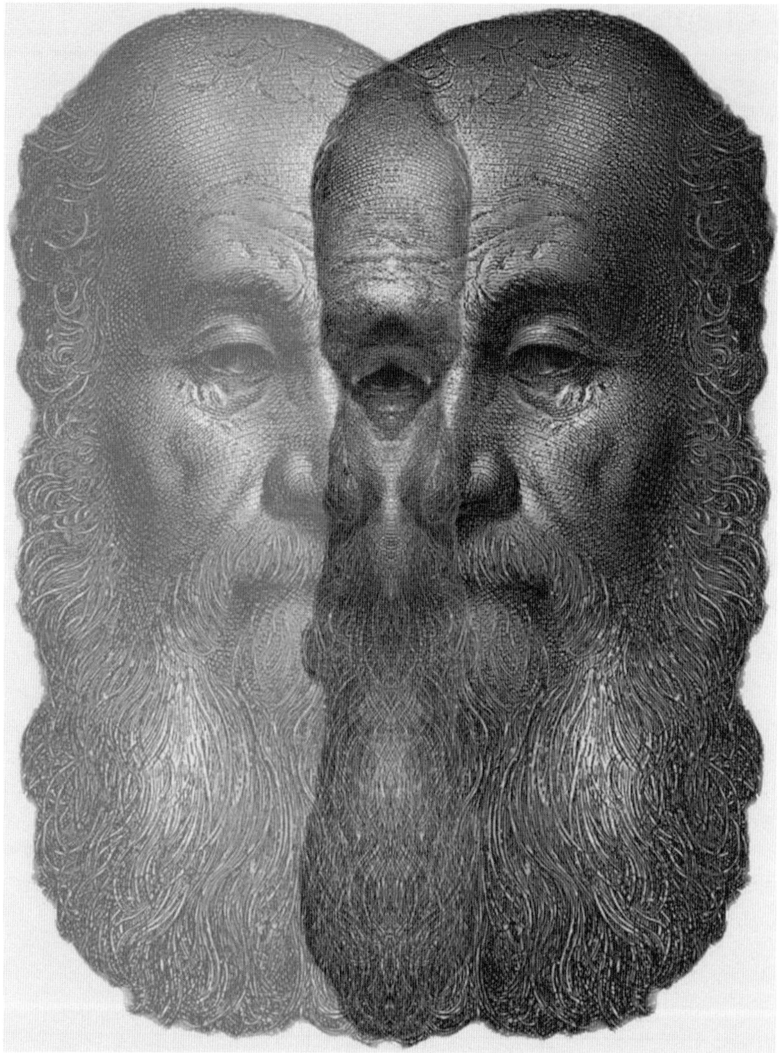

Figure V *Reflecting Galileo* by Nicholas Wade. Galileo's fascination with reflections is reflected in this dual portrait of him, derived from an engraving.

In the previous chapters we have often made reference to the mechanisms of light reflection and to the reflections occurring from irregular surfaces, like that of the earth and various terrestrial objects, and also that of the moon. Because of their irregular nature, at first view these surfaces seem unsuitable for reflection *par excellence*, the specular reflection occurring at the regular surface of a perfectly polished mirror. In Chapter 1 the difference between these two types of reflection has emerged in the natural experiment contrived by Galileo in *Saggiatore*, that of the man looking at the sunset by the seaside. The initial reflection, with the perfectly immobile water surface, corresponds to a mirror-like type of reflection capable of displaying 'the solar disc bounded as in a mirror'. As the sea surface becomes progressively more irregular, as a consequence of the wind blowing with an increasingly stronger intensity, the sea surface breaks into a multiplicity of small surfaces, as in a 'multitude of mirrors'. Accordingly, the initially well-defined image of the sun transmutes into a diffuse brilliancy, where it will no longer be possible to discern its disc. The passage is from an almost perfect specular reflection to the 'diffuse reflection', a phenomenon much more common in ordinary conditions than produced by true mirrors or perfectly still waters, i.e. by visual objects that are very rare in nature compared to most natural and artificial objects characterized by more or less irregular surfaces.

As discussed particularly in Chapters 2 and 3, the argument of diffuse reflection is of fundamental relevance for Galileo's cosmology, particularly with respect to his explanation of the luminosity of the moon, and to his views on the similarity between light reflection from the earth and moon. It is also central to his explanation of the 'secondary lumen' or 'lunar candour' visible in the dark region of the moon. By undermining the traditional conception that the moon shines on the background of the nocturnal sky because of the specular reflectivity of its surface, Galileo was breaking down one of the tenets of the old cosmology: the essential difference between the supralunar and terrestrial world. By playing on the physical aspects of light reflection from irregular surfaces, and on the psychophysiological mechanisms of perceptual contrast, he could conclude that there is no need to invoke a mirror-like reflection in order to account for the brightness of the moon. Moreover, the earth does in fact shine like the moon because in both cases the brightness comes from a diffuse type of reflection occurring from irregular surfaces. On one side, this accounts for the 'lunar candour' of the dark region of the moon (Chapter 3), and, on the other side, it explains why, in a dark room, the reflection from a wall of the light entering through a hole pierced in the opposite wall, can produce *ceteris paribus* a stronger illumination that that caused by the full moon (Chapter 2).

Because of its importance in Galileo's intellectual development, the argument of diffuse reflection is recurrent in his writings, starting from *Sidereus nuncius* (and even before), until his last published text, the letter on lunar candour of 1640. In Chapter 1 we anticipated that Galileo would deal with diffuse reflection with relation to the brightness of the moon by staging a true experiment in his masterpiece, *Dialogue concerning the two chief systems of the world*. The pages dedicated to this experiment are famous (among Galileo's readers) and also beautiful from a literary point of view and we will consider them now at length. The citations from Galileo's writings are certainly abundant in this book. However, this feature is even more accentuated in this chapter, composed almost entirely of quotations from the *Dialogue*, with rather limited interventions from our side.

5.1 The dark mirror and the bright wall

To make more evident both the mechanism underlying the moon's brightness and the argument of the earth–moon similarity, these pages contain another recurrent feature in Galileo's science.

This is the awareness and indeed the insistence he places on the surprising aspects of scientific knowledge, and particularly on its possible contrast with the immediate expectations of common sense. This attitude derives from the remark that what at first view is considered to shine more brilliantly once illuminated by sunlight (the mirror surface) is in fact less luminous than the surface of the wall of a building. Perhaps even more surprising is another consideration developed with reference to the brightness of the moon. Not only it is unnecessary to invoke a perfect specular reflection of the moon surface in order to explain its brightness, but if the moon was a perfect sphere of a crystal-like matter, it would in fact be invisible.

Let us now give the stage to Galileo, through the voice of the three debaters of the *Dialogue*, in order to assist them with the experiment of the 'dark mirror' conducted by Salviati. At the beginning, Galileo's spokesman makes clear the terms of the problem to be investigated:

SALVIATI. We are inquiring, Simplicio, whether in order to produce a reflection of light similar to that which comes to us from the moon, it is necessary that the surface from which the reflection comes shall be as smooth and polished as a mirror, or whether a rough and ill-polished surface, neither smooth nor shiny, may not be better suited. Now if two reflections should come to us, one brighter than the other, from two surfaces situated opposite to us, I ask you which of the two surfaces you believe would look the lighter to our eyes, and which the darker?

SIMPLICIO. I think without any that the surface which reflected the light more brilliantly would look lighter to me, and the other darker. (DIALOGO, p. 64; transl. p. 71)

Soon after, the rhythm of the dialogue accelerates with rapid exchanges between Salviati and Simplicio. This allows Galileo to avoid the lengthiness of a systematic presentation of the various phases of the experiment. It also allows his spokesman (Salviati) to ply Simplicio with the direct strokes of the experimental evidence with Sagredo ready to intervene with his *à propos* remarks. A possible difficulty, that of comparing two types of luminosity of inhomogeneous material (those of a mirror and a white wall) is avoided with a stratagem clearly inspired by Galileo's great familiarity with the technique of painting (where to use the darkest colour?):

SALVIATI. Now please take that mirror which is hanging on the wall, and let us go out into that court; come with us, Sagredo. Hang the mirror on that wall, there, where the sun strikes it. Now let us withdraw into the shade. Now, there you see two surfaces struck by the sun, the wall and the mirror. Which looks brighter to you; the wall, or the mirror? What, no answer?

SAGREDO. I am going to let Simplicio answer; he is the one who is experiencing the difficulty. For my part, from this small beginning of an experiment I am persuaded that the moon must indeed have a very badly polished surface.

SALVIATI. Tell me, Simplicio; if you had to paint a picture of that wall with the mirror hanging on it, where would you use the darkest colors? In depicting the wall or the mirror?

SIMPLICIO. Much darker in depicting the mirror.

SALVIATI. Now if the most powerful reflection of light comes from the surface that looks brightest, the wall here would be reflecting the rays of the sun more vividly than the mirror.

SIMPLICIO. Very clever, my dear sir; and is this the best experiment you have to offer? You have placed us where the reflection from the mirror does not strike. But come with me a bit this way; no, come along.

SAGREDO. Perhaps you are looking for the place where the mirror throws its reflection?

SIMPLICIO. Yes, sir!

SAGREDO. Well, just look at it—there on the opposite wall, exactly as large as the mirror, and little less bright than it would be if the sun shone there directly.

SIMPLICIO. Come along, then, and look at the surface of the mirror from there, and then tell me whether I should say it is darker than that of the wall.

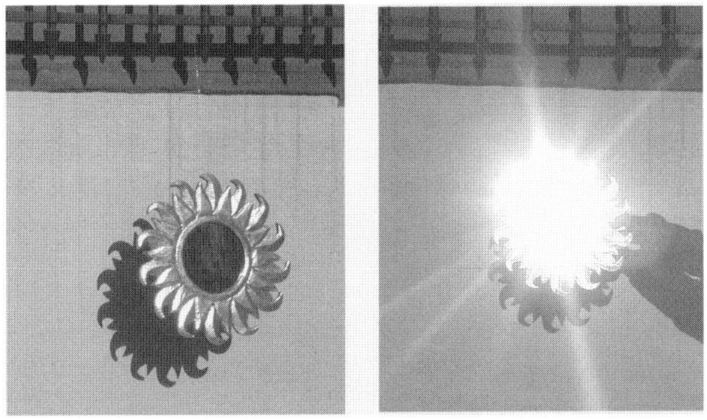

Figure 5.1 The experiment of the 'dark mirror' made by hanging the mirror on the wall of an old building of *Piazza dei Cavalieri* (Knights' square) in Pisa, a place that Galileo might have seen in conditions rather similar to the present day (this Piazza was rebuilt in the second half of the sixteenth century on a plan made by the famous architect and humanist Giorgio Vasari). On the left, the mirror, as seen for most of the time, appears darker than the wall. On the right, it was oriented such as to reflect towards the camera the direct light of the sun, appearing then extremely bright ('as bright and vivid as the sun itself'). The shadows at the right of the bright mirror correspond to the arms of the person manipulating it.

SAGREDO. Look at it yourself; I am not anxious to be blinded, and I know perfectly well without looking that it looks as bright and vivid as the sun itself, or little less so.[1]

SIMPLICIO. Well, then, what do you say? Is the reflection from a mirror less powerful than that than that from a wall? I notice that on this opposite wall, which receives the reflection from the illuminated wall along with that of the mirror, the reflection from the mirror is much the brighter. And I see that the mirror itself looks very much brighter to me than the wall. (p. 64; transl. p. 72)

What seems a winning move of Simplicio's (the brighter reflection from the mirror than the wall; see Figure 5.1) is promptly undermined by Salviati, who remarks that Simplicio's 'perspicacity' has provided an important element for the experimental demonstration. By involving his antagonist as an active player of the experiment, Salviati is adopting a similar attitude to that displayed in the discussion about the mechanism of the brightness of the moon discussed in Chapter 3. The rhythm of the discussion slows down now because Salviati needs to present the conclusion of the experiment systematically:

SALVIATI. You have got ahead of me by your perspicacity, for this was the very observation which I needed for explaining the rest. You see the difference, then, between the reflections made by the surface of the wall and that of the mirror, which are struck in exactly the same way by the sun's rays. You see how the reflection that comes from the wall diffuses itself over all the points opposite to it, while that from the mirror goes to a single place no larger than the mirror itself. You see likewise how the surface of the wall always looks equally light in itself, no matter from what place you observe it, and somewhat lighter than that of the mirror from every place except that small area where the reflection from the mirror strikes; from there, the mirror appears very much brighter than the wall. From this sensible and palpable experiment it seems to me that you can very readily decide whether the reflection which

[1] The glaring intensity of the sunrays reflected by the mirror parallels the 'very bright reflection of the sun in the surface of the sea' of the natural experiment of *Saggiatore* (see Chapter 1).

comes here from the moon comes like that from a mirror, or like that from a wall; that is, whether from a smooth or a rough surface.

SAGREDO. If I were on the moon itself I do not believe that I could touch the roughness of its surface with my hand more definitely than I now perceive it by understanding your argument. The moon, seen in any position with respect to the sun and to us, always shows the surface exposed to the sun equally bright. This effect corresponds precisely with that of the wall, which seen from any place appears equally bright; it conflicts with that of the mirror, which from one place alone looks luminous and from all others dark. Besides, the light that comes to me from the reflection of the wall is weak and tolerable in comparison with that from the mirror, which is extremely strong and little less offensive to the eyes than the primary and direct rays of the sun. It is in just such a way that we can calmly contemplate the face of the moon. If that were like a mirror, appearing as large as the sun because of its closeness, it would be of an absolutely intolerable brilliance, and would seem to us almost as if we were looking at another sun. (DIALOGO, pp. 65–66; transl. pp. 72–73)

In his final intervention Sagredo asserts the extraordinary power of scientific knowledge which is capable of being as convincing as the senses (and perhaps even more so). It is significant that he makes explicit reference to the sense of touch (already implicit in Salviati's use of the adjective 'palpable' referred to in the experiments), because in the science of Aristotle (and also according to common sense) touch appears to be the most trustworthy of the senses. In this regard, it must be also said, however, that Galileo was well aware that science exerts its power of conviction only on people prepared to receive it (like the 'very perspicacious man' of his fable of sounds). Indeed, in a letter to his pupil Benedetto Castelli written on 30 December 1610, he remarked 'that, in order to convince stubborn people [...] it will not even suffice the testimony of stars themselves which, after descending onto the earth, would narrate their history' (OG X, pp. 504–505). Stubborn people were for him 'the philosophers *ex libris*', i.e. the scholars who derived their knowledge from the books and refused to read with their own eyes the 'book of nature'.

5.2 **A bright, invisible light**

In the passage quoted earlier, Sagredo's cue closes the first part of the experiment involving the plane mirror. The second part, with a spherical mirror has some interesting peculiarities, and particularly the fact that Sagredo takes the role usually attributed to Salviati as the master of the play who puts forward the scientific explanation of the phenomenon under discussion. Before the real experiment begins, a problem is noted by Salviati as if Galileo's spokesman himself had a difficulty in going through all the intricacies of the explanation of the moon's brightness.

SALVIATI. Please, Sagredo, do not attribute to my demonstration more than belongs to it. I am about to confront you with a fact that I think you will find not so easy to explain. You take it as a great difference between the moon and the mirror that the former yields its reflections equally in all directions as the wall does, while the mirror sends its reflection to one definite place alone. From this, you conclude that the moon is like the wall and not like the mirror. But I tell you that this mirror sends its reflection to one place alone because its surface is flat, and since reflected rays must leave at equal angles with incident rays, they have to leave a plane surface as a unit toward one place. But the surface of the moon is not flat, it is spherical; and the rays incident upon such a surface are found to be reflected in all directions at angles equal to those of incidence, because of the infinity of slopes which make up a spherical surface. Therefore the moon can send its reflections everywhere and need not send them all to a single place like those of a plane mirror.

SIMPLICIO. This is exactly one of the objections which I wanted to make. (DIALOGO, p. 66; transl. pp. 73–74)

At this response of Simplicio, Sagredo intervenes by outlining the argument and providing a detailed answer based on knowledge of the physical laws involved in the reflection from spherical mirrors and on the principles of physiological optics:

SAGREDO. If it is one of them, then you must have others; but let me tell you that so far as this first one is concerned, it seems to me to be not so much for you as against you.

SIMPLICIO. You have called it obvious that the reflection made by that wall is as bright and luminous as that of the moon, whereas I think it trifling in comparison with the moon's. For 'in this matter of illumination, one must look for and define the sphere of activity.' Who doubts that celestial bodies have greater spheres of activity than our transitory mortal elements? And as to that wall, is it after all anything more than a bit of earth; dark, and unfit to illumine?

SAGREDO. Here again I believe that you are quite mistaken. But I return to the first point raised by Salviati, and I tell you that in order to make an object appear luminous, it is not sufficient for the rays of the illuminating body to fall upon it; it is also necessary for the reflected rays to get to our eyes. This is to be clearly seen in the case of the mirror, upon which no doubt the rays of the sun are falling, but which nevertheless does not appear to be bright and illuminated unless we put our eyes in the particular place where the reflection is going. Let us consider this in regard to what would happen if the mirror had a spherical surface. Unquestionably we should find that of the whole reflection made by the illuminated surface, only a small part would reach the eyes of a particular observer, there being only the very least possible part of the entire surface which would have the correct slope to reflect the rays to the particular location of his eyes. Hence only the least part of the spherical surface would shine for his eyes, all the rest looking dark. If then the moon were smooth as a mirror, only a very small part would show itself to the eyes of a particular person as illuminated by the sun, although an entire hemisphere would be exposed to the sun's rays. The rest would remain, to this observer's eyes, unilluminated and therefore invisible. To conclude, the whole moon would be invisible, since that particle which gave the reflection would be lost by reason of its smallness and great distance. And just as the moon would remain invisible to the eyes, so its illumination would remain nil; for it is indeed impossible that a luminous body should by its splendor take away our darkness, and we be unable to see it. (pp. 66–67; transl. pp. 74–75)

It is possible that by attributing to Sagredo the role of a scientific teacher, Galileo was paying a tribute to his friend, the real Giovanfrancesco Sagredo, the Venetian aristocrat who was strongly interested in science, and particularly expert in optics, although he was pleased to present himself just as a science *amateur*.[2]

[2] As we shall mention in Chapter 13, very likely Sagredo was more acquainted than Galileo with modern optical science. The self-portrait that the real Sagredo wrote in a letter addressed on 4 April 1614 to Mark Welser is particularly beautiful. Welser was the addressee of Galileo's letters on sunspots (see our Chapter 3). This is what Sagredo wrote: 'I am a Venetian gentleman. I never call myself a man of letters. I bore always an affection for *letterati* and protected them, but I do not intend to advance my fortunes, or earn praise or reputation from knowing something about philosophy and mathematics. Rather, I rest on the integrity and good administration of my offices in the governance of the Republic, to which I applied myself in my youth following the practice of my elders who in that practice have got old and consumed themselves. My studies turn toward the recognition of those things that as a Christian I owe to God, as a citizen to my country, as a patrician to my house, as a social being to my friends, and, as a gentleman and true philosopher, to myself. I spend my time serving God and my country, and, since I am free from family cares, consume a good part of my life in conversation, service, and satisfaction of friends, and all the rest I devote to my own taste and convenience; and if sometimes I speculate about sciences, do not believe, Your Excellency, that I presume to compete with the processors of those, let alone criticize them, but only to refresh my mind by searching freely, without any obligation or attachment, the truth of any proposition that appeals to me' (OG XII, pp. 43–44).

Soon after the explanation of the property of the reflection from a spherical mirror, Salviati assumes his usual role of scientific guide and prepares the experimental phase, now involving a spherical mirror:

SALVIATI. Wait a minute, Sagredo, for I see certain signs in Simplicio's face and actions which indicate to me that he is neither convinced nor satisfied by what you, with the best evidence and with perfect truth, have said. And now it occurs to me how to remove all doubt by another experiment. I have seen in a room upstairs a large spherical mirror; have it brought here. And while it is on its way, Simplicio, consider carefully the amount of light which comes from the reflection of the flat mirror to this wall here under the balcony.

SIMPLICIO. I see that it is little less lighted than if the sun were striking it directly.

SALVIATI. So it is. Now tell me; if, taking away that little flat mirror, we were to put the large spherical one in its place, what result do you think that would have upon the reflection on this same wall?

SIMPLICIO. I think it would produce a much greater and broader light.

SALVIATI. But what would you say if the illumination should be nil, or so small that you could hardly perceive it?

SIMPLICIO. When I have seen the effect, I shall think up a reply.

SALVIATI. Here is the mirror, which I wish to have placed beside the other. But let us first go over there, near the reflection from the flat mirror, and note carefully its brightness. You see how bright it is here where it strikes, and how you can distinctly make out these details of the wall.

SIMPLICIO. I have looked and observed very closely; now place the other mirror beside the first.

SALVIATI. That is where it is. It was placed there as soon as you began to look at the detail, and you did not perceive it because the increase of light over the rest of the wall was just as great. Now take away the flat mirror. See there, all the reflection is taken away, although the large convex mirror remains. Remove that also, and then replace it as you please; you will see no change whatever in the light upon the whole wall. Thus you see it shown to your senses how the reflection of the sun made from a spherical convex mirror does not noticeably illuminate the surrounding places. Now what have you to say to this experiment? (pp. 66–67; transl. pp. 75–76)

Simplicio appears to be disconcerted by the fact that he has not been able to notice the presence of the spherical mirror, which should have produced 'a much greater and broader light' than the flat one. He thinks of possible trickery (*giuoco di mano*), particularly because he cannot understand how no evident increase of the room illumination is produced by the mirror, despite the fact that the mirror itself, when looked at directly, 'gives out a dazzling light' capable of almost blinding him.

SIMPLICIO. I am afraid you have introduced some trickery. Yet I see, in looking at that mirror, that it gives out a dazzling light that almost blinds me; and what is more significant, I see it all the time, wherever I go, changing place on the surface of the mirror according as I look at it from this place or that; a conclusive proof that the light is reflected very vividly on all sides, and consequently upon the entire wall as upon my eyes. (p. 67; transl. p. 76)

Salviati grasps the occasion for warning Simplicio of the fallacies incurred by giving assent to what is demonstrated only by logical reasoning (*il solo discorso*). Simplicio's amazement in realizing that the light of the mirror, despite its apparent splendour, appears in fact incapable of illuminating the room, is indeed comprehensible. Salviati then makes reference to 'sensible experiences' (*sensate experienze*). As already remarked, this is a recurrent and important expression in Galileo's scientific prose, which can mean both sound experiences based on the senses and issues of trustworthy scientific experiments.

SALVIATI. Now you see how carefully and with what reserve one must proceed in giving assent to what is shown by argument alone. There is no doubt that what you say is plausible enough, and yet you see that sensible experiences refutes it. (p. 67; transl. p. 76)

Simplicio's intellectual frustration has the positive effect of leading him to abandon his stubborn adherence to traditional science and of inducing him to be more receptive to the new science announced by the other debater. In developing his explanation of the surprising phenomenon, Salviati makes reference to another important aspect of Galileo's elaboration on senses, that concerning the problem of the great perceptual errors that can occur when looking at small luminous bodies (like stars and many planets, but also 'the flame of a candle at some distance').

SIMPLICIO. How, then, does this business proceed?

SALVIATI. I shall tell you what I think about it, but I do not know how it will satisfy you. First of all, that brilliance which you see so vividly on the mirror, and which seems to you to occupy such a large part of it, is not such a big piece. It is really very tiny, but its extreme brightness causes an adventitious irradiation of your eyes through the reflection made in the moisture at the edges of your eyelids, which extends over the pupils. It is like the luminous hair (*capillizio*) that seems to be seen around the flame of a candle at some distance; or you may want to compare it with the apparent rays around a star. For example, if you match the little body of the Dog Star as seen in the daytime through the telescope, when it is without irradiations, with the same seen at night by the naked eye, you will perceive beyond all doubt that with its irradiations it appears thousands of times larger than the bare and real starlet. A similar or larger augmentation is made by the image of the sun which you see in that mirror; I say larger, because it is more vivid than that of the star, as is obvious from one's being able to look at the star with less injury to one's vision than at this reflection in the mirror. Thus the reflection which has been imparted over this entire wall comes from a small part of the mirror, while that which was coming a little while ago from the flat mirror was imparted and confined to a very small part of the same wall. What is the marvel, then, that the first reflection shone very brightly, and this other remained almost imperceptible? (p. 69; transl. pp. 76–77, revised)

It is clear from Salviati's words that 'sensible experiences', like those resulting from the experiments with both the plane and spherical mirror, can account for some surprising observations and they can go both against common-sense expectations and the apparently immediate sensory data.

We are not going to discuss how the 'adventitious irradiation' invoked by Salviati could account for the visual magnification of bright bodies seen at a distance. We will deal with this phenomenon in later chapters, particularly Chapters 8 and 13. We limit ourselves to remark that, being aware of the possible fallacies, Galileo makes Salviati estimate the luminosity by means of a more objective parameter: the potential capacity of a light beam to injure one's eye. A star which appears very bright does in fact irradiate much less light than the reflection of sunlight from a mirror, even though it seems incapable of illuminating a wall opposite.

At this point Salviati provides his explanation of 'diffuse reflection', the surprising phenomenon whereby 'the wall, being of so dark a material and so rough a surface, is able to reflect light more powerfully and vividly than a smooth and well-polished mirror'. We will find here elements similar to those expounded by Galileo in *Saggiatore* with reference to the observation of the reflection of the sun from the sea.

SIMPLICIO. I am more perplexed than ever; I must bring up the other difficulty. How can it be that the wall, being of so dark a material and so rough a surface, is able to reflect light more powerfully and vividly than a smooth and well-polished mirror?

SALVIATI. Not more vividly, but more diffusely. As to vividness, you see that the reflection of that little flat mirror, where it is thrown there under the balcony, shines strongly; and the rest of the wall, which receives

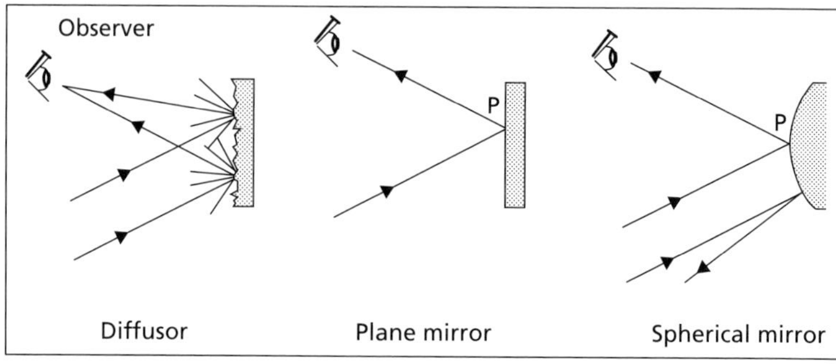

Figure 5.2 Comparison of diffuse reflection (as in a wall), specular reflection in a plane mirror, and specular reflection in a spherical mirror. In the first case since the surface, because of its irregularities, can be considered as made by a myriad of small plane mirrors, it reflects the light rays towards various directions, and the eye will receive a substantial part of them from most points of view. In the case of the plane mirror, the rays will arrive at the eye only in a single position, which depends on the spatial arrangement of light source, mirror, and observer. In the case of the spherical mirror, from several points of view the eye will just see a single light ray (or a very narrow light beam). Reproduced from Galilei, G., Frova, A., and Marenzana, M., *Thus spoke Galileo: the great scientist's ideas and their relevance to the present day*, © 2006, Oxford University Press.

a reflection from the wall to which the mirror is attached, is not lighted up to any great extent (as is the small part struck by the reflection from the mirror). If you wish to understand the whole matter, consider how the surface of this rough wall is composed of countless very small surfaces placed in an innumerable diversity of slopes, among which of necessity many happen to be arranged so as to send the rays they reflect to one place, and many others to another. In short, there is no place whatever which does not receive a multitude of rays reflected from very many little surfaces [*moltissime superficiette*] dispersed over the whole surface of the rough body upon which the luminous rays fall. From all this it necessarily follows that reflected rays fall upon every part of any surface opposite that which receives the primary incident rays, and it is accordingly illuminated. It also follows that the same body on which the illuminating rays fall shows itself lighted and bright all over when looked at from any place.

Therefore the moon, by being a rough surface rather than smooth, sends the sun's light in all directions, and looks equally light to all observers. If the surface, being spherical, were as smooth as a mirror, it would be entirely invisible, seeing that that very small part of it which can reflect the image of the sun to the eyes of any individual would remain invisible because of the great distance, as we have already remarked. (p. 69; transl. p. 77: see our Figure 5.2])

5.3 In the goldsmith's shop: producing brilliancy with a darkening tool

Although at this point Simplicio claims to have understood Salviati's argument clearly, nevertheless he presents other objections to the general conclusion of his adversary. They are based on one of the traditional arguments of the peripatetics in support of a mirror-like reflection from the moon. This allows Galileo to continue his discussion (through Salviati's words) on the comparison between mirror-like reflection and diffuse illumination, again with the recourse to some demonstrative experiments.

It is relevant to note that a part of the following discussion is concerned with the modifications of reflectivity from a metallic surface induced by the various phases of the process of 'burnishing' (*brunitura*), following the technique normally used in Galileo's day. In order to make the surface of precious metals shine, silversmiths and goldsmiths first treat them with various types of chemical solutions capable of removing rust and oxidation products. These treatments produce small irregularities on their surface. To eliminate these irregularities and make the surface perfectly polished, they then treat it mechanically with a particular instrument called a burnisher (*brunitoio*). The initial treatment is called 'bleaching' (*bianchimento*), because it results in a white colour of the surface. As Salviati explains, after the bleaching process, silver vases appear white as snow (*candidi come la neve*), because the fine irregularities in their surface make them capable of reflecting the light in all directions at the minute scale of their fine-grained roughness. In other words, after the bleaching process the surface of metals does not reflect an image as mirrors do.

As the surface is made more and more regular through the polishing action of the burnisher two things happen in parallel. The surface becomes progressively more capable of reflecting a well-defined image in a mirror-like fashion, and, at the same time, it loses the white colour, becoming dark. This last effect accounts for the terms, *brunire* (in Italian) or *burnish* (English), both derived from the old French *brunir* which means to make brown. Among the variations proposed by Salviati is the suggestion of taking a large plate of metal and bleaching it. Afterwards, with the burnisher one should polish only a localized portion of its surface so that 'the minute inequalities are levelled by burnishing'. In the presence of an appropriate source of light, the burnished zone appears luminous only if viewed from a position receiving the reflected rays, while the rest appears white. If the observer moves, the bleached zone will continue to appear white while the other becomes dark. The conclusion of this experiment is congruent with the remarks made before with relation to the experiment with the plate mirror which appears darker than the white wall under most viewing conditions.

At this stage, convinced by the arguments of Salviati (and Sagredo) we might have lost the totally counterintuitive character of the phenomenon. Normally, we would have agreed with Simplicio and his colleague that a mirror (and a perfectly polished surface) should shine more than an irregular surface, and to call the first bright and the second opaque. But things are different, and if we were not under the misleading influence of common sense we should have realized this through a natural experiment to which we are exposed almost every day of our lives. Simply look at the windows of a building and compare the brightness of the glass panes with that of the adjacent walls. In most viewing conditions, the polished surface of the glass panes appear 'surprisingly' darker than those of the adjacent surfaces. As in the case of the plane mirror, only in the rare conditions of a perfect triangulation between the sun, the windows, and ourselves would the glass panes appear bright and shining, and much clearer than the irregular surfaces of the adjacent walls (see Figure 5.3).

As a justification for the old authors and their followers, we could perhaps say that mirror panes were much less frequent in old cities and thus this 'natural' experiment was not so natural for them as it is now for us. However, in their time, there was the surface of the sea and lakes which could provide a proper 'reflection' on the mechanisms of reflection which could have led them to different conclusions on the cause of moon brightness, and thus perhaps to a different vision of the cosmos.

As Galileo points out in many of his writings, the surface of a still water seen at a distance should appear less brilliant than that of the adjacent earth regions. The problem of the difference between mirror-like and diffuse reflection is returned to in the *Dialogue* by Salviati; he describes a simple experiment that is stimulated by a difficulty expressed by Simplicio with these words:

SIMPLICIO [...] Another trouble originated in my believing that the reflection from the seas ought to be stronger, on account of the evenness of their surface, than that from the land, whose surface is so rough and dark. (DIALOGO, p. 90; transl. p. 97)

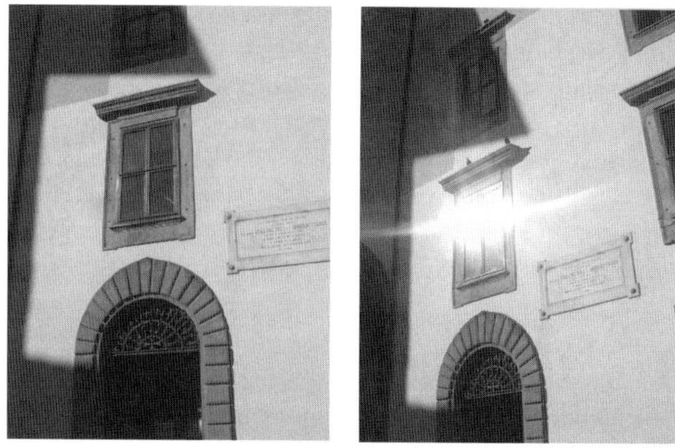

Figure 5.3 Left, a window as it appears on a sunny day, in most of the viewing conditions, and right from the particular point of view in which it reflects in a specular way the sunlight towards the observer. As in Figure 5.1 these pictures were taken in *Piazza dei Cavalieri* in Pisa.

This is the way Salviati upsets Simplicio's common sense, but apparently justified, opinion (maintained, among others, even by Kepler—see Chapter 11):

SALVIATI. [...] Concerning the other question, it seems to me that from our having considered events that take place in mirrors we can understand quite well that the reflection of light coming from the seas would be less than that coming from the land. I mean here its general reflection, for as to the specific reflection from a quiet sea toward one certain place, I have no doubt that anyone located in that place would see from the water a very strong reflection. But from all other places, the surface of the water would be seen darker than the land. And to show this to your own senses, let us go into that hall and pour a little water on the pavement. Tell me, now, doesn't this wet brick look darker than those dry ones?

Of course it does, and it looks so from every place but one; namely, where the reflection of light from that window strikes. Therefore move gently backward a bit.

SIMPLICIO. From here I see the wet part brighter than the rest of the pavement, and I perceive that this happens because the reflection of the light from that window is coming straight toward me.

SALVIATI. All that this wetting has done is to fill the little pores in the brick and reduce its surface to a smooth plane, from which the reflected rays then come unitedly toward a single place. The rest of the pavement is dry, and keeps its roughness; that is, that is, an innumerable variety of slopes in its minute particles, from which the reflections of light go out in every direction but are much weaker than if they were all to go united together. Therefore the appearance of this part varies little or none when observed from various directions, but looks the same from everywhere—and much less bright than that one particular reflection from the wet part.[3] (DIALOGO, pp. 90–91; transl. pp. 97–98)

[3] As we know from a Jean Tarde, a French ecclesiastic interested in astronomy who visited Galileo on various occasions during his journey in Italy in 1614, Galileo used to perform the demonstration of the moistened brick to his visitors in order to make clear the mechanism by which the moon reflects sunrays: '*Et, entre autres choses, le Seigneur Galilei nous a fait voir que la surface du corps lunaire éstoit autant raboteuse que celle de la terre. Que, si elle éstoit uniforme, bien unie et polye comme un miroir, elle ne renvoyeroit pas les rayons du soleil vers la terre, ains qu'elle nous seroit invisible au ciel. Ce que il a montré par l'exemple d'un peu d'eau éspandue sur le pavé qui ne réverbère la lumière du corps apposé que le long de la ligne de réflection qui faict l'angle égal à celui qu'on appelle* incidentiae,*hors laquelle ligne on ne voit point de réflexion*' (Tarde, 1984, pp. 64–65; a more faithful transcription of the original text is available on the website: <http://moro.imss.fi.it/lettura/LetturaWEB.DLL?AZIONE=UNITA&TESTO=EaZ&PARAM=175-339356-26547&VOL=19>).

We will discuss in detail the theme of the reflections from water in Chapters 11 and 13. It suffices here to say that the observation on the darkening effect of moistening was well known, being discussed among others in a treatise entitled *De coloribus* attributed to Aristotle.[4]

5.4 **Looking to the Americas through the moon face**

What immediately follows shows Galileo's extraordinary long-sightedness and his deep conviction that the same physical and perceptual laws hold for near objects and for astronomical objects: following a simple experiment based on the moistening of a brick of the pavement, he is able to predict that, seen from the moon, the oceanic regions of the earth would appear darker than the lands. Or said otherwise, and with a more technical and modern astronomical language, that the reflectivity or albedo of the seas is much lower than the albedo of deserts or of mountains not covered by trees.

SALVIATI. I conclude therefore that just as the surface of the ocean seen from the moon would appear level (except for islands and rocks), so it would appear less bright than that of the land, which is uneven and mountainous.

He would even go so far as to suppose that the difference in the reflection between the lands and the oceans of the earth might produce slight variations in the 'secondary lumen' of the moon, i.e. in the illumination of the dark part of the moon that he attributes to the reflection from the earth:

SALVIATI. And if it were not that I do not wish to seem too eager, as they say, I should tell you of having observed the secondary light of the moon (which I say is a reflection from the terrestrial globe) to be appreciably brighter two or three days before the conjunction than after. That is, when we see it before dawn in the east it is brighter than when we see it in the evening after the setting of the sun in the west. The reason for this difference is that the terrestrial hemisphere opposite to the moon when it is in the east has fewer seas and more land, containing all Asia But when the moon is in the west, it faces great seas—the whole Atlantic Ocean up to America—a very plausible argument for the surface of the water showing itself less brilliantly than that of the land. (pp. 91–92; transl. p. 98)

Nowadays, due to the extreme importance of the albedo of earth in meteorological and climatic studies, the earthshine, i.e. the light reflected from the earth, is studied with satellites and other monitoring systems. Its variations for a simulated lunar observer are registered and analysed. If we consider all that, we cannot but recognize the extent to which Galileo was intellectually long-sighted.

Although the 'secondary lumen' of the earth can vary as a consequence of accidental factors (like the extensive cloud coverage of large regions of the globe), there is—exactly as Galileo remarks through Salviati's words—a periodical variation connected to the moon phases. The weak light on the dark zone of the moon appears to be slightly more intense in the phase of waxing lunar crescent visible in the morning compared to the waning lunar crescent visible in the evening. The effect is largely due to the bigger proportion of land reflecting the sun rays towards the moon in the phase of waxing crescent compared to the second condition. To have an idea of

4 Kepler dealt with this theme, with reference also to the arguments raised in *De coloribus*, both in 1604 (in his *Optical part of astronomy*) and in his posthumous work, *Somnium seu Opus posthumun de astronomia lunari*.

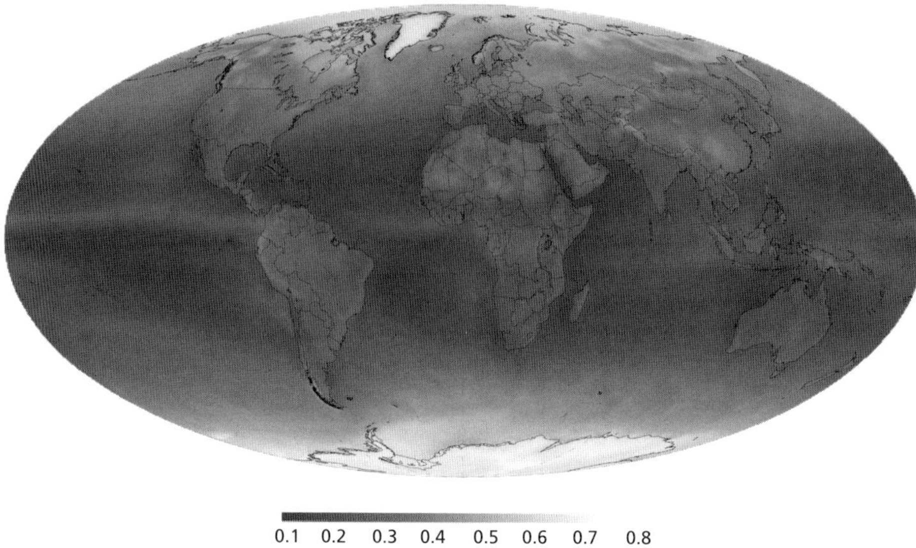

Figure 5.4 An illustration of the reflectivity of different regions of the earth based on satellite data. As shown below the planisphere image, the darker colours indicate regions with low albedo, while the regions with smaller albedo are represented by lighter colours. The zones with higher albedo are the glacial regions due to the very high albedo of snow (0.8–0.9) and iced oceans (0.5–0.7), while the zone of smaller albedo are the oceans (because of the very low albedo of water, near zero with obliquely incident light). In their ensemble the regions situated at the east of Italy (Galileo's observation point) have more lands compared to the western regions of this planisphere. Among the land regions, a particularly high average albedo is in the desert and mountainous regions of Africa and Asia, and the eastern regions of Asia. Image source: NASA—Clouds and the Earth's Radiant Energy System.

the extraordinary perspicacity (both visual and intellectual) of Galileo, one should keep in mind that, in the absence of any recordable measurement of the phenomenon, he should keep in his visual memory the track of the two slightly different brightness for about two weeks (the time span elapsing between a waxing and a waning crescent). Under another perspective, we could say that by noting the difference of the intensity of lunar candour under the two conditions, Galileo might be able to know, even before actually discovering the Americas, that the most western regions of earth (relative to his observation point) were relatively richer in waters, compared to the Euro Asiatic regions (see Figure 5.4)

Benedetto Castelli was inspired by what Galileo reports in his *Dialogue*, i.e. the earlier quoted passage of Salviati on the more intense secondary lumen of the moon in the condition or morning crescent. In a letter dated 14 November 1637 he wrote to Galileo that he had noticed a particularly bright secondary lumen in a condition in which 'the moon happened to be southern' (i.e. facing the southern regions of earth). He added that, within the framework of Galileo's explanation of the cause of the secondary lumen of the moon, it came to his mind 'that the southern regions [of the earth] unknown to us, should have very vast lands, and this is why they reflect a vigorous lumen of the moon' (OG XVII, p. 217). Galileo seems to have approved of Castelli's supposition as we learn from another letter from Castelli written on 12 December of the same year. Castelli's observation has been interpreted as evidence of the existence of a southern continent, still to be discovered, Australia (see Millosevich, 1919).

5.5 Astronomia lunaris

In order to understand why the earth shines more light towards the moon in the condition of (moon) waxing crescent (the crescent visible in the morning before sunrise, compared to the symmetric condition of the evening waning crescent, visible after sunset) we need to imagine the aspect of the moon seen from the earth and that of the earth seen from the moon at the same time. The second situation requires an imaginary journey to the moon. Before Neil Amstrong and his crew of the Apollo 11 spacecraft landed there, Kepler had contrived such a journey in a book published in 1634, four years after author's death (but conceived in 1593 during his studentship years in Tübingen). Interestingly, Kepler's aim in elaborating his imaginary voyage was very similar to that which is pushing us to go there, that of visualizing the appearance of the sky (and particularly of the earth) from such a remote location, i.e. to contrive a lunar astronomy, as indicated by the title of his fiction: *Somnium seu Opus posthumun de astronomia lunari* ('The dream, or posthumous work on lunar astronomy').

Among the remarkable aspects of the very dark night sky observed from the moon during the very long nights (lasting about one half of our month) there is the presence of a very big celestial body (about 13 times bigger in surface than the moon observed from the earth, and shining about 80 times more intensely with a coloured appearance dominated by blue). It is nothing else than our familiar earth, although its aspect looks somewhat strange from this unusual observation point.

There are important asymmetries in the imaginary vision of the earth from the moon compared to our familiar vision of the moon from the earth. Let us suppose that we observe the moon from Galileo's place (Florence or Pisa), and the lunar observer is located at the centre of the moon (i.e. the part of the moon visible from the earth). From any terrestrial point of view the moon is seen to change its position in the sky continuously, i.e. to rise from orient, arrive near the zenith, and eventually to set towards occident. If we repeat the observations at different moments of a terrestrial month, we would become aware that the moon appears to repeat its movement from orient to occident every day. There is, however, a progressive change of the time it rises and sets during the day. Since, for geometrico-astronomical reasons, in the phases near the new moon it occupies a position on the vault of the sky near the sun (see Figure 5.5), it will rise around sunrise and will set about sunset. For analogous reasons, in the phases near the full moon, it will rise about sunset, and set about sunrise.

For lunar observers looking at the earth, the situation is different regarding the two main respects just considered. First they will see the earth always in the same location in the sky: for them, the earth never rises, never sets. Since we have assumed that they have the earth near its zenith, the earth would maintain indefinitely its high location on the sky. However, in contrast to what happens to the terrestrial observer looking at the moon, they would see a continuous and relatively rapid change of the image of the earth face, due to the daily rotation of the earth around its axis. This is why Kepler called it Volvania in his *Astronomia lunaris* (from the Latin *volvere* meaning to turn). Suppose that the lunar observers start looking at the earth when the Pacific Ocean is the centre of the earth phase. They would see (in sequence) the eastern regions of Asia and Australia, central Asia with Siberia, the high mountains of Himalaya, India, the desert part

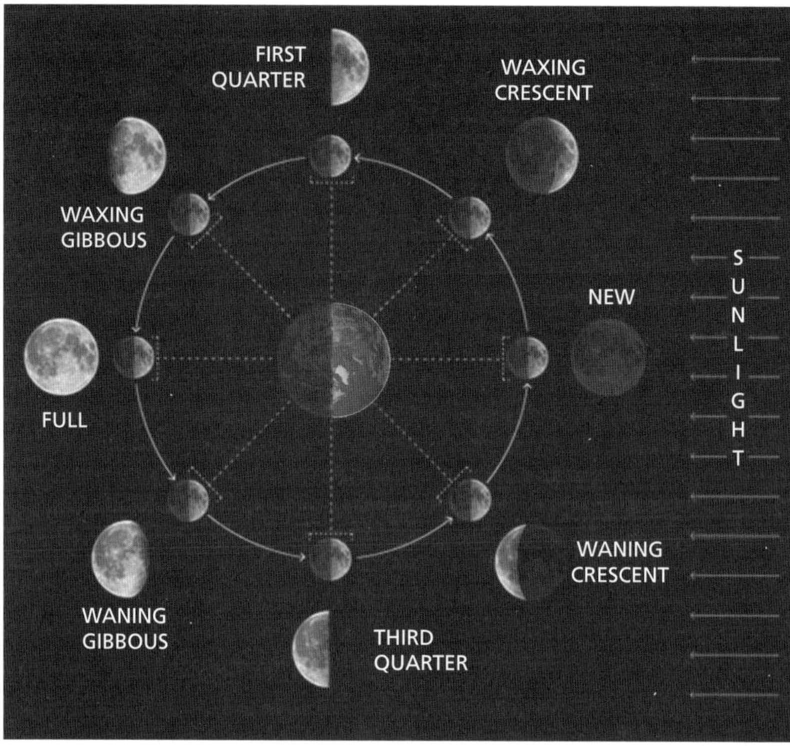

Figure 5.5 Diagram of the moon phases to aid understanding of the variations of the 'secondary lumen' of the moon in the two conditions of waxing or waning moon crescent. As indicated, the sunrays are supposed to come from the right of the figure and the cycle to occur in an anticlockwise way. The earth is seen from the top. Notice first the complementarity between the phases of the moon with those of the earth. When the moon is new, the earth (seen from a lunar position) is full, and vice versa. By comparing the two conditions of moon crescent, it appears that in the phase of waxing crescent (relative to an observer situated in Tuscany), the dark region of the moon is facing mainly the land-rich regions of Asia, whereas in the phase of waning crescent, it faces mainly the Atlantic Ocean. © Moonconnection.com, modified.

of Asia, Europe, and Africa, the Atlantic Ocean, the Americas, and eventually the Pacific Ocean again. It would take only one (terrestrial) day to observe all these mutations on the earth face (even without a telescope, because, due to the larger size of the earth globe, some details can be seen even with an unaided eye).

This is all we need to know for the moment concerning the similarity and difference of the vision from the two points of view, the lunar versus the terrestrial one. Let us now introduce, in the play between the two globes, the sun as the main origin of light in the solar system. Relative to our location on the earth (Tuscany), when the sun starts rising and is therefore very low on our horizon it is high in the sky of Asia. The same would be for the moon in the phases near the new moon, when it is located in the sky near that of the sun. At sunset, the sun (and the moon near the new moon) would be centred about the Atlantic Ocean and Americas.

We have now enough information to understand why (through Salviati's words) Galileo could advance his explanation of the dimmer secondary lumen of the moon based on the greater earth reflection from the Asiatic regions compared to the 'whole Atlantic Ocean up to America'. The best condition to see the secondary lumen of the moon is to look at it during the dim illumination of the sky near sunrise and sunset. This is a condition near the new moon, as when only a thin crescent appears at the border of the moon (this is the condition in which the earth appears full when looked at from the moon). We would not see the secondary lumen during the day because the intense sunlight would make it invisible (and possibly also the directly illuminated part of the moon) due to physiological light adaptation processes in the visual system. On the other hand, we would not perceive the secondary lumen of the moon during the night. This is because the excessive apparent luminosity of the moon part directly struck by sunrays would make the secondary lumen appear darker due to visual contrast effects.

We have two apparently symmetrical conditions of lunar crescent in which we should see the best secondary lumen of the moon. One in the morning, when the moon rises a little earlier than the sun from the east (being at the west of the sun separated from it by about eight degrees, with the convex rim on the left, towards the sun); the other in the evening, when the moon sets a little later than the sun (being in this case at the east of the sun, and with the convexity pointing towards the west, again of course towards the sun). Although symmetrical from a geometrical point of view, these two situations are not perfectly symmetrical with regard to the secondary lumen of the moon. This is because the moon in the east faces the land-rich regions of Asia, whereas the moon on the west side is directed at the water-rich region of Atlantic Ocean. From which it would ensue that in the first situation the secondary lumen would be a little more intense than in the second circumstance. This is the basis of Galileo/Salviati's explanation in the *Dialogue*.

Before ending this section, and coming back to our usual conversation between Salviati, Simplicio, and Sagredo, a remark seems appropriate here. Although the secondary lumen of the moon (or lunar candour) is very dim, Galileo was probably in a favourable position to see it and notice differences in the two moon crescent conditions considered earlier in this chapter, because he was using a telescope. Most likely this was not so much due to the light-collecting properties of the telescope because Galileo's telescopes allowed in much less light than modern ones. Probably the main reason was that he was trying to resolve the details on the moon (craters, mountains) in both its luminous and dark regions. He was particularly interested in the phenomena visible at the rim separating the two regions (the terminator) with variable play of small luminous or dark points which changed with the change of the relative inclination of sunrays during the period of observation (see Chapter 6). As often remarked in this book, the brightness of a visual object or scene is a very fallacious clue to their luminance. However, the possibility to resolve details in a visual scene is a much more dependable criterion for evaluating the illumination of an object. This Galileo knew well, and it is indeed for this reason that he makes frequent remarks based on this criterion when he wishes to compare the luminosity of different objects or environments (he insists often on the ease of reading a text as a dependable test of the illumination conditions).[5]

Salviati makes his argument about differences in the secondary lumen of the moon in a somewhat doubtful way. There is a possible reason for this. The reflectivity of the earth can vary considerably in an accidental way due mainly to changes in the cloud coverage of the earth. It is possible that, having contrived his explanation for the difference in the secondary lumen of the moon

[5] This interpretation is consistent with a remark made in *Sidereus nuncius* where, in dealing with the secondary lumen of the moon, he writes that this is relatively bright 'so bright indeed, that with the help of the good spyglass (*ope exacti Perspicilli*) the great spots can be distinguished in it' (SIDEREUS, p. 14; transl. p. 68).

based on the differences on the relative positions of moon–earth–sun, he could not verify it in all the observations he made, because of fortuitous variations of the earth's reflectivity.

After the death of Galileo, his (and Castelli's) conclusions on the different intensity of the secondary lumen during the moon's cycle were largely confirmed by Johannes Hevelius (the founder of modern selenography), and by various astronomers and physicists in the eighteenth century (like Johann Heinrich Lambert—of the Lambert and Beer photometric law—and Johann Hieronymus Schröter). In the following century François Arago suggested that a photometric analysis of the variable intensity and colours of the moon's secondary lumen could be useful to establish the atmospheric conditions of the earth, and particularly the variable presence of clouds in the regions of the earth surface sending their diffuse reflection onto the dark part of the moon (Arago, 1865, pp. 475–485; see Millosevich, 1919).

5.6 Reflections in a clothes shop

After this long explanatory digression, let us return to the direct dialogue between Salviati and Simplicio. Following a question raised by Simplicio about the possibility that the large dark spots on the moon might be seas, Salviati then gives a lesson in method largely inspired by the motifs expounded in the fable of the sounds (nature can produce its effects in a variety of ways which may be unknown and unimaginable to us). Afterwards, he returns to the argument of the different brightness of seas and lands by making a comparison with the visual effects that can be produced in different cloths depending on their fine structure. This makes clear his great perceptual skill and, moreover, his deep conviction that similar physical and perceptual laws can be applied to objects of different scale and different observation distance, with no difference between sublunary and supralunar world:

SIMPLICIO. [...] But do you believe then that those great spots which are seen on the face of the moon are seas, and the brighter balance land, or some such thing?

SALVIATI. What you are now asking me is the first of the differences that I think exist between the moon and the earth, which we had better hurry along with, as we are staying too long on the moon. I say then that if there were in nature only one way for two surfaces to be illuminated by the sun so that one appears lighter than the other, and that this were by having one made of land and the other of water, it would be necessary to say that the moon's surface was partly terrene and partly aqueous. But because there are more ways known to us that could produce the same effect, and perhaps others that we do not know of, I shall not make bold to affirm one rather than another to exist on the moon. We have already seen that a bleached silver plate changes from white to dark by the touch of the burnisher; the watery part of the earth looks darker than the dry; on the ridges of mountains the wooded parts look much gloomier than the open and barren places because the plants cast a great deal of shadow while the clearings are lighted by the sun. Such a mixture of shadows is so effective that in sculptured velvet the color of the cut silk looks much darker than that of the uncut because of shadows cast between one thread and another; and plain velvet is likewise much darker than made of the same silk taffeta [actually *ermisino*, i.e. the precious silk cloth fabricated in Hormuz]. So if on the moon there were things resembling dense forests, their aspect would probably be like that of the spots we see; a like difference would be created if they were seas; and, finally, there is nothing to prevent these spots being really of a darker color than the rest, for it is in that way that snow makes mountains appear brighter. What is clearly seen in the moon is that the darker parts are all plains, with few rocks and ridges in them, though there are some. The brighter remainder is all full of rocks, mountains, round ridges, and other shapes, and in particular there are great ranges of mountains around the spots. That the spots are flat surfaces we are certain, from observing that the boundary which separates the light and dark parts makes an even cut in traversing the spots, whereas in the bright parts it

> looks broken and jagged. But I do not know whether this evenness of surface is enough by itself to cause the apparent darkness, and I rather think not. (DIALOGO, pp. 92–93; transl. pp. 98–99)

In Chapter 6 we will discuss how Galileo used his telescopic observations to conclude that there were mountains, craters, and other form of irregularity on the surface of the moon, and how he succeeded in calculating with astonishing precision the altitude of lunar mountains. Moreover, we will concentrate on his reflection of the 'visibility' of lunar irregularities as an elaboration of the meaning and limit of visual processes.

What seems sure to us from what has been said in this chapter is that a reflection on vision, its subtleties, and possibly fallacious appearances, was a very relevant aspect of his interests, and a formidable tool in his astronomical investigations. Several pages of the First Day of the *Dialogue* can be considered as a discussion on vision and on its possible importance in a cosmological and astronomic context.

Chapter 6

Seeing mountains on the moon

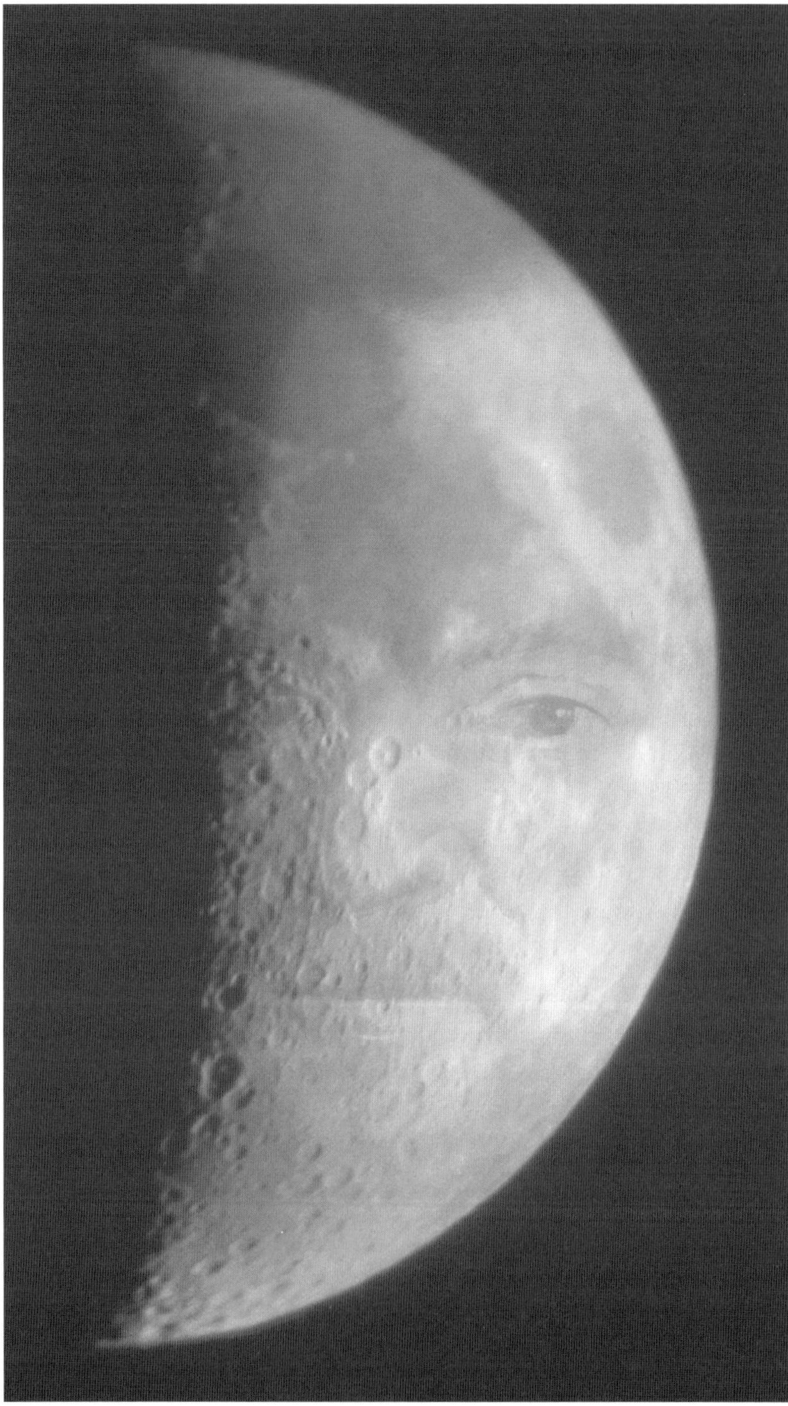

Figure VI *Galileo's mountains on the moon* by Nicholas Wade. The bright crescent of the moon contains a youthful portrait of Galileo.

Galileo's first telescopic observations for which we have a written record were on the presence of high mountains and deep craters on the moon's surface. They are documented in an important letter bearing the date 7 January 1610 (i.e. about two months before the publication of *Sidereus nuncius*) and addressed to an unknown correspondent (probably Antonio de Medici, one of the members of the Florentine court). This letter is rather detailed and accompanied by a series of images of the moon prepared by Galileo so that his description of the appearance of the lunar surface could be better understood (OG X, pp. 273–278).[1]

Because of this chronological priority we should perhaps have dealt first with Galileo's announcement that the moon 'is full of eminences and cavities, similar, but much bigger, to the mountains and valleys spread on the earth surface', as he put it in this letter (OG X, p. 273). The presence of irregularities on the moon's surface logically precedes Galileo's elaboration on the similarity between the mechanism of light reflections by the moon and the earth as well as the interpretation of the 'secondary lumen' of the moon.

This notwithstanding, we will now examine the way Galileo arrived at his conclusions about the moon's uneven surface having dealt with the light reflected from the moon and its 'secondary lumen'. This is because it is with relation to the problem of the presence of mountains and craters on the moon that he proceeds to his more perceptive analysis of vision and of the reasons why one can reach sound conclusions about the reality of the world despite the possible fallacies of vision.

It is not by chance that this happened in the context of the interpretation of astronomical ideas in three dimensions. This is because three-dimensionality is one of the attributes of the real world which is more difficult to translate into the sensory world, and more prone to ambiguities for the vision of distant objects. This is especially the case for observation and representation of celestial bodies. For such objects we lack a number of cues which normally help to resolve the depth of objects within reach. In particular we lack the depth information provided by vision with two eyes (stereopsis) which is effective only within the range of metres; and of course we lack the information provided by other senses. In many respects, perceptual inferences concerning three-dimensional reality of celestial objects are even more difficult to achieve than for the evaluation of their physical luminosity (one of the sensory arguments central to Galileo's intellectual elaboration that we have considered in the previous chapters).

The most important text concerning the nature and limits of the visual process in the context of the three-dimensional characteristics of distant objects, and particularly of the moon's surface, is a long letter addressed by Galileo to the Jesuit, Christoph Grienberger, in September 1611. Grienberger was the pupil of Christoph Clavius, a famous astronomer of the age and first professor of mathematics at the Roman College (the main educational institution for Jesuits and the forerunner of the present Pontifical Gregorian University of Rome). He was known for an important commentary on the most current textbook of astronomy, the *Sphaera* by Sacrobosco (i.e. by the English monk, John of Holywood, generally known as Johannes de Sacrobosco) (Figure 6.1). Because of his astronomical competence, in 1579 Clavius had been involved by Pope Gregory XIII

[1] A brief allusion to the irregularity of the moon is also contained in a letter written to Belisario Vinta, the secretary of the Grand Duke of Tuscany. Although dated 30 January 1610 (and thus later than the earlier mentioned one) it refers to conclusions about the irregular nature of the moon's surface obtained with the telescope from an earlier observation. Galileo writes that he had already had the opportunity to show to the Grand Duke that 'the moon is a body very similar to earth' during his previous sojourn in Florence (that is, during the Christmas holidays of 1609: OG 10, p 280).

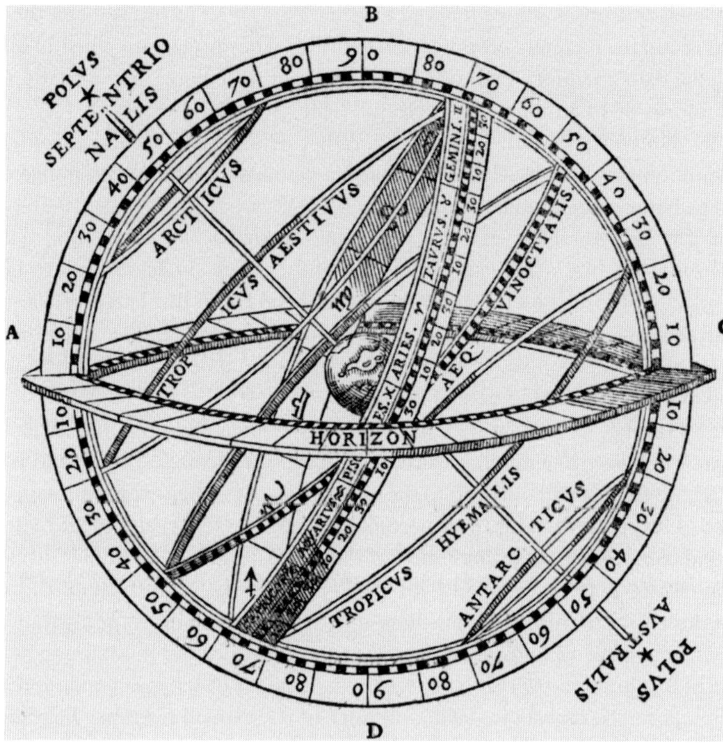

Figure 6.1 The armillary sphere from the Sacrobosco's *Sphaera* in the 1602 edition edited and commented on by Christoph Clavius (Clavius, 1602). Galileo held two editions of this opus in his private library.

in the reformation of the calendar.[2] The presence at the Roman College of Clavius and his team of experts, forming the so-called 'Mathematical Academy', of which Grienberger was a member, made this institution the reference centre for astronomical studies of the age.

6.1 **Jesuit mutations**

Grienberger had been following Galileo's astronomical discoveries closely, not only for his personal interest in the field but also because in the spring of the same year he had been one of the members of a committee charged by Cardinal Roberto Bellarmino (a Jesuit himself and eminent member of the Roman Inquisition) with verifying Galileo's astronomical discoveries, among which was 'whether the moon has the surface rough and uneven'. The other members of the committee, all belonging to the Mathematical Academy of the College, were Clavius and two other brothers (Odo van Maelcote and Paolo Lembo). This team of experts reached their conclusions very quickly and these were made public. They were largely favourable to Galileo, although with some reservations about the irregular nature of the moon's surface, expressed particularly by

[2] Clavius' commentary on Sacrobosco, together with others of his astronomical works (*Gnomonices*, *Astrolabium*), were brought to China by one of his students, the famous Jesuit Missionary, Matteo Ricci, who also helped to translate them into Chinese.

Clavius (who still adhered to an old theory which attributed the spotted aspect of the moon to an unequal density of lunar matter). Galileo was in Rome at that time, visiting many members of the Roman intelligentsia in order to promote his discoveries. He had had the opportunity of discussing them personally with Clavius, Grienberger, and Maelcote who he visited at the College on 30 March, just one day after his arrival in Rome from Florence.

On 13 May, i.e. about one month after the conclusions of the Jesuit astronomers had been published, opinions even more favourable to Galileo were expounded by Maelcote (possibly with Grienberger's support), during a public and sumptuous assembly held at the College, in a conference which was later given the title of *Nuncius sidereus Collegii Romani*. Because of the great authority of the Roman College in astronomical matters, the conclusions of the committee and the public attitude expressed on this and other occasions by the mathematicians of the Jesuit institution were of paramount importance in supporting Galileo's discoveries. Due to their revolutionary character with respect to the traditional cosmology and astronomy, from their onset Galileo's telescopic observations encountered many difficulties and objections and were still the target of criticisms, sometimes very harsh, particularly on the part of the most conservative exponents of the culture of the age.

Initially the Jesuits of the College had expressed serious doubts about these discoveries, particularly because, due to the low quality of the telescope used in their first observations, they had not been able to repeat some of them, as Grienberger noted in a letter addressed to Galileo on 20 March 1611. While communicating to his correspondent that he and his fellows Jesuit astronomers (and notably Clavius) agreed now with most of his discoveries, Grienberger pointed to the initial difficulty encountered in accepting, in the lack of trustworthy data, conclusions that went 'against opinions introduced since so many centuries and consolidated by the authority of so many scholars' (OG XI, p. 33). It was the use of a new and more precise instrument that had allowed the team of Jesuit astronomers to verify Galileo's discoveries, and this was why they were ready to express a favourable opinion when summoned by Bellarmino.

In 1612, when Grienberger published an updated sky catalogue containing newly discovered stars (*Catalogus veteres affixarum longitudines ac latitudines conferens cum novis*), he indicated that even more new celestial entries could be inserted in future catalogues, thanks to the 'new Machines' that 'with the guide of Galileo, a very powerful and successful leader' paved the way for the discovery of new stars in the most remote regions of the universe. Interestingly in his catalogue the Jesuit had inserted the novae of 1572, 1600, and 1604, an indication of his open-mindedness towards the new astronomy and the possible occurrence of changes in the immutable sky of classical cosmology (see Figure 6.2). It is likely that Grienberger, who was not inclined to appear publicly as the author of the texts he wrote or contributed to, was the real author of the lecture on the 1604 nova delivered at the College on that occasion by Maelcote.

The competence, intelligence, and intellectual honesty of Grienberger made him an ideal correspondent for Galileo in his discussion about his astronomical discoveries and the contrasting reception they had been receiving in various cultural milieu of the epoch. In point of fact, he would remain on Galileo's side in the controversy on sunspots that, starting from 1612, set Galileo in opposition to Scheiner, despite their common Jesuit affiliations.

6.2 The immaculate circle of the moon

In May 1611, while Galileo was still in Rome, Grienberger played a role in a controversy between Galileo and another member of the Jesuit order; it occurred following a conference held in Mantua by a Jesuit from the College of Parma. The conference concerned the celestial novelties announced

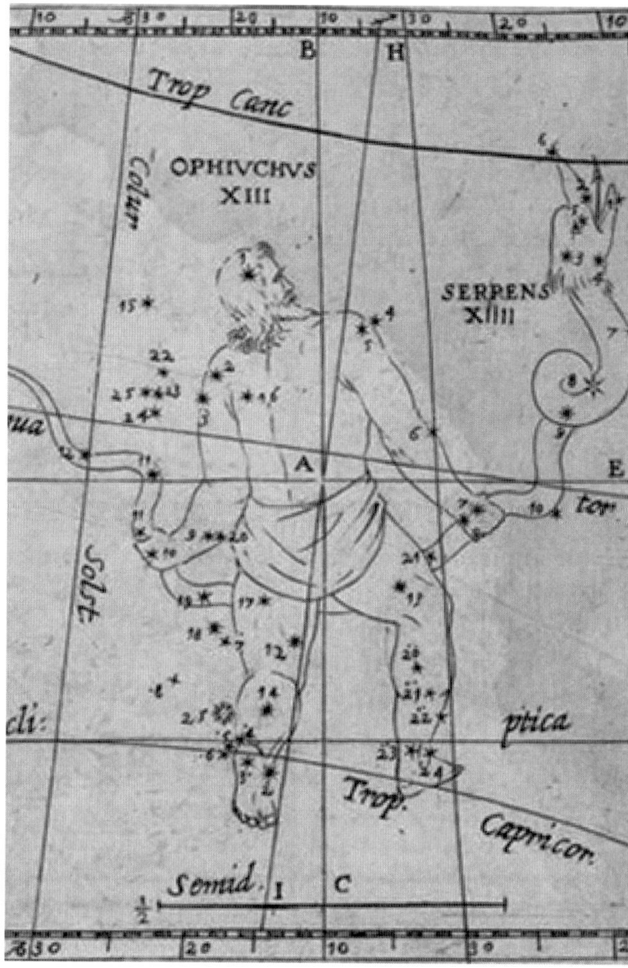

Figure 6.2 The constellation of the Ophiucus from the Catalogue of stars published in 1612 by Christoph Grienberger. The very intense new star (supernova) of 1604 is the star no. 25 represented in large size, and emanating many light rays, near the left foot of the mythological figure.

by Galileo. It was initially held before the public in the Church of Trinity of Mantua (a dependency of the local Jesuit monastery). It was later repeated in other locations and with different audiences, first in the presence of Duke Vincenzo I, then in the presence of Cardinal Ferdinando Gonzaga. Generally known as the 'Problem of Mantua', the text of the conference was circulated in a manuscript form with the title *De lunarium montium altitude* ('The heights of lunar mountains') and with no indication of the author (as was often the case with writings by Jesuits). The author was Mario Bettini, professor of mathematics (and also of moral philosophy) at the College of Parma, although Galileo (as well as Grienberger) initially ascribed it to another member of the Jesuit Society, Giuseppe Biancani (an old acquaintance of Galileo since his time in Padua) and an important astronomer.[3] Bettini's authorship of the Problem of Mantua would be recognized later

[3] The lunar crater, Biancanus, is dedicated to him; it is situated near Clavius, another 'Jesuit' crater. There is little wonder that so many lunar craters are dedicated to Jesuits, since many of them were named by

by the author himself, in an encyclopaedic two-volume work entitled *Apiaria universae philosophiae mathematicae*, first published in 1642. In this work, dealing with various mathematical and astronomical issues and curiosities, he mentions having argued against the opinions of moderns with relation to the presence of mountains on the moon (Bettini, 1642, II p. 73).

Although generally recognizing the importance of Galileo's discoveries, the author of the Problem of Mantua disagreed with one of the conclusions expounded in *Sidereus nuncius*, that concerning the presence of mountains in the extreme rim of the lunar circumference.[4] Galileo maintained that the circumference of the moon was mountainous despite the fact that through the telescope the lunar border appeared devoid of any irregularity. Using an acerbic tone, the Jesuit used this to give Galileo a lesson in scientific methodology:

> In the extreme periphery of the part of the moon which we can see, i.e. that the astronomers call visible, no such mountains can be found. This is for the obvious reason that there is no reason, no visual appearance, no phenomenon that would force us to assert its presence. As a matter of fact if, either with the naked eye or with the telescope [*tubospecillum*] you look very carefully at the extreme circle of the moon when it shines in full splendour, nothing you would detect salient, nothing jagged, nothing serrate. [On the other hand] do not protuberances (tumores) appear, as we showed, in the moon face that looks toward the earth? There is therefore reason why we should assert their presence there. Do they appear in the extreme periphery? There is therefore no reason why we should assert their presence there. Indeed, if protuberances were there, there would be indeed no reason forbidding their appearance. Why then, speaking philosophically, multiply entities [*entia*] with no real necessity and assume they are certain? The very learned man Galileo Galilei fell in this error, if we do not error ourselves, This is because, without any constraint by important arguments, he wished to encircle everywhere the lunar globe with a mountainous surface. Finding himself trapped into the greatest difficulties, he tried to respond with answers that, far from freeing him, have indeed cast him even more in the traps. (OG III, p. 304)

Facing this criticism from the author of the Problem of Mantua, in a letter to Grienberger written on 1 September 1611, Galileo first develops arguments to support his ideas that, contrary to the assertion of his antagonist, if mountains are present in the extreme circumference of the moon they would not be seen, even with the help of the telescope. For Galileo the main reason for this is that the appropriate viewing conditions that allow for the detectability of mountains for the main part of the visible face of the moon are lacking for the lunar periphery. This argument had indeed already been expounded in *Sidereus nuncius* in order to propose the presence of mountains and craters on the facing part of the moon. In *Sidereus* Galileo had also considered the possibility that the invisibility of irregularities on the extreme circumference of the moon could

Giovanni Battista Riccioli, another Jesuit, in his *Almagestum novum*, first published in 1651. Among these craters there were those dedicated respectively to Grienberger, Scheiner, and Bettini. As to Clavius, it is perhaps worth mentioning here that his name was used to indicate a lunar settlement (Clavius base) in Arthur C. Clarke's fiction, *2001: A Space Odyssey*, which served as reference for Stanley Kubrick's famous movie of the same name.

[4] As we shall see in Chapter 7, in his *Apiaria*, Bettini denies even the presence of mountains in the main part of the moon and attributes the telescopic appearances suggesting their presence to the variable transparency of the lunar matter, along an explanation current in the most conservative philosophical milieu of the age. It is to be recalled that, between the time of the Problem of Mantua and 1642 and the epoch of the publication of the *Apiaria*, Galileo had been condemned by the Church, and Jesuits had moved more and more towards traditionalism, due to intensified internal censorship of their religious Order and to the general cultural politics of the Vatican.

be due to the optical effects of a lunar atmosphere. The idea of a lunar atmosphere, based on old astronomical view, was, however, soon abandoned.[5]

In the letter to Grienberger, by addressing his discourse to the Jesuit as 'H[is] R[everence]', and quoting the Latin form of the question raised by the Jesuit of Parma (indicated as the author of the Problem or the Father), Galileo writes:

> The author of the Problem answers: *Apparent in ea Lunae facie, quae terras aspicit, tumores? est igitur ratio cur eos inibi esse affirmemus. Non apparent in extrema periphaeria? non est igitur ratio cur eos inibi esse affirmemus; cum si inibi essent, nulla sufficiens ratio prohibeat quin apparerent.*[6] But I ask the Father, how can he see that in the middle parts of the moon there are eminences? He answers in the Problem: because he sees some illuminated cusps in the dark part, near the boundary of the light, even though entirely disconnected from the luminous part. Now I bring to the consideration of H. R. why this effect cannot occur in the extreme circumference, nor in the parts near it, and this for two reasons. First because when the boundary of the light is near to the extreme circumference and the dark part of the moon points toward us, then the mountainous parts of the moon have their illuminated part adverse from us, and offer to us the dark part; from which would ensue that only their peaks, a little on their sides, could make them visible to us. But also this is impossible, even if they were intensely brilliant, for the following, second reason: the low and dark spaces and intervals separating the cusps illuminated by the boundary of the lumen, remains invisible to us in the extreme parts of the moon because their lowness and elusiveness [*sfuggimento*] and because the last parts of the moon toward the extreme periphery are seen, as perspectivists say, in foreshortening. For this reason the said cusps must appear attached and united to the lights placed on the same term and boundary of the light. This does not happen when the said boundary passes across the most internal parts of the lunar disc. There the rays of the eye, falling in a more oblique way, resolve [*comprendono*] well the separations of such cusps from the boundary of the darkness. It is therefore of no moment the inference of the Father: *Apparent tumores in medio? ergo ibi sunt: non apparent in circumferentia ergo inibi non sunt.*[7] This is because there is no reason why they should appear in the periphery. (OG XI, p. 182) (See Figures 6.3 and 6.4.)

In this passage, Galileo accounts for the presumed invisibility of mountains at the extreme circumference of the moon on the basis of foreshortening effects and the impossibility of resolving the peaks of the illuminated cusps of mountains in the dark part of the lunar surface from the nearby illuminated region. On the other hand, he says that, in contrast to what happens at the extreme circumference, we can detect the illuminated cusps (and other details of the lunar surface) near the dark–light boundary when this boundary 'passes across the most internal parts of the lunar disc' (ideally near the half-moon phase as in Figure 6.4).

5 The idea of lunar atmosphere had a long history, starting at least with the *De facie* of Plutarch (see Chapter 11). In the epoch of Galileo's the optical effects of this presumed lunar atmosphere had been a matter of discussion between Kepler and his former teacher Michael Maestlin. Maestlin assumed that the apparent diameter of the moon was increased by this atmosphere. Kepler, who held a different view of the phenomenon, discussed the problem in various works and notably in his *Astronomiae Pars optica* and in the *Somnium*.

6 We have already translated this passage earlier in the chapter: 'do not protuberances appear, as we showed, in the moon face that looks toward the earth? There is therefore reason why we should assert their presence there. Do they appear in the extreme periphery? There is therefore no reason why we should assert their presence there. Indeed, if protuberances were there, there would be indeed no reason forbidding their appearance'.

7 'Do not protuberances appear in the middle? Therefore they are there: do they appear in the circumference? Therefore they are not there.'

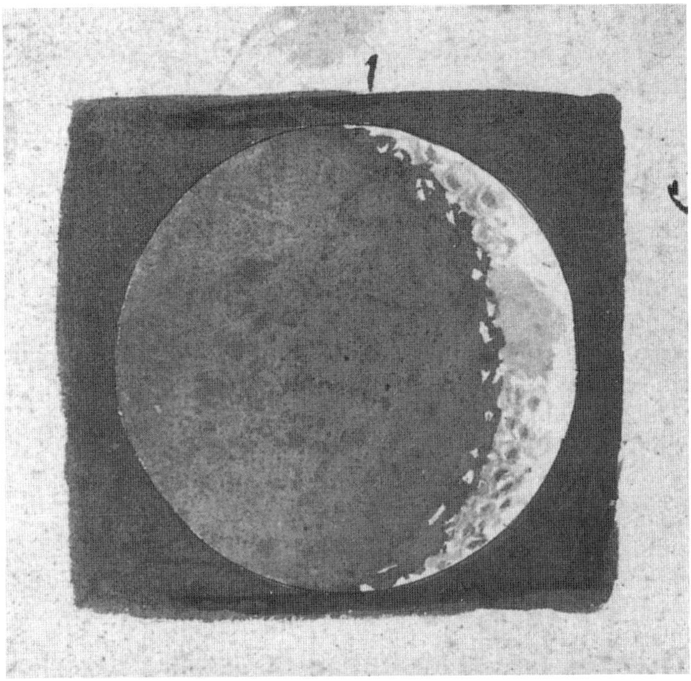

Figure 6.3 One of the original watercolour images prepared by Galileo for the illustration of *Sidereus nuncius*. The bright spots visible on the dark part of the moon, near the boundary with the illuminated part, are the tops of mountains which receive the sunlight (coming obviously from the right) somewhat before the nearby plains. Notice the non- mountainous, and apparently regular, aspect of the lunar circumference, where, according to Galileo, mountains (and craters) are present but remain invisible for the reasons expounded in the letter to Grienberger. Another interesting aspect of this image is the relative visibility of the dark part of the moon because of the rather intense 'secondary lumen' shone from earth towards the lunar body in the phase of lunar crescent—see Chapter 5 (BNF GAL 48, F28r; © Biblioteca Nazionale of Florence, Italy).

6.3 **The invisibility of mountains on the face of the moon**

Soon after, Galileo arrives at the affirmative part of the Jesuit's objection. Paradoxically, he negates what seems obvious (and what the Jesuit is ready to concede), i.e. that mountains are seen in the main part of the lunar surface. It is here that the Tuscan scholar further develops his discourse on the nature and limits of vision. In the particular case of the lunar mountains, the argument is specifically concerned with the three-dimensional character of distant objects. However, Galileo's reflection has more far-reaching implications for visual science. Again he starts quoting the Latin form of the question raised by the Jesuit father:

> The Father writes: *Apparent in Lunae facie, quae terras aspicit, tumores*? I answer not [i.e. they do not appear], and I say that protuberances and eminences of the moon (as eminences) not only cannot be seen from such a long distance, but that they could not even be seen from as close as 100 miles; similarly to our hills and to the major mountains which by no means would be discerned to arise from the flat regions from an altitude and distance of 50 miles, and even less. How then could we say that the moon is mountainous? We do not know it simply with the sense, but by coupling and joining the [logical] discourse with the observations and the sensible appearances, by arguing in such way. (OG XI, p. 183)

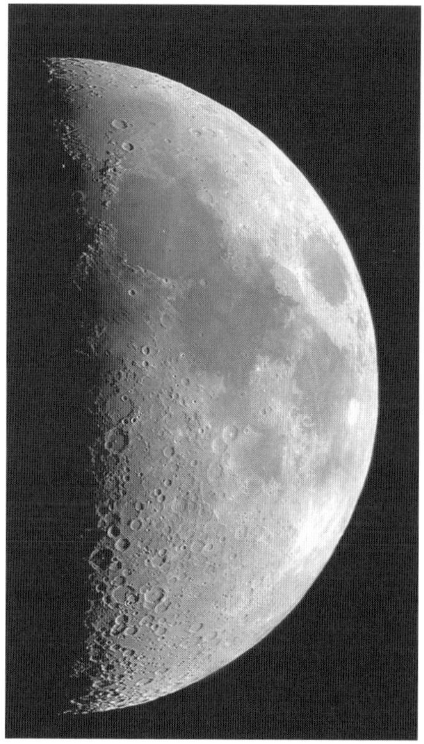

Figure 6.4 A modern image of the lunar surface near the half-moon phase, which again shows how irregularities are particularly visible at the boundary between the dark and bright part of the moon (because of shadowing effects), while the border appears regular. Image by courtesy of Paolo Beltrame.

For Galileo, the existence of mountains and craters on the moon is not simply the outcome of the act of vision. It is, instead, the result of a complex visual experiment, based on accurate comparisons derived from a series of observations made under different conditions. These comparisons take into account the change of the relative position of the sun and moon responsible for different aspects of the moon spots, due to the shadowy and bright parts which vary in their appearance because of the change of their position relative to the direction of sunrays. The interpretation is based on previous visual experience and depends on knowledge of the mathematical laws of perspective and optics. It also makes recourse to the knowledge concerning the importance of shadows and chiaroscuro in suggesting the three-dimensionality, as elaborated particularly by the painters of the Renaissance in their attempt to conjure up the impression of relief in the two-dimensional surface of their paintings (see Figure 6.5).

Let us hear from Galileo in his own words how we can resolve the inherent ambiguity of visual images 'by coupling and joining the discourse with the observations and the sensible appearances', and thus arrive at the knowledge that there are indeed mountains on the moon:

> The arched line separating the dark from the illuminated part of the moon is seen crested, sinuous, crenellated and, in sum, very uneven. Therefore it cannot be the termination of the illumination in a spherical surface, terse and even, but on the contrary mountainous and uneven. Moreover, in the illuminated part are seen very many black small spots; these are more numerous near the boundary

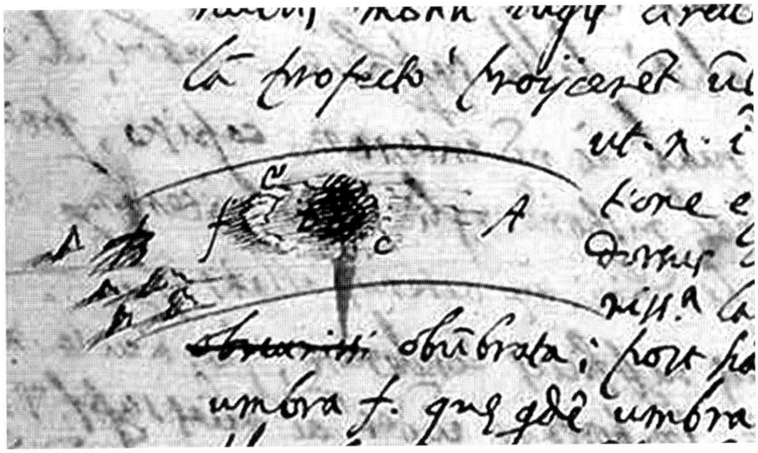

Figure 6.5 A detail of a letter sent to Mark Welser in which Galileo illustrates to his correspondent of the play of shadow and light on the craters and mountains of the lunar surface (BNF GAL 53, F40v; © Biblioteca Nazionale of Florence, Italy).

> than farther away. Furthermore, the said dark spots are seen spreading themselves toward the part not exposed to the sun irradiation, and surrounded, in the sun part, by some borders more clear than the nearby parts. Other similar borders are seen on the opposite part, after some dark projections follow. These spots go on decreasing as the boundary of the illumination goes on forward, i.e. as the sun get more elevated above them. Finally they get lost altogether, and annihilate, as in the full moon every part become illuminated. On the contrary, while the sun revolves and the moon decreases, other similar, very black spots are seen again near the boundary of the moon. While the sun gets lower above them, go on by getting longer, and showing themselves similarly surrounded by very luminous borders. Finally, inside the non illuminated part of the moon, rather far from the termination of the light, appear, in the guise of stars, some luminous specks. By growing little by little they eventually join the termination of the light, which similarly goes toward them, when, however, the moon is waxing. On the contrary in the waning moon such small stars get separated more and more and finally they get lost. On the other hand such accidents and appearances cannot occur in a spherical surface which is smooth and even, and correspond *ad unguem* [i.e. perfectly] to an uneven and mountainous. This is why, with a necessary demonstration one concludes that the lunar surface is full of eminences and depressions [*bassure*]. (pp. 183–184)

To summarize what Galileo writes in the preceding passage from the letter to Grienberger, we can say that the conclusion that the moon is uneven and irregular is the issue of a complex mental process based on a kind of sensory experiment, and depends on the conceptual framework and visual skill and education of the observer. The main elements of this process are: firstly, the irregular aspect of the line that separates the illuminated from the dark part of the moon (the terminator of the astronomers).[8] Secondly, near this boundary bright spots are visible in the dark

[8] In this context it is important to note that Galileo was aware of the irregular nature of the moon surface long before his telescopic observations. This is apparent from an already mentioned text that he published in 1606, under the pseudonym of Alimberto Mauri, with relation to the new star of 1604. In the 'Consideration XXVIII', by comparing the moon and the earth, he wrote about the lunar surface: 'It is not inconsistent to think that it is likewise not entirely even, but that there are also on the moon mountains

part, and dark spots in the illuminated part; the former correspond to the cusps of mountains that receive the light from the sun when it is low on the horizon, and thus incapable of illuminating the nearby plains; the latter are the depth of craters, which remain for a while in the dark, even when the surrounding parts are illuminated by sunlight, due to the small elevation of the sun above the horizon. The bright spots eventually merge with the illuminated part of the moon as the sun rises above the horizon such as to flood the plains around the mountains with its light. Conversely, the dark spots eventually merge with the dark part of the moon as the sun sets below the horizon and its rays cannot reach the flat zones around the craters (see Figure 6.6). These variations correspond nicely (*ad unguem* in Galileo's words, meaning literally 'to the nail') to the changes with the variable play of light and shadows on an irregular near-spherical surface.

Despite the soundness of this reasoning, Galileo's previous assertion regarding the apparent absence of mountains in the main part of the moon might appear paradoxical: 'protuberances and eminences of the moon (as eminences) not only cannot be seen from such a long distance, but that they could not even be seen from as close as 100 miles; similarly to our hills and to the major mountains which by no means would be discerned to arise from the flat regions from an altitude and distance of 50 miles, and even less'.

The matter might appear paradoxical mainly for a naïve observer, accustomed to believe that things are just like we see them, and vision is a simple act capable of transporting external reality to our perceptual world with a minimum of transformation. We have a ready example to illustrate Galileo's assertion by viewing the images of the earth's surface provided by satellites which are now easily accessible on the Internet.

Figure 6.7 refers to Monte Pisano, the mountain separating Pisa from Lucca, a place familiar to Galileo who was born in Pisa and spent long periods of his life in the town of the leaning tower. Only those who know these places very accurately might have the chance to recognize whether the dark parts of the image are peaks of mountains or valleys or forests. People who would look at this zone from high for the first time might possibly arrive at a correct conclusion about its three-dimensional characteristics by observing it from different viewpoints and making observations at different times of day. They should pay particular attention to the variable play of light and shadows, with reference to the relative position of the sun and of the luminous and dark parts.

With less distant objects our three-dimensional perception of external objects is based on many cues that are lacking in astronomical observations: the slight spatial disparities of images on each eye, the state of convergence of the eyes, lateral motion of the head, as well as those

of gigantic size, just as on earth; or rather, much greater, since they are [even] sensible to us. For from these, and from nothing else, there arises in the moon that scabby little darkness, because greatly curved mountains (as Perspectivists teach) cannot receive and reflect the light of the sun as does the rest of the moon, flat and smooth. And for proof of this I shall adduce an easy and pretty observation that can be made continually when she is in quadrature with respect to the sun [i.e. in the half-moon phase]; for then the semicircle is not smooth and clean, but always has a certain boss in the middle. For this, what more probable cause will ever be adduced than the curvature of those mountains? By that, and particularly in that [middle] place, she comes to lose her perfect rotundity' (MAURI, F15v; transl. p. 104). Another indication of Galileo's previous awareness of the irregular nature of the lunar surface comes from *Sidereus nuncius*, where, in the context of the mutual light reflection between earth and moon (a phenomenon which presupposes the moon irregularity) he writes: 'In this place I wish to explain the cause of another lunar phenomenon worthy of notice. This phenomenon was observed by us not recently but rather many years ago, shown to some close friends and pupils, explained and given a causal explanation' (SIDEREUS, p. 14; transl. p. 53).

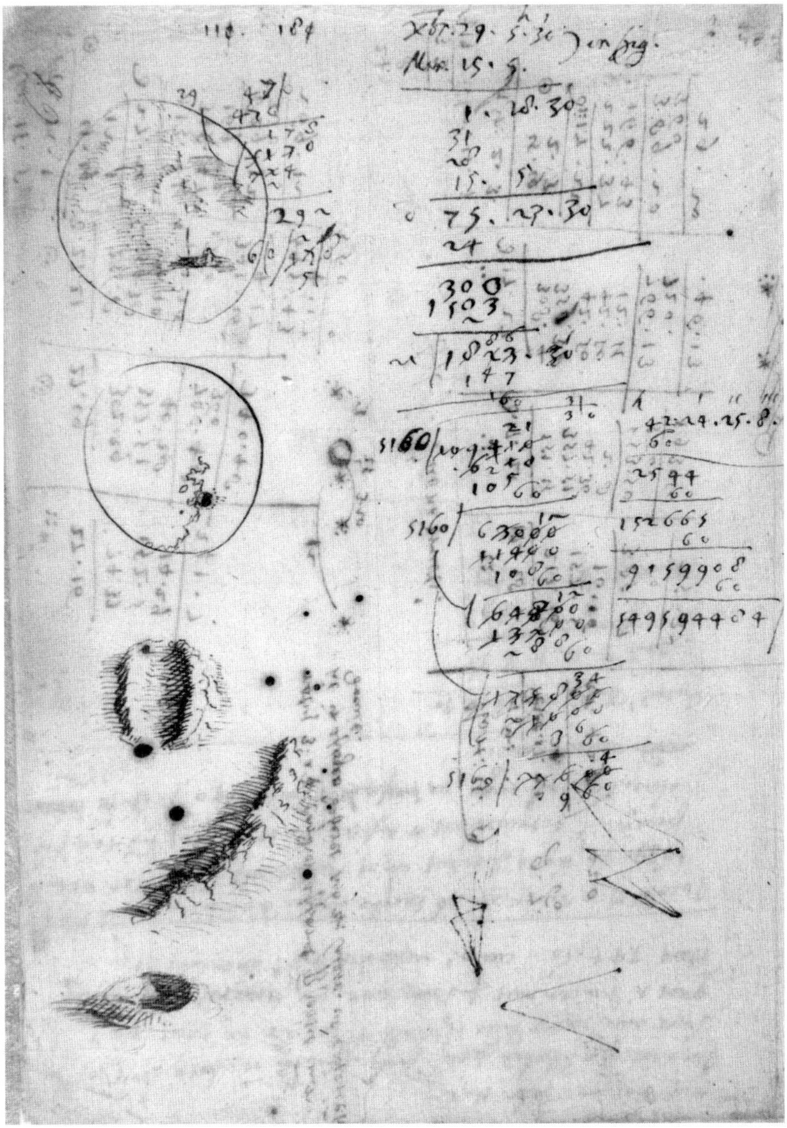

Figure 6.6 Details of a page of Galileo's handwritings with drawings illustrating mountains and craters and their relation with the terminator (the irregular line separating the dark from the luminous part of the moon). Of particular interest is the detail of the moon face in the upper part of the panel on the left, which is illustrated on the right at magnification scale. It is rather likely that, drawing a bird-like view of the mountain in the lower part of this image, Galileo wished to show why the terminator appears irregular, and, in particular, why the dark zone invades the luminous zone in the presence of mountains near the terminator (BNF GAL 50, F68r; © Biblioteca Nazionale of Florence, Italy).

used by painters—interposition, relative size, texture, changes of colour due to the presence of variable layers of terrestrial atmosphere (the so-called 'aerial perspective'). As we know now (but was unknown to Galileo) stereoscopy is based on the small differences in the images of an object formed in the two eyes and it only operates for objects that are relatively close (less than 20

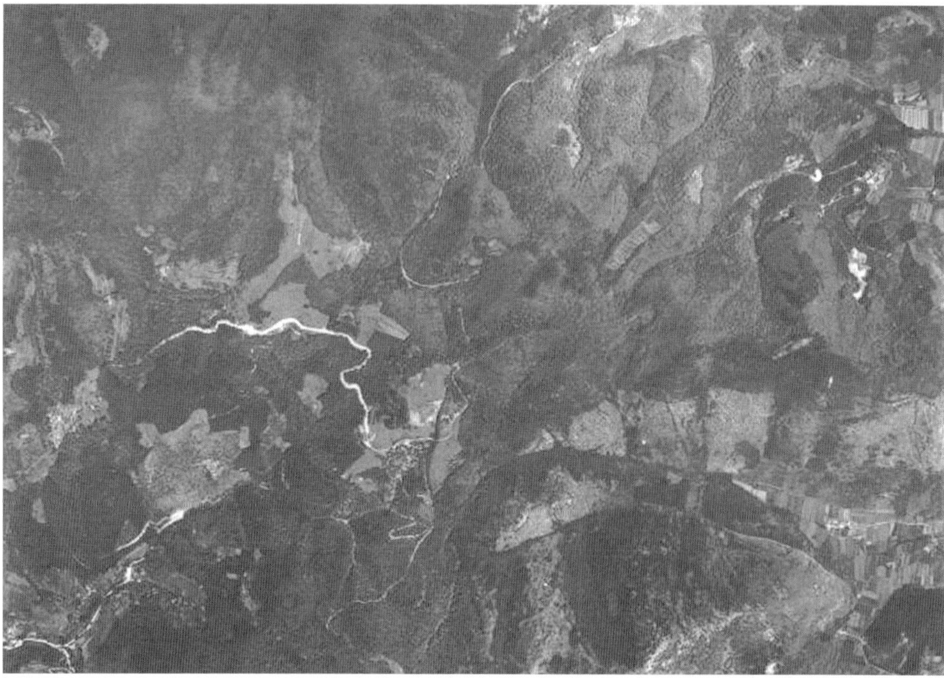

Figure 6.7 An aerial view of Monte Pisano taken from an airplane. The black and white version of the image better simulates the condition of the observation of the moon where there is virtually no chromatic contrast. The detectability of mountains and valleys, would improve by a small degree with a colour image.

metres). Stereoscopy could not have been a factor in Galileo's telescopic observations because the instrument is used by a single eye and the objects were far beyond the limits of stereoscopic acuity.

6.4 **Playing with shadows and resolving the moon's ambiguities**

Besides the lack of these and other cues to solidity, there is another important difficulty in the case of astronomical observations (at least those made in Galileo's time) which derives from the unfamiliar character of the lunar surface. The identification of the shape, dimensions, and of the solidity of ordinary objects is indeed facilitated by the familiarity we have with them, which contributes to their recognition and plays an important part in perceptual constancy. Accustomed as we are to seeing pictures of the lunar surface obtained with powerful telescopes and with complex image manipulations, we say normally (in a similar way to the Parma Jesuit) that we see, for instance, craters on the moon when looking at the circular figures characterizing the lunar images at the top of Figure 6.8. In other words, we have no doubts that these figures represent a depression of the lunar surface with, possibly, a relatively thin elevated border. We could not imagine that exactly the same appearance could be produced by, say, a protuberance of the moon surface, seen from a slightly different viewing condition. All that is needed is to rotate the image by 90 degrees anticlockwise to achieve this visual transformation, from a predominant concavity to a substantial convexity of the features (see Figure 6.8a). On the other hand, the opposite rotation results in a reinforcement of the concave aspects of the craters (compare (c) with (a) and (b)).

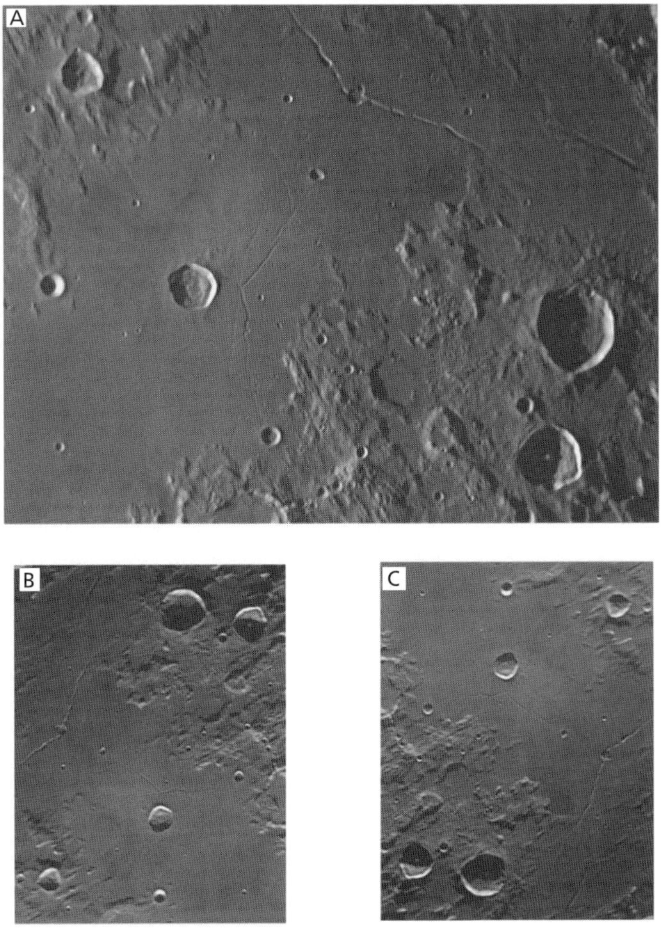

Figure 6.8 A picture of the lunar surface in the region of the Triesnecker crater and Rima Hyginus. To most observers the craters in the image (a), appear as craters, i.e. as characterized by a substantial depression of the lunar surface with their rim at the right illuminated on their left side by the sun coming from the left hand of the figure. In (b), the image has been rotated anticlockwise by 90 degrees, resulting in a predominantly convex appearance, whereas the opposite occurs in (c), where the rotation was clockwise. Notice, moreover, that whatever would be the appearance of the craters in (b) (in terms of convexity or concavity), the opposite appearance would result in observing (c) soon after, and vice versa. Image by courtesy of Paolo Beltrame.

The reason for this visual transformation, which a modern Simplicio could perhaps impute to a sort of trickery, is due to a well-known effect and depends ultimately on the intrinsic spatial ambiguity of visual features. Exactly the same visual appearance as the craters of Figure 6.8a can be produced when the source of light (the sun) illuminates the concave forms of real lunar craters from the left; or, when a light, coming from the right side, illuminates a reverse, convex variety, of the crater-like features. Untrained observers might have difficulty in producing the perceptual shift from concavity to convexity with the image in Figure 6.8a (by virtually assuming a different direction for the source of light). On the other hand, as terrestrial beings we are accustomed to the light of the sun coming from above. When an image has a chiaroscuro effect along the vertical

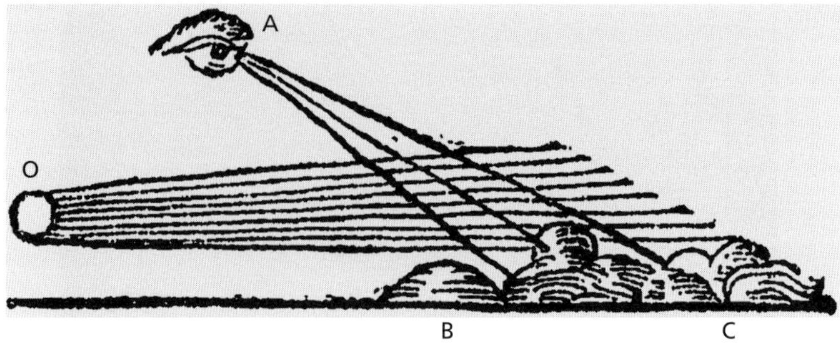

Figure 6.9 The image by which, in the letter to Grienberger, Galileo illustrates the necessity that the line of sight does not correspond to the direction of the luminous rays if the relief of a surface is to be perceived through the play of light and shadow. Reproduced from OG XI, Galilei, G. (1890–1909). *Le opere di Galileo Galilei. Edizione nazionale*. A. Favaro ed., 20 vols. Firenze, Barbèra, p. 185.

direction, we normally resolve the ambiguity by attributing to the feature the shape consistent with an illumination from above: in the case of Figure 6.8b this corresponds to the impression of convex round feature, whereas in the case of Figure 6.8c light coming from above would produce that particular light-shadow effect in the case of concave circular features.

In the letter to Grienberger, Galileo reiterates the reasons for the impossibility of seeing irregularities on the border of the moon despite the presence of mountains, and other types of unevenness extending up to the extreme periphery of the moon. He does this by making recourse to another figure pointing to the conditions required in order to perceive the interplay of light and shade when drawing conclusions about the lunar surface. As he shows, it is necessary that particular spatial relations exist between the source of light, the moon surface, and the observer. These relations can be encountered easily for the middle part of the moon in phases different from the full moon, but cannot be achieved for the extreme border:

> I say therefore that every time an uneven surface is illuminated by the sun or other particular lumen (such as the eminences are illuminated and the low zones tenebrous), the sun (or whoever were to be situated in the sun) would in no way see the zones in the shadow, but only the illuminated ones. This is because in this case the rays of the sight and those of the illumination proceed along the straight lines;[9] and there would be no shadow where the illuminating ray arrives. This is why none of the obscure parts can be seen. In order to see them, it is necessary that the visual ray would be higher on the said surface than the ray of the sun: as it can be seen in the present figure [our Figure 6.9] where O is the place of the light source, BC the mountainous surface, whose eminences are illustrated, while the lower parts remain in the shadow. It is manifest here that the eye situated in O would see none of the shadows of the surface BC, because its rays proceed as those of the light source. I say more. When the light source were more elevated on the surface to be illuminated, and the eye less so (as for instance if the eye were in O and the sun in A), then the parts in the shadow of the said surface would remain more hidden to the sight. The rays impinging on the extreme visible circumference have no elevation above it, but touch in them the surface of the moon. It ensues in a manifest way that, wherever the sun would be,

[9] The wording here (and in other texts by Galileo) suggests that Galileo adhered to the old extramission theory of vision, i.e. to the theory held by Euclid and other classical mathematicians and philosophers, which considered that light was emitted from the eyes and returned with images of objects. We will consider this topic later in this book and particularly in Chapter 13.

never could be seen by us the low places very close to the said circumference; on the contrary, since the obscure parts remain hidden among the nearby illuminated eminences, we would detect nothing else than a totally luminous continuity. (OG XI, pp. 184–185)[10]

6.5 Artistic reliefs

Galileo was well aware of the visual difficulty of providing immediate information about the three-dimensional aspects of the objects, particularly when they are very distant. It is mainly the interplay of light and shadow (together with some other cues like the variation of brightness, colour, and spatial detail in the visual images) that can contribute to an apprehension of the third dimension in the case of distant objects. This is well known to painters who, besides using perspective effects, use the chiaroscuro and the play of light, shade, and colour in order to contrive the appearance of solidity on a flat surface of a canvas.

However, in order for these to be effective—in both vision and artistic representation—it is necessary to be in a situation in which the shadows are well defined and the observer in a position to perceive them. In the case of the moon we cannot effectively change our location in order to perceive the separation between light and shadows more sharply. What we can do is to wait for the particular zones of interest to be located at the boundary between the light and dark parts of the moon. There the sun rays are low enough and the shadows well developed and easily detectable. Understanding this, astronomers seek such conditions to resolve the details in which they are interested. They are well aware, for instance, that the full moon is not suitable for observing reliefs and depressions on the moon's surface because there is the almost complete correspondence between the line of sight and the sun rays under these circumstances.

Chiaroscuro and the interplay of light and shade had been particularly important for the Italian artists of the Renaissance and were still pursued during Galileo's time. Ludovico Ciardi (known as Cigoli, from his native village near Pisa) was an important painter and a great friend of Galileo; he described it in his treatise *Prospettiva pratica*, circulated in a manuscript form, and most probably known to Galileo:[11]

> The objects seen on the luminous part have no relief because of the scarcity of shadows, and, when seen on the excessively shadowy part appear unpleasant; when the view is situated in the middle, between the light and shadow, they show themselves of a more proper colour and have more relief. (Cigoli, folium 82)

The use of shadows to represent the solidity of objects is central to a famous letter addressed by Galileo to Cigoli on 26 June 1612. Upon a request from his friend, Galileo establishes a comparison (*paragone*) between sculpture and painting, along a well-established literary tradition by which different artists and humanists attempted to praise the superiority of their respective endeavours:

> A statue does have relief not because it is wide, long and deep, but because it is light in some parts and dark in others. As an evidence of that, one should be aware that of the three dimensions, two only are submitted to the eye, i.e. the length and the width (these make the surface, which was said by Greeks *epiphany*, that is periphery or circumference); of the things that appear and are seen we see but the

[10] Since at least the epoch of Leonardo it was a common teaching in the treatises of painting or perspective that no shadow can be seen when the direction of illumination correspond to the direction of sight. As we shall discuss, particularly starting from Chapter 11, Galileo was well acquainted with the ideas of Leonardo and more generally with the principles of perspective.

[11] Cigoli's *Prospettiva* has recently been published (see Camerota, 2010).

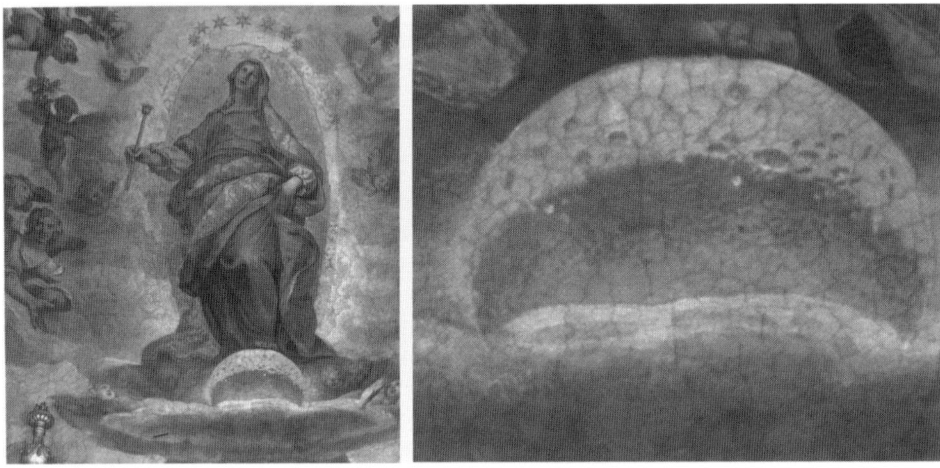

Figure 6.10 *The Virgin of the Immaculate Conception* by Cigoli, in the dome of the Pauline chapel in Santa Maria Maggiore in Rome. Notice the irregular surface of the crescent under the feet of the Virgin and the dim illumination of the dark part of the moon, particularly visible in the detail on the right. Notice, moreover, that due to the increasing brightness along a vertical direction, from top to bottom, of the dark part of the moon, this appears somewhat concave (which is another aspect of the three-dimensional ambiguity already discussed in Figure 6.7).

> surface; the depth cannot be comprehended by the eye, because our sight does not penetrate inside the opaque bodies. The eye sees the long and the wide, but not the deep, that is never the bulkiness. Therefore, because the depth is not exposed to the sight, we could comprehend of it only the length and the width. From that it appears manifest that we see but the surface, which is nothing else then length and width. We know therefore the depth, not as an object of vision by itself and absolutely, but by accident and with relation to the clear and obscure. And all this is in the painting not less than in the sculpture, I say the clear and the obscure, the length and the width. However, the clear and the obscure is given to the sculpture by the nature; to the painting by the art. Therefore, also for this reason it is to be more admired an excellent painting than an excellent sculpture. (OG XI, p. 341)

In another part of the letter to Cigoli, Galileo writes that if a statue is coloured in such a way that it is deprived of the natural chiaroscuro 'by darkening it where it is clear, such as that the colour is all unified, then it would remain entirely devoid of relief' (OG XI, p. 340).

Galileo's belief that even the three-dimensionality of a near object like a statue could be perceived only on the basis of chiaroscuro might be an indication that, because of a problem with his right eye, he had difficulty with stereoscopic vision. It is, however, possible that by praising the power of painting to contrive the appearance of solidity he was simply using a rhetorical tool to favour his painter friend, who had asked him for a text aimed at vindicating the primacy of painting over sculpture.[12]

Cigoli, besides being a painter, was also an amateur astronomer himself and he was collaborating with Galileo in observing sunspots. He did this particularly when he was in Rome, decorating the Pauline chapel of the Church of Santa Maria Maggiore (Figure 6.10). There, in the

[12] In addition to the works of Leonardo and Cigoli, the idea that we see relief by the play of light and shadow is expressed in a particularly clear way in the *Pensieri* of Paolo Sarpi that we will consider in detail in Chapter 12.

fresco of the *Immaculate conception* on the dome of the chapel, he was the first to paint the moon with mountains and craters on its surface, according to the new discoveries made by his friend Galileo. In this period he exchanged many letters with Galileo (among which was the one requesting the *paragone*), and he was informing his friend of the reactions of the Jesuits to the astronomical novelties announced in *Sidereus nuncius*. In a letter addressed to Galileo on 11 August 1611 (shortly after Galileo's return to Florence following his visit to Rome), Cigoli complained that Clavius was not willing to accept the idea of the irregularity of the lunar surface. In that regard he remarked:

> I have now thought about it, and I could find only one excuse to his defence; that a mathematician, how great he could be, if he lacks the drawing competence [*trovandosi senza disegnio*], is, not only a half-mathematician, but even a man without eyes. (OG XI, p. 168)

If we keep in mind that, at that time, 'mathematician' was the term commonly used to designate an astronomer, the painter's remark reflects an acute insight into the importance of being a visual artist in order to understand and decipher the elusive complexity of the new astronomical images.

Chapter 7

Visible and invisible luminous peaks of lunar mountains

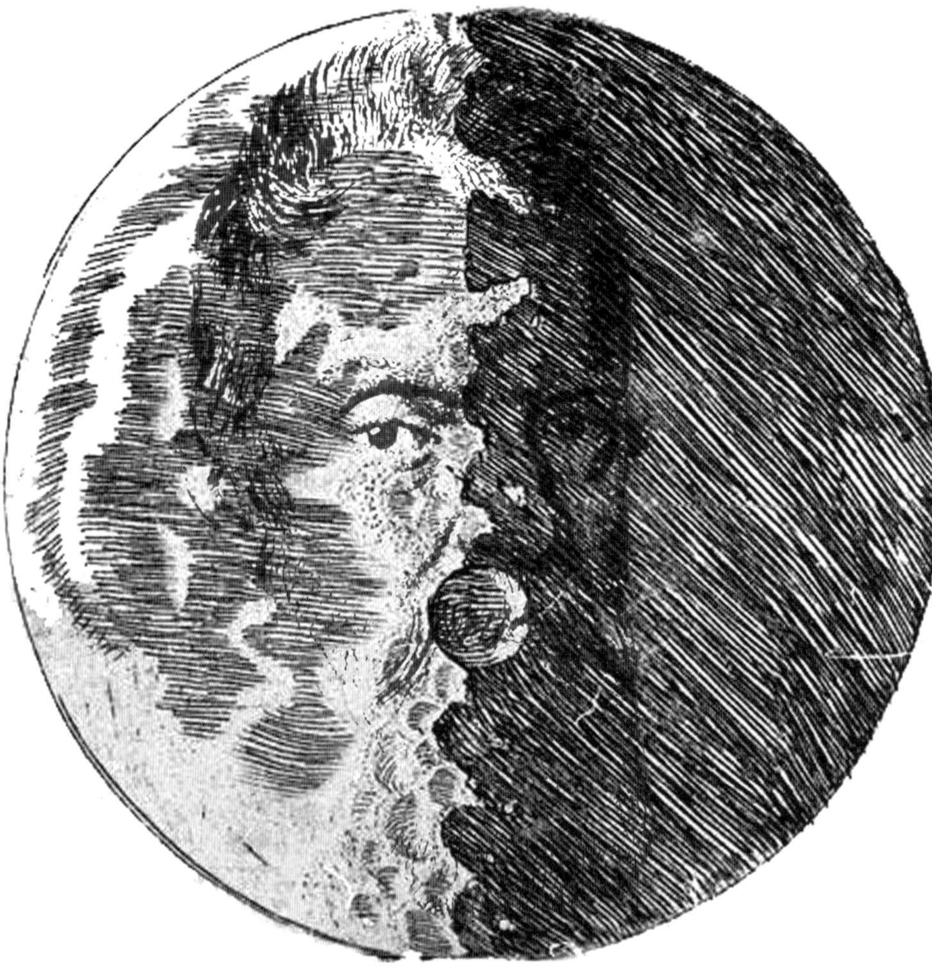

Figure VII *Galileo's moon* by Nicholas Wade. Galileo's portrait, derived from the engraving by Ottavio Leoni in 1624, is enclosed within an illustration of the moon from *Sidereus nuncius* (Galileo, 1610).

In the letter to Christoph Grienberger examined in Chapter 6, Galileo demonstrated why mountains at the extreme circumference of the moon could not be seen by a terrestrial observer even with the aid of a telescope. However, the arguments adduced in the first part of the letter were just supporting the idea that, if mountains were really there, they would be invisible to us. They did not prove the positive part of his conviction, i.e. despite their invisibility, mountains were actually there, on the extreme circumference, as they were in the main part of the moon.

7.1 **The power of tips**

In order to prove this assertion, Galileo invites his correspondent (and through him the author of the Problem of Mantua, as well ourselves) to consider the telescopic appearances of the moon in the condition of the thin crescent, paying particular attention to its extreme tips. From an accurate consideration of these appearances, we could—in his view—gather positive evidence that mountains are also in the extreme circumference of the moon.

But let us listen again to his own words (while keeping an eye on the modern image of the thin tip of the lunar crescent of Figure 7.1):

> Finally the third reason which not only has persuaded, but even forced me to put mountainousness up to the extreme circumference of the moon, is the following. When the illuminated part of the moon shows itself to us as a thin crescent, the internal circumference of the crescent is not parallel to the other, external and convex, periphery; on the contrary, it is quite large in the middle parts, i.e. those that could be called the belly of the crescent; toward the horns of the lunar crescent it grows narrow, so that, in both extremities it terminates into two, very sharp and thin tips. In these tips, the concave and the convex circumference, in merging together, tighten and close the luminous part between two very narrow spaces. It is in these extreme horns that the boundary between shadow and light becomes almost the same as the extreme circle

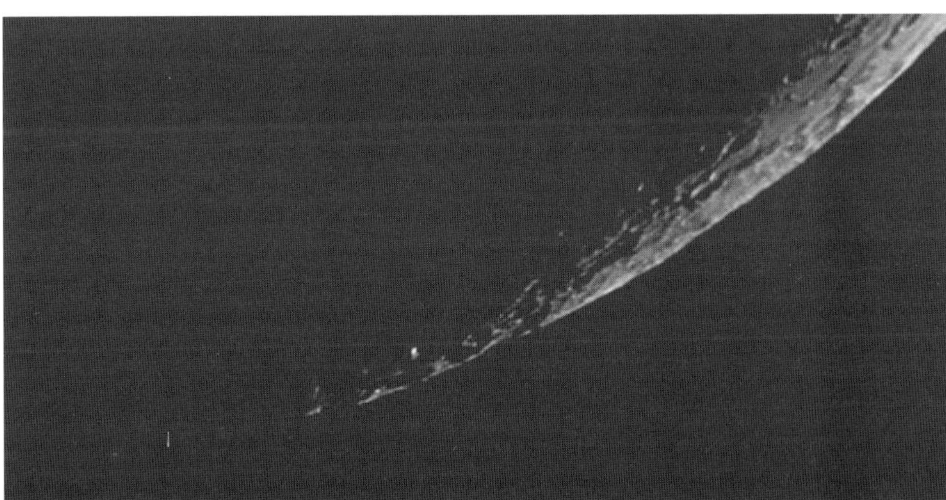

Figure 7.1 A modern telescopic image of the moon near the lower horn of the waxing crescent. Notice that the illuminated spots in the dark part near the dark–light boundary extend to the very tip of the horn, and, moreover, that the rim there seems to be interrupted by the presence of tenebrous gaps due to the impossibility of the sun's rays penetrating the intervals between the more elevated regions of the lunar surface. Similar interruptions are not visible far from the tip of the horn. Photo by courtesy of Paolo Beltrame.

> itself which surrounds the visible hemisphere of the moon. Indeed we could not find in the sky this circle, if we were without the help of the more spacious and luminous belly, which drives and guide us to it. Look now, in either the waning and waxing moon, to both the superior and inferior horn. You would see, toward the one and the other horn, and for rather long distances, two or three illuminated cusps, situated in the extreme circumference, not only separated from the tip of the horn, but also distinct and divided the one from the other. This effect would in no way occur if the exterior and ultimate visible circumference of the moon were even and not mountainous. Such illuminated cusps separated by great intervals are seen only at the extremities of the horns. They are not so at the boundary of the shadow in front of the middle part, i.e. in front of the belly. The reason of this will be manifest to those who are capable of figuring the different views by means of the perspective. He should also consider that the cusps in front of the belly not only offer us the part adverse to the sun, and therefore tenebrous, but that the shadowy spaces, separating them from the luminous part, are lost because of the foreshortening. On the other hand, the cusps and the peaks situated in front of the extremity of the horns, not only show us, at least by side, their illuminated part, but it also occurs that that the spaces between them and the boundary of the light are represented to us, not by foreshortening, but by profile, and along their maximum distance from the said boundary; and the gaps, i.e. the spaces between the one and the other of the cusps, are there not because they are really discontinued and separated, but because the lunar surface interposed among them remains shadowy, and thus invisible. (OG XI, pp. 189–190)

Up to this point of his letter to Grienberger, Galileo's discourse on the invisibility of the peripheral mountains deals almost uniquely with the theme of light and shadow and on considerations of perspective. Afterwards it moves gradually to other considerations which have an even more direct relevance with vision. In *Sidereus nuncius* Galileo had estimated by trigonometric methods the heights of lunar mountains and, on the basis of these measures and other considerations, he assumes an average height of the mountains situated at the extreme rim of the moon to be about 2 miles (i.e. *c.* 3000 metres: see Chapter 9).[1] In his view the elevation of these mountains from the lunar surface, being about 1/1000 of the available measure of moon diameter, would not be large enough, due to the magnification limits of the available telescopes (and mechanisms of vision), to make them visible even if they were aligned in a single file along the moon circumference. As Galileo remarks, the problem would be even more difficult by considering that the peaks of the majority of lunar mountains do not rise abruptly from the flat lands of the moon; and, moreover, that 'not only one order of mountain is found there [i.e. near the extreme circumference] but many and many files, one opposed to the other; these mountains, by interposing one to the other alternatively, and the ones with their eminences making obstacle to the grooves of the others, would somewhat arrive to straighten and level off the vertex, along the same line' (p. 192).

Galileo's conclusion is largely justified even though the value of moon diameter on which he bases his calculation (the accepted value in his age) is underestimated (2850 km against the average modern diameter of 3476 km), and the height of lunar mountains at the moon circumference

[1] The (Italic) mile used by Galileo corresponded to about 1478 metres. Galileo's estimate corresponds rather well with the range of the heights of lunar mountains which, in the visible face, go from few hundreds of metres to more than 5.5 km (of Mons Huygens), in the long chain of lunar Apennines, in the northern hemisphere. Galileo concluded that the estimated height of 2 miles in the mountains of the lunar circumference was about 1/1000 of the moon's diameter; this was based on the then current value of the lunar diameter estimated to about 2000 miles (i.e. *c.* 2956 km). This value is rather different from present-day measurement of the mean lunar diameter (3474.2 km). Nevertheless, Galileo's deduction that 'mountains which would ascend to the perpendicular height of 2 miles, would elevate themselves above the said [lunar] circumference by one thousandth of the lunar diameter' (p. 191) is justified.

is particularly underestimated. This can largely exceed 3000 metres. Some of the highest mountain ranges are indeed found at the extreme rim of the moon, in the south south-west region, like the chains of Montes Doerfel and Leibnitz, the heights of which can exceed 7000 metres. The proportion of the height of these mountains to the moon diameter is therefore nearer to about 500 times rather than to the 1000 times calculated by Galileo. Nevertheless, as Galileo had argued, the elevation of the peaks from the immediately surrounding regions is not so dramatic; this is the case for other high mountains (and particularly for the highest peak, lunar Mount Everest at 8848 metres). For the isolated peaks emerging from flatlands the figure of *c.* 3000 metres given by Galileo is reasonable if we consider that on the visible face of the moon the values are between 500 metres (Mons Rümker) to 4600 metres (Mons Hadley). It can also be justified for a single chain of mountains seen in profile but is largely overestimated for multiple mountain chains set at different distances.

If we follow Galileo's reasoning, assuming about 3000 metres as the elevation of peaks from the surrounding lunar border, and if we take into account that the magnification factor of most of the telescopes he was using was 20 times, then the irregularities at the border of the moon would have been hardly detectable in his astronomical observations. This is because at the distance of the moon from earth, a detail of 3000 metres size, magnified by 20 times, would subtend an angle of about 1.4′, that is an angle just a little larger than the 1′ limit of human visual resolution (see Chapter 8). We should consider, moreover, that Galileo's telescopic observations were not under ideal viewing conditions. This was both because of the optical aberrations of his telescope and of a variety of physiological factors and particularly the conditions of adaptation to low light levels typical of astronomical observations which—as we shall see particularly in Chapters 8 and 13—involve a substantial decrease in visual resolution. It would be necessary to produce better telescopes, with higher magnifications and smaller optical aberrations in order to detect the presence of irregularities at the extreme periphery of the moon.

Among the first to directly observe these irregularities with an improved telescope were Gian Domenico Cassini, a famous Italian astronomer, and Giuseppe Campani an instrument maker and astronomer himself. In *Ragguaglio di due nuove osservazioni* ('Report of two new observations') published in 1664, Campani reports on various telescopic observations made with his improved telescopes, some of which were carried out in the company of Cassini, 'the celebrated professor of Mathematics at the University of Bologna'. After describing the first observation concerning the appearance of Jupiter, Campani writes:

> The second concerns the Moon, whose circumference with my Telescopes is seen to be not perfectly circular, but rough and tortuous [*anfrattuosa*] in the shape; as our horizon, when it is terminated by thick and far mountains appears if viewed from a high place. And the inequalities, due to the prominences and lownesses, are seen so sharp and distinct, such as they can be easily drawn, and transferred one by one to the drawing from the correspondent places. (Campani, 1664, pp. 39–40)

7.2 **The shining mantle of a lamb and a dormouse**

In the letter to Grienberger, after having argued for the impossibility of seeing the irregularities around the circumference of the moon, Galileo imagines a possible objection by an adversary which involves another visual problem. The adversary could point out that Galileo assumes the invisibility of the elevated peaks or cusps at the extreme lunar circumference while at the same time arguing for the presence of mountains in the main part of the moon near the dark–light boundary.

Let us follow Galileo's response to this possible objection:

> I hear now a person of very acute mind and exquisite perspicacity raising a very robust question, and saying to me: You have been asserting that those bright small islands which, almost as small stars, on the surface of the not-yet-illuminated moon are seen far from the boundary of the lumen are the peaks of eminences already illuminated by the sun which elevate themselves above the smaller mountains, and, little by little, extend themselves, as the lower and more spacious parts get illuminated. Now, if those small outgrowths make them visible in the middle part of the lunar surface, why should they not be visible in the extreme circumference, were this really mountainous?
>
> Suppose that I will answer to this objection by saying that such luminous points make themselves visible in the middle parts because here they are surrounded by an obscure and tenebrous field, which makes them spring out, and that this does not happen in the over-eminences of the extreme periphery, which are implanted over the very bright range of nearby mountains. I will then hear [the adversary] to argument, in an acute way, that, although in the extreme circumference the supreme cusps are not entirely divided from the other, lucid parts, over which they emerge, nevertheless they are, at least for their external half, surrounded by the tenebrous field of the nocturnal sky, not less obscure that the shadowy part of the moon; from which it should ensue, either that these last ones should be visible, or that the interior ones also remain invisible because of their smallness, as the others do. (OG XI, p. 192)

Soon after Galileo introduces his answer to this last objection with a philosophical consideration of great importance in his general approach, which we will address later (see Chapter 11):

> The reply is no less ingenious and subtle than the first motion; nevertheless (this being the privilege of truth) I do not believe that I will be lacking a powerful response apt to remove any doubt. It must be remarked anyhow that nature has no obligation and convention whatever with humans, and particularly with me, to make its own works and effects existent as far as I understand them and can support them against whomever would like to negate and destroy them. And my [possible] ignorance of the cause why we do not see roughness on the moon circumference does nor argue for the absence of such cause. (pp. 192–193)

He elaborates his reply with two different arguments. The first based on perspective and foreshortening effects, and a second one (more important from our point of view) introducing the theme of the particular behaviour of the visual system in the presence of small, bright light spots on a dark background. This normally applies to celestial bodies with the notable exceptions of sun and moon. This second argument is of fundamental importance within the framework of the visual elaborations of Galileo, and we will discuss it in some detail in Chapter 8 and later chapters (particularly Chapters 13 and 14). Here we will consider mainly how it arises in the letter to Grienberger with relation to the problem of the lack of apparent irregularities at the moon's border.

In this letter, addressing the first of the two arguments Galileo writes:

> Nevertheless I respond twice. First I say that the luminous tops situated in the middle parts of the moon are, just for their position, of a much greater size than those situated in the circumference. The difference comes from the fact that, in the first case, they are seen in face, whereas they are in profile in the second case. In a similar way the spherical surface comprised within the two polar circles would appears as a perfect circle to an observer having the eye perpendicularly erected on the pole; whereas, to somebody having the eye on the line that touches the said sphere in its pole, the same circle would represent itself under the figure of an extremely subtle portion of circle comprised under the arc of about 47 degrees. (p. 193)

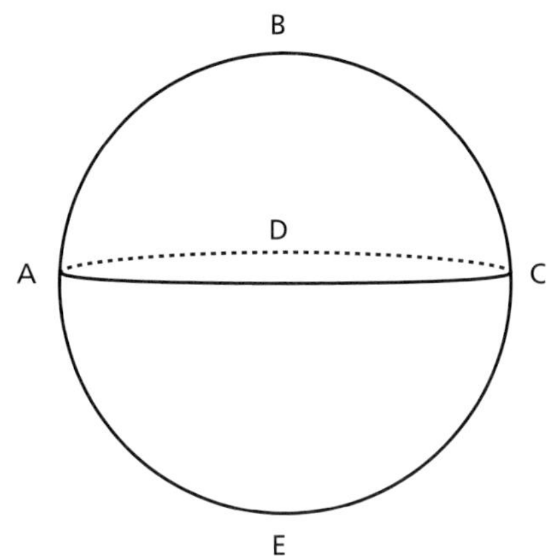

Figure 7.2 The image used by Galileo to explain why the top of a mountain (assumed to be roughly of a spherical form) should be seen better at the centre of lunar surface than in the extreme periphery of the visible moon face where it appears foreshortened.

After supporting his argument with a geometrical demonstration based on a figure inserted in the letter (Figure 7.2), Galileo entertains the second, more genuinely visual consideration, where stars and terrestrial lights are treated in a similar way and submitted to the same physical and perceptive laws:

> But let's now establish with a better firmness the foundations of the truth of our assertion, by saying: any luminous body, when seen from near, shows itself to us under its true and real figure; but from far it seems like garlanding itself with some accessory [*ascitizi*] rays, among which the boundaries of its figure get lost, and it seems then that its size gets bigger. A sensible experience of such a phenomenon is given us by any lamp and by the stars too. As to the first ones, which—from near—show their small flames sharply outlined as small brilliant tongues, from far they appear much larger and irradiant, and their figure gets completely lost among such very big irradiation. Concerning the latter ones, at the moment the sun sets, or a little later, they are seen very small; however, as the darkness grows greater, also they grow in size and coronate themselves of rays [*di raggi s'incapellano*], hiding among these the boundaries of their features. (pp. 193–194)

As mentioned, we will discuss in detail in Chapter 8 and later chapters the problem of irradiation which modifies the perception of small luminous objects, particularly in the presence of a dark background. That luminous sources tend to appear larger than the geometrical dimensions of their images was a long-held notion. Also Kepler was well aware of the phenomenon. It is, however, only Galileo who fully develops the argument with reference to the vision of celestial bodies, and particularly the stars, such as to support the new cosmology.

In order to substantiate his argument concerning the vision of stars and flames, in the *Dialogue* Galileo makes reference to one of his most important astronomical discoveries, i.e. the demonstration that the planet Venus also shows phases corresponding to the variable positions it occupies with relation to the sun and the earth (i.e. new Venus, waxing crescent, quarter, waning gibbous, etc.; see Figure 7.3):

> To what extent these features get altered, one can infer from the star of Venus. Near its vesper set or its morning rise, it shows itself, as the other stars, round and radiating, even though its real figure is a

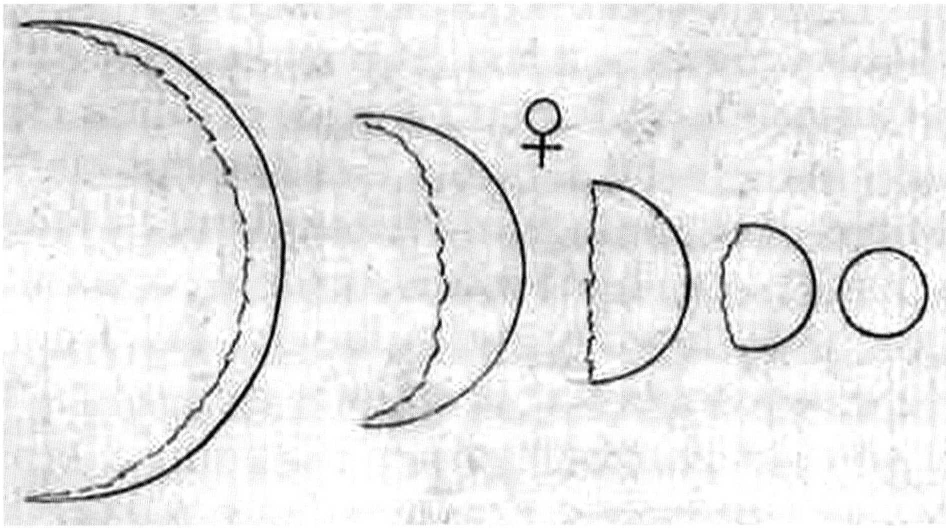

Figure 7.3 The phases of Venus in an illustration from *Saggiatore*. These appearances were observed by Galileo with the telescope in December 1611. For astronomical reasons, to terrestrial observers the planet appears of larger size when it is in the phase of thin crescent, being nearer to the earth. Its angular size is smaller in the phase of full Venus (corresponding to the astronomical condition of 'opposition'). The argument of irradiation allows Galileo to explain why with the unaided eye it appears always globular, and (during the night) of an angular size much bigger than that expected from pure geometrical considerations. It must be remarked that the similarity of the phases of Venus to those of the moon was by itself important evidence for the Copernican system[2] (p. 217).

> very thin crescent, similar to the moon when this does not exceed the age of two days. This irradiation makes itself larger or smaller as the light is more or less intense.[3] (p. 194)

After discussing the extent to which the same effect applies to other planets (and particularly to Mercury, due to the very strong illumination it receives by its proximity to the sun), Galileo returns to the moon, where he notes the specificity of the phenomenon connected to the large image size of the moon:

> The moon is not exempt from such an accident; on the contrary, also it crowns itself with a similar garland, and particularly in those parts where it receives the solar irradiation more directly. It is indeed true that its figure is not deformed, and this is because of its big size. The reason is that hairs [*crini*] of the same length, when they encumber a small figure, alter it more than a large one: This is the same

[2] Also the Ptolemaic system predicted, however, that the aspect of Venus should change with a monthly cycle, although in a less prominent way than within the framework of the Copernican system. Alhazen attributed the absence of variations of the shape of the planet to a self-luminosity of its body, analogous to that of the fixed stars.

[3] People acquainted with Galileo's texts know the curious episode of the anagram by which, before publishing his discovery of Venus phases, Galileo announced it to his colleague (and possible competitor) Kepler, through the mediation of Giuliano de' Medici, the Tuscan ambassador in Prague: '*Haec immatura a me iam frustra leguntur o y*'. After the rearrangement of the characters this becomes: '*Cynthiae figuras aemulatur Mater Amorum*' (The Mother of Love [Venus] imitates the figures [that is the phases] of Cynthia [the moon]) (OG XI, p. 12).

guise that hairs hide and remove totally the boundaries of the skin and the musculature of a small dormouse while they only little hide the features of a horse.[4]

Now, because, like any other luminous body, also the moon crowns itself of its rays, what would be the wonder if the very tiny tops and concavities, potentially capable of notching its circumference, would remain hidden within the hair of the moon? Venus should be an argument for that, because when horned, nonetheless it appears to us as a radiating circle, as if its hairs originated from a small round light. Then, if the very big concavity of the crescent gets hidden and lost among the rays of Venus, it is reasonable to assume that small asperities, possibly caused on the lunar perimeter by some peaks more elevated than the others, would remain encumbered and hidden by its own irradiation. (pp. 193–194)

7.3 A brilliant terrestrial experiment and the capitulation of Jesuits

There is an important point stressed in this passage, as well as in all Galileo's treatments of the problem of the irradiation from luminous bodies, which is indicated with a variety of expressions, some of which are difficult to translate into English (*raggi ascitizii*, or *stranieri*, *irradiazione ascitizia*, *capellatura*, or *capillizio*, or *capellizio*, *ghirlanda*, *crini*). It is that, all other conditions being equal, irradiation does not increase with the size of the luminous object but remains substantially constant in its spatial extent. As we shall see in Chapter 8, this is a consequence of the mechanisms whereby the main components of the irradiation are produced. Because of this, it has a relatively greater effect on the perceived size of small objects (like most luminous stars and planets) than large celestial bodies (like the moon). In the case of the moon one of the consequences is—for Galileo—a very small increase in the apparent circumference of its illuminated part 'which elevates itself over the circumference of the obscure part, such as this one seems to have a smaller circle, and the other a slightly bigger one (*alquanto maggioretto*)' (p. 196).[5] The other consequence has already been mentioned: the invisibility of the small cavities among the cusps situated on the most peripheral mountains which is the central argument of the letter to Grienberger.

In the letter, Galileo develops various arguments with relation to the accessory rays capable of increasing the perceived size of luminous bodies and changing the appearance of their visual contours. They are discussed with reference to celestial bodies (and especially the moon with its mountains). There is, however, also concern and attention to sources of terrestrial lights. These

---

4 In *Saggiatore* the same theme is rendered with a similar zoological metaphor: 'What happens here is precisely what would happen if you were to dress an ant in the hide of a lamb—the ant's tiny members would be completely lost in the length of the hairs, and the resulting appearance would be merely that of a fleece of wool, but the lamb is large enough so that its members may be clearly discerned under the same clothing' (Galileo, 1623, p. 215/Drake and O'Malley, 1960, p. 322). The problem of the apparent size of small luminous bodies like stars and planets had already emerged in *Sidereus nuncius*, but without the metaphorical argument derived from the animal world. As we shall see in the next chapter, it will also be considered by Galileo in the *Dialogue*. Moreover, it was also present in the *Discorso delle comete* published in 1619 under the name of Galileo's student, Mario Guiducci, but largely due to Galileo himself (OG VI, pp. 37–105). Finally, it would be central to one of Galileo's last scientific texts, *Le operazioni astronomiche*, probably composed in 1637 and left unfinished and unpublished (see OG VIII, pp. 449–466).

5 A similar observation had been also made by Kepler who reports it in his *Astronomiae, pars optica*. He attributes the phenomenon to the larger appearance of luminous bodies compared to dark ones (see our Chapter 13).

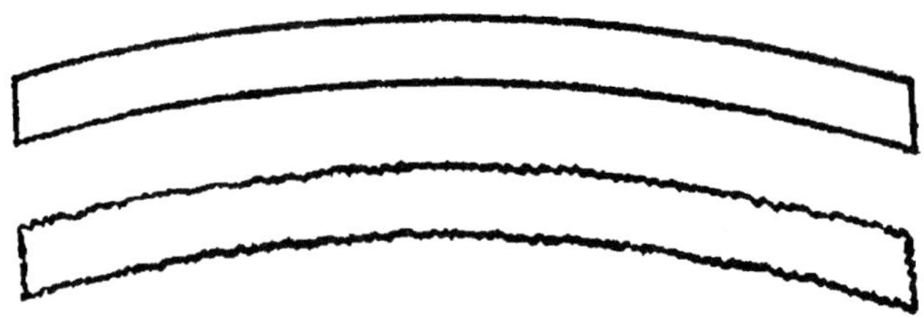

Figure 7.4 The drawing used by Galileo in his letter to Grienberger to demonstrate the invisibility of the mountain at the extreme circumference of the moon. The experiment, which is very easy to replicate, is described in the text.

are considered as providing the opportunities for visual experiments that could replicate issues concerned with the appearances of stars and planets. Among these is the effect of the spurious luminous rays when the luminous body is particularly bright and small. Moreover, Galileo notices that the effect of the spurious rays is particularly strong when the light (either issuing from a celestial body or from the flame of a candle) is surrounded by a dark field, and tends to disappear when the background illumination is increased:

> The small flame of a candle, seen from 4 or 6 cubits, is seen terminated and profiled by its own figure; but in the distance of 100 or 200 [cubits] it appears quite bigger, magnified by many rays, among which its form gets lost: this variation occurs more in tenebrous than in clear places; and any star (with the exception of the moon) during the day, or until the air is still very clear, is seen extremely small and with very few rays, but in the darkness of the night it appears very big and radiating. The planets more near to the sun irradiate more than the most remote, because they receive from the sun a most lively and powerful light. (p. 195)

In the last part of the letter to Grienberger, after asserting why peripheral lunar mountains are invisible, Galileo supports his argument with a 'terrestrial' experiment:

> Let's take a rather thin iron plate, and let's cut into it two fissures, similar to those sketched below [our Figure 7.4]; suppose that one of them is contained between two evenly drawn lines whereas the other between tortuous and rough lines; let's put the said plate in a dark place, and let's situate, behind it, a flame, large enough to cover the space between the two fissures and hide the splendour of this flame such as no other light is seen besides that passing across the fissures. If we now look these fissures from near, we will see distinctly two luminous strips, one terminated between clear-cut lines, and the other all rough similar to the fissure; if, on the other hand, we distance ourselves by 100 or 150 steps, both would appear irradiated at their contour in the same way; the inequalities of one of them would be lost among the rays, so that both make us the same appearance. Eventually, if we distance ourselves by 1000 or 1500 cubits, not even the telescope will suffice to make their images[6] [*specie*] so near that we could see them outlined in a different way; nor could we see the roughness and asperities of the one which really has got them. (pp. 198–199)

The importance of Galileo's considerations on the apparent size of luminous objects, and especially of small luminous spots on a dark background, has other important cosmological implications besides the argument of the invisibility of mountains (and craters) at the extreme boundary of the moon. We will deal with these aspects of Galileo's thought in Chapter 8, as well

[6] The original word used here by Galileo is *specie* (species), a term largely used in both classical culture and the tradition of perspectivists during the Middle Ages to denote the presumed immaterial images emanating from the objects and making them visible.

as considering the physical and physiological constraints on visual resolution from a modern perspective (this last aspect will be also discussed in Chapters 13 and 14). We will see how Galileo, without reference to any theory of image formation in the eye, is able to capture the essentials of the problem. He would show that the true angular subtenses of stars and most planets are much smaller than the values accepted for millennia on the basis of a naïve confidence in the immediate power of perception. It is another important instance of his extraordinary capability of critically analysing visual appearances, disclosing their possible fallacies, and, despite these, deriving important information in his attempt to read correctly the 'book of the universe'. In other words, it is another instance of his astonishing ability to see more, and well beyond the limits of the immediate sensorial world.

7.4 **Jesuit variations and Bettini looking at the peripheral lunar mountains**

With regard to the extant but invisible mountains at the extremities of the moon, in *De lunarium montium altitude* the Jesuit Mario Bettini (the author of the Problem of Mantua) wrote that the mountains do not appear (*non apparent*). In other words, he criticized Galileo for placing mountains where they could not been seen, while he was more inclined to accept their presence where they could be seen, i.e. in the main visible part of the moon. Several years later, in his book of mathematical curiosities *Apiaria* (first published in 1642), Bettini not only persisted in refuting Galileo's arguments on the existence of peripheral lunar mountains but he also doubted the existence of any mountains on the moon. Reasoning ad hoc, he accounted for the astronomical data by assuming that telescopic observations could be accounted for by assuming a non-homogeneity of the deep lunar matter which would simulate the appearance of mountains and valleys. Indeed, in the section of his work dealing with this problem he wrote that he had used the adjective *apparentibus* (apparent) to mountains on the moon seen through the telescope: 'because, to tell the truth, there are no mountains at all in the Moon, as it will appear in the following propositions' (Bettini, 1642, II, p. 72).[7] This changed attitude was perhaps the consequence of the more conservative cultural politics of the Catholic Church, and particularly of the Jesuit Society, after the explosion, in 1632, of the Galileo affair.

The great opus by which the official catholic culture attempted to undermine and constrain the new astronomical science of Copernicus, Galileo, and Kepler was the *Almagestum novum* published in 1651 by another Jesuit, Giovanni Battista Riccioli (Figure 7.5). Confronted with the novelties of the revolutionary new science of Galileo and his followers, and obliged to abandon the old system of Ptolemy, they were still reluctant to accept the idea of earth dethroned from the centre of the universe and revolving around the sun. In its place the Jesuits adopted the system proposed by Tycho Brahe. This retained a stationary and central earth but assumed that sun, moon, and stars revolve around it, while the other five planets revolve around the sun. Tycho's system was at the core of *Almagestum novum*, as indicated at the outset by the allegorical frontispiece image, where the muse of astronomy, having abandoned the system of Ptolemy, ponders the system of Copernicus and that of Tycho (in a variation proposed by Riccioli himself), giving the preference to this last one, on the base of 'their own weight'.

---

7 The full title of the section is *Paradoxa, et nova phenomena in Luna, sive de montibus in Luna per tubum dioptricum apparentibus* ('Paradoxes and new phenomena in the Moon, that is concerning the mountains apparent on the Moon through the telescope').

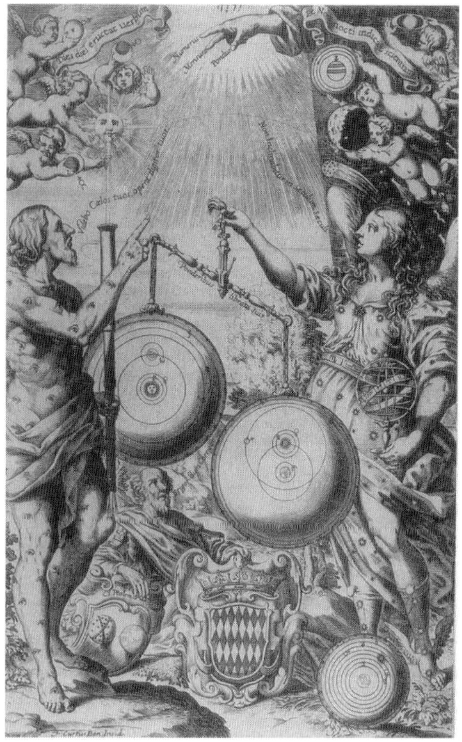

Figure 7.5 The frontispiece image of the *Almagestum novum* where the system of Tycho (in Riccioli's variation, that is, with Jupiter and Saturn revolving around the earth instead than around the sun as in the system of the Danish astronomer) prevails over that of Copernicus.

Credit: Frontispiece to 'Almagestum Novum' by Giovanni Battista Riccioli, published in 1651 (engraving), Italian School, (17th century) / Private Collection / The Bridgeman Art Library.

When dealing with the problem of lunar mountains, Riccioli makes extensive reference to Bettini and to the other opponents of a mountainous moon. However, despite the general anti-Galilean character of his work, he is honest enough to say that, 'with a very good telescope' he had not infrequently seen the external rims of the moon, on both the oriental and occidental side, 'rough and uneven because of parts protruding in them' (Riccioli, 1651, IV, p. 207½), thus somewhat vindicating the long-sightedness of the Tuscan scholar. Moreover, in the beautiful lunar cartography prepared by another Jesuit, Francesco Maria Grimaldi (an important physicist and astronomer), and inserted in the *Almagestum novum*, craters and peaks appear to penetrate until the extreme tips of the lunar crescent (Figure 7.6). This was just as Galileo had remarked in his letter to Grienberger as crucial evidence to support the peripheral mountainous nature of the moon, despite visual appearances to the contrary.

In the lunar map of Grimaldi, however, the main part of the outer circumference of the moon is drawn regular and sharp, and a long time would pass before selenographic representations in which the profile of mountains is drawn on the extreme circumference of the moon would be seen. This occurred with the lunar map prepared in the first half of the nineteenth century by the German cartographer Wilhelm Lohrmann, and published in 1878 by another German selenographer, Julius Schmidt (Figure 7.7). It is perhaps an irony of history that the moon crater dedicated to Bettini (Bettinus) in the south-west part of the visible moon is very near where the most prominent mountains of the lunar circumference appear (the peaks of the Doerfel and

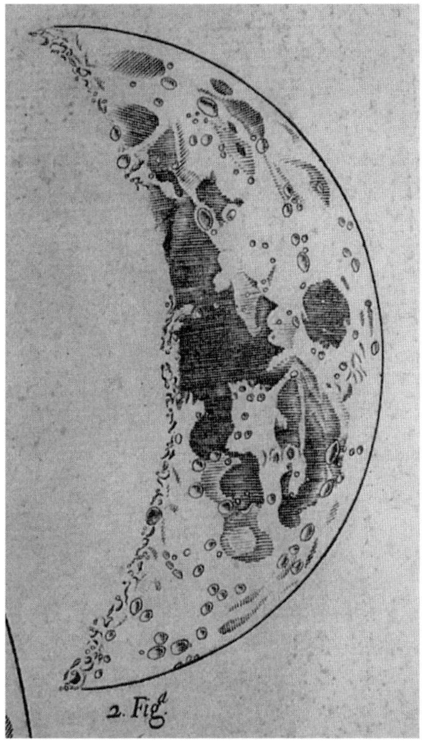

Figure 7.6 The lunar crescent in the cartographic map of the moon prepared by Francesco Maria Grimaldi for the *Almagestum novum*, published in 1651 by Giovanni Battista Riccioli. Notice the presence of irregularities at the extremity of both horns of the crescent, suggesting the presence of mountains and craters even at the extreme periphery of the moon. Reproduced from Riccioli, G. B., *Almagestum novum astronomiam veterem novamque complectens*. Bononiae, 1651, Victorii Benatii.

Leibnitz Ranges). It is rather as if, by a law of retaliation, the stubborn Jesuit is condemned to look permanently at the mountains, not only where they were apparent, but also where they could not be seen!

Lohrmann was a cartographer, and as cartographers know well, a map is never a simple copy of reality and it does not correspond to the immediate visual aspect of the object to be represented. Besides being based on prolonged observations and measurements made under different viewing conditions, it introduced distortions in the representational phase in order to accentuate the relevant details. In order to give a pictorial representation of the peripheral mountains Lohrmann has exaggerated their size and accentuated their profile somewhat.

Perhaps more realistic representations of the moon are those obtained with modern photographic techniques, as illustrated in Figure 7.8. Of especial importance are the high-quality images obtained through the use of sophisticated technology and spacecraft facilities, as, for instance, those of the Lunar Reconnaissance Orbiter Camera (LROC) NASA programme. As shown in three of these images illustrated in Figure 7.9, the lunar circumference appears sharp and well delineated, and would appear largely so even at magnifications comparable to that of Lohrmann's chart. Nevertheless, the NASA images confirm fully the arguments expounded by Galileo in his letter to Grienberger. This is because, while Figure 7.9a is a picture of the ordinary

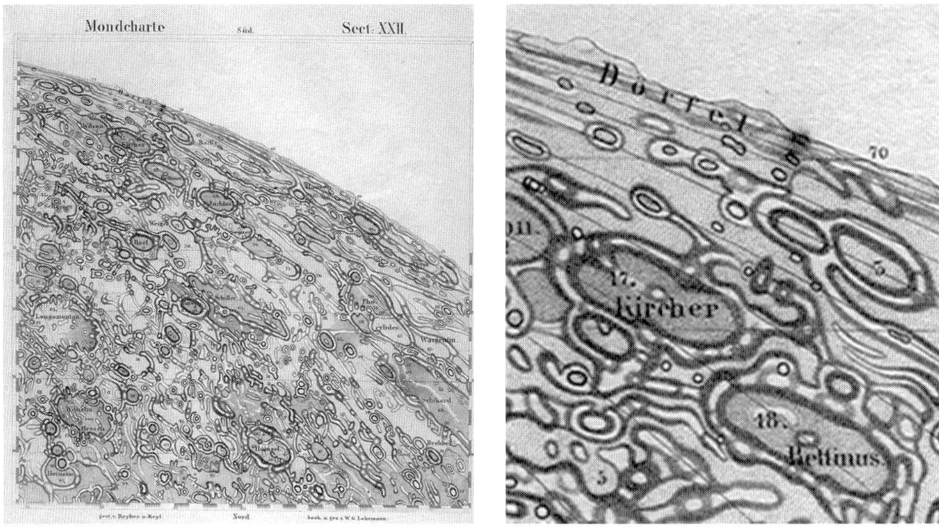

Figure 7.7 Section XXII of Lohrmann's *Mondcharte* ('Moon chart') with, at the right, a magnified detail showing the profile of two mountains on the extreme moon circumference, and, among others, the crater Bettinus (from Lohrmann and Schmidt, 1878). This map is inverted with relation to the normal view of the moon, and the south-west regions are represented by the sections on the top and right of the global map.

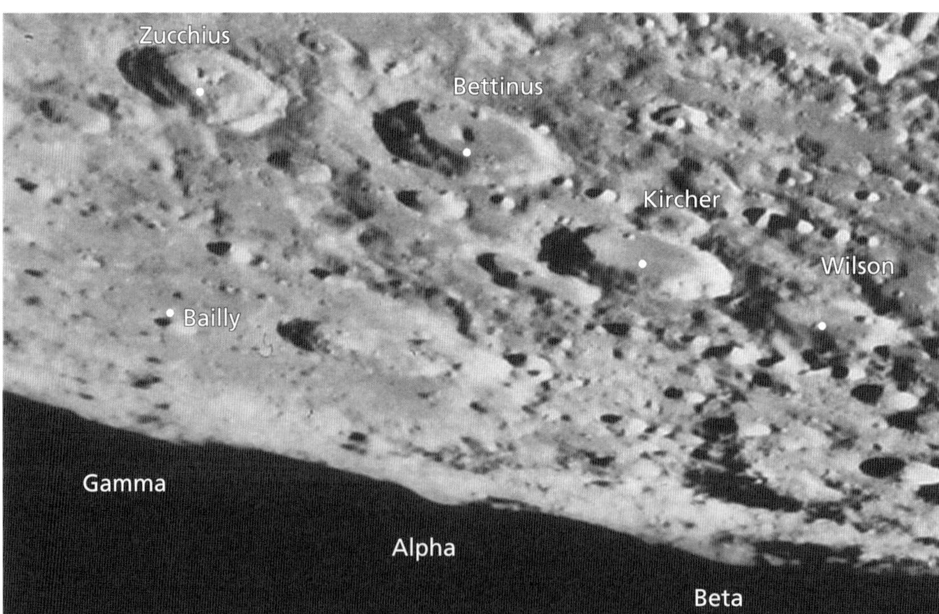

Figure 7.8 A high-magnification picture of the south-west rim of the moon showing the mountains indicated as Doerfel in Lohrmann's *Mondcharte*. Notice how, in the photographic view the mountain profile is less prominent than in the cartographic representation of the *Mondcharte*. Reproduced from *Monthly Notices of the Royal Astronomical Society*, Vol. 39, p. 266, 1879, Oxford University Press.

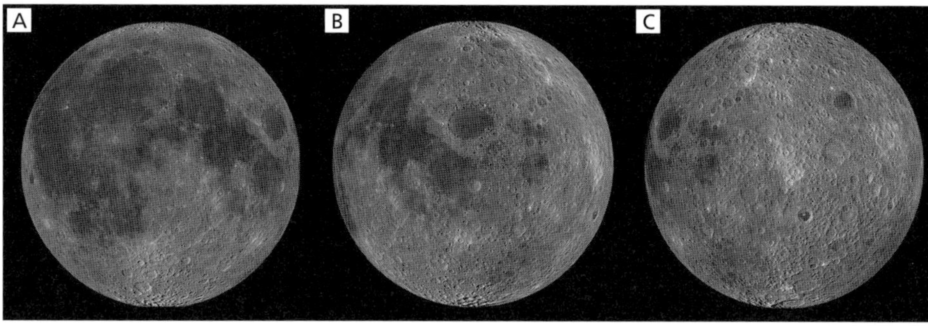

Figure 7.9 Images of the moon based on the superposition of a mosaic of photos obtained with a wide-angle orbiting camera, and arranged as to represent orthographic view centred respectively at 0° longitude and 0° latitude (a), at 60° longitude and 0° latitude (b), and at 120° longitude and 0° latitude (c). Source: NASA; reproduced with permission under the Creative Commons Attribution-Share Alike 3.0 Unported License.

face of the moon (recognizable by the large size and radiated crater Copernicus in the upper left quadrant), parts (a) and (b) are pictures representing the moon seen from, respectively, 60° and 120° longitude. In particular, Figure 7.9b is centred on the lunar meridian that in the ordinary view (Figure 7.9a) corresponds to the 'extreme circumference' of the moon. As Galileo had anticipated, there are mountains there as in all the other parts of the moon.

To say whether these mountains and craters are there simply because they are 'seen' by the NASA high-performance camera is perhaps another story. This is because not only are vision and cartography complex processes, but also photography is far from being a simple copy of reality. The NASA images appear to our eye so detailed and informative because they are the result of a complex superposition of many different photographs, taken by the orbiting camera from different points of view and with different arrangement of colour filters.

At variance with the opinions of the author of the Problem of Mantua, and in agreement with the results of modern science, lunar mountains and craters occur both where we 'see' them and where we fail to 'see' them. We could perhaps better say that, following the steps of Galileo, we can demonstrate the presence of lunar mountains where ambiguous visual cues suggest their presence, and also where visual appearances seem fallaciously to suggest their absence.

In conclusion, we should perhaps be indebted with the stubborn Jesuit of Parma for having obliged, with his apparently sound objection, Galileo to go deeply into the complex mechanisms of visual perception as well as into deciphering the appearances of the moon.

Chapter 8

Visual limits and the visibility of infinitesimals

Figure VIII *The many moons of Galileo* by Nicholas Wade. Galileo can just be discerned in an array of crescent moons.

For Galileo, the predominant sense of science was the eye, and vision itself was an integral part of his scientific endeavour. What the eye saw could be described, catalogued, and even subjected to mathematical analysis. He pursued the awe of the eye and vision as it was expressed by Plato: 'Vision, in my view, is the cause of the greatest benefit to us, inasmuch as none of the accounts now given concerning the Universe would ever have been given if men had not seen the stars or the sun or the heaven. But as it is, the vision of day and night and of months and circling years has created the art of number and has given us not only the notion of Time but also a means of research into the nature of the Universe' (1946, p. 107). However, Galileo was also aware of the limitations and fallacies to which vision is prone, and it is the former that will be examined in the present chapter.

As anticipated in Chapter 7, the theme of the visual magnification of luminous bodies is one of the most significant aspects of Galileo's elaborations on vision. Its importance arises with reference to the vision of stars. We will return to this theme in the last part of our book because it helps to define Galileo's observational approach to vision in contrast to the optical theories developed by Kepler and Scheiner (Figure 8.1). The former described the dioptric properties of the eye and

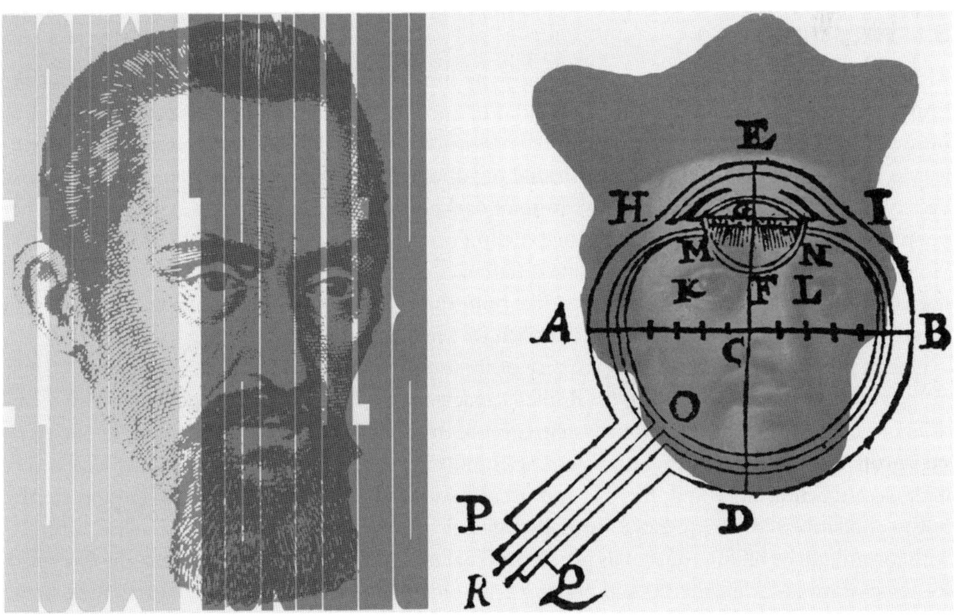

Figure 8.1 *Kepler's retinal image and Scheiner's eye* by Nicholas Wade. Johannes Kepler is portrayed in the letters RETINAL IMAGE which are inverted and reversed. In addition to his *Ad Vitellionem Paralipomena* of 1604, Kepler wrote *Dioptrice* in 1611. In the first of these he added many things to Witelo's perspective, both experimentally and theoretically. Amongst them was the formulation of the basic principle of photometry that the intensity of light diminishes with the square of the distance from the source. Kepler did not have available to him an adequate account of the anatomy of the eye. This was provided by Christoph Scheiner in 1619. Scheiner's portrait is shown in the diagram of the mammalian eye published in his *Oculus*: the lens and its curvatures are appropriately represented and the optic nerve leaves the eye nasally. This figure has frequently been reprinted, and it is often claimed that it represents a human eye, even though Scheiner stated that he did not have the opportunity of dissecting one.

the latter married this with its correct gross anatomy. Kepler provided an optical background potentially capable of accounting for the visual magnification of point light sources. Despite that, he had to realize that an explanation based only on optical causes was far from being exhaustive; and was obliged to invoke (at least in a metaphorical way) other elements, of a more physiological and perceptual dimension. Galileo's approach to the problem was of a completely different nature; it was of an operational and experimental character, and, notably, was totally independent of considerations based on geometrical optics. With regard to the specific problem of visual appearances of the stars it was more successful than that of the German astronomer.

In order to appreciate the differences in approach between Galileo and Kepler we need to deal with certain aspects of the visual function as they emerge from modern visual science. This is mainly because the vision of stars involves the limits of visual spatial resolution and detection. Some of these limitations are of a physical nature, like those relating to the physical properties of light and its undulatory nature. Others have to do with the optical properties of the eye. Yet other constraints are related specifically to the biological aspects of the eye and visual system, and to the neural mechanisms of visual information processing in the retina and more central sites in the nervous system. Finally, others are perceptual in nature.

8.1 Why limits?

Although visual performance is subject to many limitations, in general interest in most of the limits is restricted to specialists in the field. For most of us, the inability to detect infrared or ultraviolet radiations is of little concern. This does not mean that, in principle, it would be worthless to have a specific sensibility for infrared or ultraviolet radiations. If we were equipped with eyes capable of detecting infrared rays in total darkness we could perceive the presence of other people or animals based on the variable emission of infrared rays from their bodies. With ultraviolet detecting eyes we could appreciate differences of colour between objects that appear to be the same hue to our sight. Some species, like honeybees, have ultraviolet photoreceptors and can detect characteristics of some flowers of which we are unaware.

One of the main reasons for the existence of these and other kinds of limits in the performance of the visual system has to do with the limited capacity of the nervous system to handle large quantities of information. In the nervous system most of the information is coded in the form of electrical signals, largely (but not exclusively) of an impulsive nature. However, nerve fibres have a very high electrical resistance and, for this and other reasons, they are capable of discharging electric pulses at relatively low frequency (normally well below 1000 impulses per second). This contrasts with the million or billions of signals per second that modern electric devices can handle (we speak for them of mega- or gigahertz) and per se sets a fundamental constraint to the functioning of the nervous system in general, and to the sensory systems in particular, and especially to vision.

The impossibility of resolving fine details of a visual scene is evident to most of us. For those with normal vision, however, this limitation appears to be relatively unimportant for close objects. This is probably because our survival and evolutionary success did not depend on resolving the fine details of objects. Moreover, modern manufactured items have been made with knowledge of our visual performance. This is the case for the letters of the book you are now reading, their font size is such that the text can be read comfortably at the normal viewing distance. Another reason for our relative lack of concern for objects below the resolution limits of our vision is simply that we have never seen them except when using microscopes or other means of magnification. We have therefore neither direct awareness of them nor an immediate grasp of the possible advantages we could derive from their visibility.

It is when viewing distant objects that we become aware of the limits of our spatial resolution, As Euclid put it in Proposition 3 of his *Optics*, 'every object seen has a certain limit of distance, and when this is reached it is seen no longer'. Seafarers experience this when trying to identify the coastline or other distant ships. They can, however, ascertain the nature of the objects when on land. Such confirmation is not available to astronomers looking at stars and planets. This is a principal reason for the interest that astronomers have shown in the limits of visual resolution. Observations of astronomical bodies with the naked eye were even used as tests of visual acuity. In particular, normal vision was related to the ability to distinguish the faint star Alcor in the constellation of *Ursa Major* (Big Dipper) from its brighter companion Mizar. The interest did not decrease when astronomical observation passed from those with the naked eye to those based on more sophisticated telescopic devices. This is because as the magnification power of telescopes increased, new reasons emerged for the difficulties of improving their visual resolution.

Over the centuries, many investigators became progressively aware that people with normal vision have difficulty in discerning objects that subtend a visual angle of less than 1′, that is, 1/60 of a degree. The resolution limits of vision have been discussed with relation to the structure of the retina, and particularly the dimensions and spacing of the retinal cells. It became evident that the measured limits of visual resolution were dependent upon the type of stimulus used for testing vision and on the conditions of illumination. An isolated stimulus, like a spot or a line, could be resolved at smaller angular subtenses than the gap between two spots or lines. In the last case the minimum resolvable distance in the optimal conditions of observation (high mean luminance, strong contrast) was generally found to be about 1′ whereas for isolated spots or lines the minimum angular size could be of the order of few seconds of arc.

When modern telescopic techniques enabled accurate estimates of the angular size of stars, it was clear that our ability to detect a luminous object can apparently go even beyond these limits. Suffice it to say that the angular size of the star which appears as the biggest in the Northern hemisphere, Sirius (the *Cane* or *Canicula*, i.e. the Dog star in Galileo's terminology), subtends 0.0059″ and we can perceive many stars much smaller than this. The apparent size of the stars is much larger than their calculated geometrical size (Sirius being perceived as a light globule subtending an angle of about 3′, i.e. about 500 times bigger than its physical dimension). Under appropriate viewing conditions we would be able to see any luminous object, as small as it could be, irrespectively of its true angular size, provided that it irradiated a 'sufficient amount' of light.

In order to understand why and how this could happen we have now to consider various physical and physiological aspects of vision. Despite the fact that any one of them could influence vision, they do not necessarily act independently. An interesting and somewhat unexpected consequence of this is that some physical imperfections of the optical mechanisms of our eye might turn out to be advantageous for vision.

8.2 The physical and physiological expansion of point light sources

A fundamental limitation to imaging faithfully a point light source irrespective of the optical system (artificial or natural) has to do with the physical nature of the light. Since the time of Euclid, vision has been analysed in terms of geometrical optics and visual rays which travelled in straight lines. We know now that, because of the undulatory nature of light that this is just an approximation. Even in the most perfect optical system (i.e. one with no aberration) a point light source would be imaged as an expanded and complex spatial pattern due to this undulatory nature of light which results in the phenomenon of diffraction. In an aberration-free system

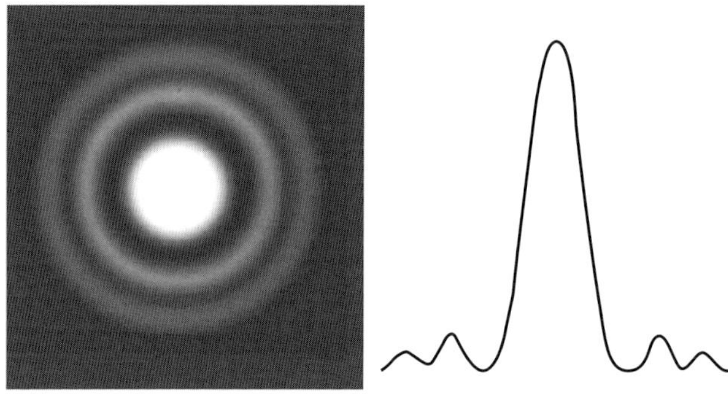

Figure 8.2 The diffraction pattern (Airy disc) on the left, with (on the right) the profile of luminance along a one spatial dimension. An image like this is seen when looking at a star with a high magnification telescope of good optic quality and in conditions of small atmospheric turbulence.

(generally indicated as 'diffraction-limited'), the image of a point source (generally referred to as 'point transfer function' of the system) corresponds to a concentric circular pattern, with a central, intense, blurred disc (containing a large amount of the total luminous energy), surrounded by a series of rings of progressively larger and rapidly decaying intensity (Figure 8.2). This pattern is called an Airy disc after the Astronomer Royal, George Biddell Airy, who dealt theoretically with the phenomenon in 1835. The diffraction limitations depend on the optical aperture of the apparatus and on the wavelength of the light. Large optical apertures and shorter wavelengths result in sharper images. With apertures sufficiently large, the order of magnitudes of the central disc and the distances of the most immediate peripheral rings is that of the wavelength of the light (hundredths of nanometres, nm).

Because of diffraction, the most perfect light microscope based on normal lenses cannot resolve details of less than about 200 nm; similarly a traditional light telescope of, say, 1-metre length having ideal optics cannot resolve details subtending less than about 0.1″ (i.e. one-tenth of a second of arc); the resolution improves with the length of the telescope, and it can approach 0.02″ for one having a length of 8 metres, but since stars subtend angles much smaller than these values they cannot be properly imaged even with the most powerful optical and most perfect traditional light telescopes.

Another important limitation rooted in the physical nature of light has to do with its corpuscular nature, which comes out particularly in the case of its interaction with matter. As we shall see, in the case of vision the corpuscular, or quantal, nature of light plays a role at low light intensities.

The dioptric apparatus of the human eye is far from being perfect due to a number of imperfections of various types.[1] Some of these imperfections (like spherical aberration) derive from the defective geometrical design of the refracting surfaces (mainly those of cornea and crystalline

[1] It is perhaps appropriate to quote here what the great German scholar Hermann von Helmholtz used to say about the optical quality of the human eye in his popular lectures: 'If an optician wished to sell me an instrument with all these defects, it would not be exaggerated to say that I will feel myself perfectly justified in blaming, with the strongest expressions, the carelessness of its work, and in giving him back the object by protesting' (Helmholtz, 1895, I, p. 194). This notwithstanding, Helmholtz recognized that the optic imperfections of the human eye exceeds only by a small extent the anatomical and physiological constraints of the visual process.

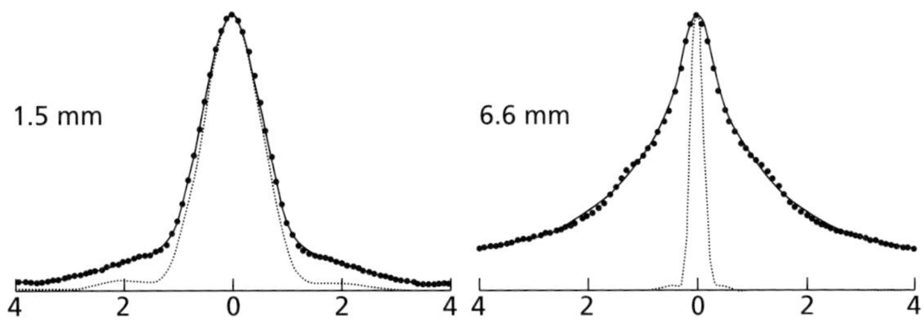

Figure 8.3 The distribution of light on the human retina in the presence of a thin line source (line spread function) at two different pupil diameters (indicated in each panel). The thinner lines represent the diffraction image of the line at that given pupil diameter. Reproduced from Campbell, F.W. and Gubisch, R. W., Optical quality of the human eye, *Journal of Physiology*, 186, pp. 558–578 © 1966, John Wiley and Sons, with permission.

lens). These aberrations become important with large pupil apertures. With small pupil sizes (of about 2 mm diameter) the limitations due to spherical aberration are reduced and the optical performance of the eye approaches that of a diffraction-limited system. Because of the pupillary dilatation induced by dim light, this relatively ideal behaviour is found exclusively in conditions of high ambient illumination (i.e. during the day or under intense artificial illumination). It must be noted, however, that, although at small pupil sizes the eye approaches the diffraction-limited optical behaviour, the amount of diffraction increases when the pupil diameter decreases (Figure 8.3). This is the reason why the optimal optical behaviour of the eye is found at pupil sizes slightly exceeding those corresponding to the diffraction-limited behaviour. In other words, the best optical performance of the eye is achieved thanks to a trade-off between two opposite conditions: small pupil sizes in order to avoid spherical (and similar) aberrations, and large pupil sizes in order to reduce diffractions phenomena.

Spherical aberrations are only one of the many types of optical defects influencing visual performance. Other types of aberrations result from the different focusing of rays of different wavelengths. These are called chromatic aberrations, an optical imperfection that is normally corrected in artificial optical devices but not in the human eye. Optical limitations also come from the imperfect transparency of the ocular media and from internal reflections at the different surfaces delimiting them. There are, moreover, limitations which are midway between the physical and physiological optics like those due to imperfect focusing. These become significant at low light levels. Also important for visual performance in normal conditions are the small amplitude movements of our eyes which persist even if we make an effort to block them by fixating steadily on a target. These involuntary eye movements are of various types, but the most significant for their possible influence on the visibility of the tiny detail of the visual scene are the so-called microsaccades. The generally have a frequency of a few hertz and an amplitude that can achieve many minutes of arc.

Due to the various forms of physical imperfections that affect the optical performance of the eye, the image formed on the retina in the presence of a sharp point source of considerable intensity is degraded to a relatively smooth distribution, of variable shape and dimensions according to the prevailing optical limitation. With pupil sizes of 2 mm or less the lateral spread of the luminance follows the diffraction pattern rather faithfully, which is rather wide (because of the prominence of this kind of imperfection at small optical apertures). At large pupil sizes, the lateral distribution of light becomes smooth (because of the predominance of spherical aberration) and considerably expanded compared to the diffraction pattern (which is narrower than in the previous condition). This behaviour is illustrated in Figure 8.3 which portrays the results of experiments in which the optical quality of the dioptric mechanism of the human eye was measured by using a thin luminous slit rather than a point source. The information provided by this method (resulting in the determination of the 'line spread function') is basically similar to that obtained with point source, and the results are generally more reliable. Although the spatial extent of the light distribution is considerably larger with the large pupil size, in both circumstances the order of magnitude of the central part of the image is in the range of minutes of arcs. This happens even with the smallest light sources capable of irradiating enough light such as to produce a sufficiently intense image in the eye. If we apply these considerations to the vision of stars, and take into account the large size of the pupil in night vision, we could easily understand why the image of a sufficiently intense star might be of the order of magnitude of minutes of arc, even if the geometrical angle subtended by the star at the observer's eye is much less than seconds of arc. Said otherwise, the dimensions on the retina of the image of a point light source is, by far, more a measure of the effects of various intra-ocular optical phenomena, than of the physical dimension of the light source.[2]

Having considered mainly the physical factors capable of limiting the resolution and detection of the fine details of the visual scene, it is time now to briefly survey the anatomical and physiological factors that enter into play in this context.

The first consideration necessary to transform a physical pattern like those of Figures 8.2 and 8.3 into a seen image has to do with the intensity of light. Other things being equal, we would see a larger image with a more intense light. This is because retinal photoreceptors are excited only when the physical stimulus impinging on them exceeds a minimum 'threshold' value. If we consider the pattern at the right of Figure 8.3 (large pupil size) this could result in an image seen as several tens of arc seconds at low intensities (when only the cusp of the central lobe might exceed the threshold) or of several minutes at strong light intensity (when also the luminosity of lateral 'skirts' is above the threshold for the underlying photoreceptors).

In physiological circumstances what normally happens is that at high levels of light intensity the pupil size decreases. Moreover, the retina undergoes a series of other, complex, functional modifications, which make it less sensitive to light and more capable of discriminating the finer details of the visual scene. These modifications are of various types. First they involve a shift from one to the other of the two main types of photoreceptors present in our retina, the rods (the most sensitive receptors) and the cones (the less sensitive). Besides being intrinsically less sensitive to light, the cones exist in three chromatic types (this being the basis of our capability of discriminating colours: see Chapter 10). They work exclusively in conditions of high ambient (or retinal) illumination (i.e. in conditions referred to as photopic). Cones are finely spaced and are abundant in the central part of our retina (the macula), being the exclusive photoreceptors present in the small pit existing in the middle of the macula (the fovea), the region where our visual acuity attains its maximum.

The average distance between a cone and its neighbours in the fovea is of the order of about 2.5 microns, and this contributes an important limit to the possibility of resolving the spatial details of the visual scene. This is the consequence of a fundamental theorem of information science which stipulates that the spacing of elements in the detecting array sets an important limit

---

[2] As we shall discuss later, in telescopic observation a factor that might influence the observation of the stars is atmospheric turbulence. In conditions of clear sky the effects of atmosphere on vision of stars with the naked eye are, however, very limited.

(Nyquist limit) to the resolution of the system. On the basis of the photoreceptor spacing in the fovea, and of the dimensions and optical parameters of the human eye (one degree of angular size corresponding in the retina to a surface of about 300 micron linear dimension), we can calculate the finest pattern that the human fovea can discriminate. This corresponds to a striped spatial gratings containing about 60 complete cycles of light and dark alternations within one degree of visual angle. This is indeed the optimal performance of the central vision of a normal human eye in conditions of high ambient illumination (i.e. when vision depends on cones, and especially on foveal cones).

In order to have an idea of how big is a one-degree visual angle we can follow the rule introduced centuries ago by astronomers: one degree corresponds to the visual angle under which we see our little finger when looking at it with the arm fully stretched. Alternatively, and still within the astronomical field, a degree is twice the visual angle under which we see the moon. This means that the theoretical limit of spatial resolution set by photoreceptor spacing in the human fovea corresponds to about 60 cycles of light and dark alternation in the field of our small finger seen with a stretched arm, or to 30 cycles within the lunar disc.

It is mainly since the pioneer studies started about half a century by the Scottish physiologist Fergus W. Campbell, that physiologists use gratings in order to evaluate the spatial performance of vision. In these patterns the luminance changes in a sinusoidal way along one direction of space. Of these 'spatial sinusoids' one can modify the number of cycles within a given visual angle, the average luminance, and the contrast between the light and dark peaks (Figure 8.4).

Investigating visual resolution with these visual patterns is more precise than the letter-based tests of visual acuity. The plot of the results obtained from such investigations shows that we are most sensitive to patterns with three to five cycles per degree, and that, with highest maximum contrast, we come near to the limit of 60 cycles per degree, set by the spacing of photoreceptors in the retinal array (Figure 8.5, uppermost plots).

The fact that in the optimal viewing conditions our visual performance comes near to the Nyquist limit of the retinal sampling means that the optical imperfections of the eye (spherical and chromatic aberrations, light scattering due to defective transparencies of the ocular media) and other physical or preretinal factors (light diffraction due to the undulatory nature of light, instability and tremors of the eye) do not interfere much with the spatial performance of the visual system. As to the optics of the eye, this does not mean that its quality is particularly good, but simply that it is adequate enough with reference to other, non-optical limitations. Indeed, experiments in which spatial sinusoids were produced on the retina by bypassing the optics of the eye, based

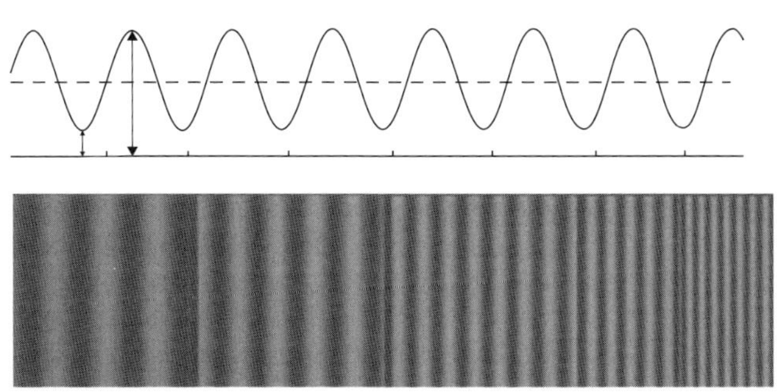

Figure 8.4 Top: profile of luminance along one direction of the space in a spatial sinusoid. Bottom: five gratings with increasing spatial frequencies from left to right.

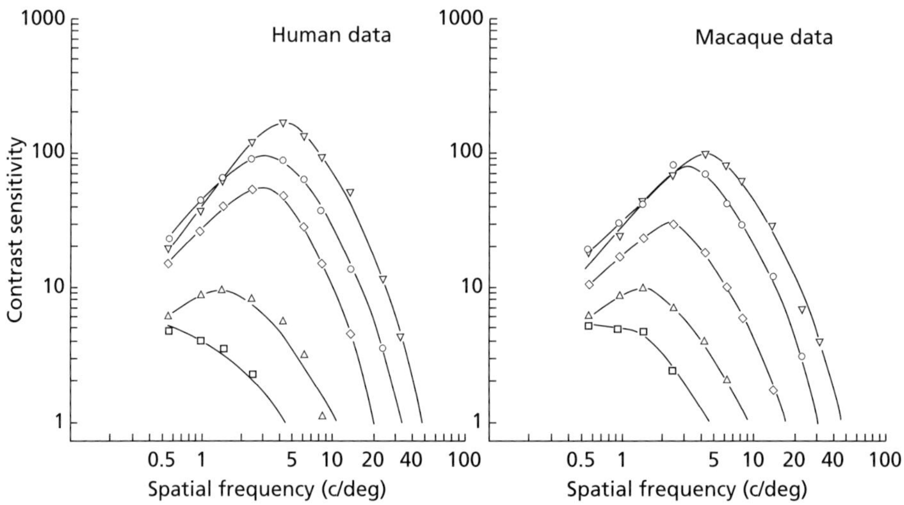

Figure 8.5 A measure of the capability of humans (left) and monkeys (right) to detect the presence of a striped pattern of spatial sinusoids as a function of number of sinusoids with a degree of visual angle (spatial frequency). The different curves were obtained at different levels of mean luminance (with the less intense—lowermost curve—being 10,000 weaker than the maximum—uppermost curve). The 'contrast sensitivity' in the ordinates, measures the reciprocal of the minimum contrast at which each sinusoidal is perceived as different from a uniform visual scene. Notice the substantial similarity between the macaque and human data which makes the monkey a good model for the study of the human visual system. Reprinted from *Vision Research*, 14 (1), Russell L. De Valois, Herman Morgan, and D. Ma Snodderly, Psychophysical studies of monkey vision. III. Spatial luminance contrast sensitivity tests of macaque and human observers, pp. 75–81 Copyright (1974), with permission from Elsevier.

on the production of interference fringes on the eye fundus, showed that the visual performance with high-frequency sinusoids was only slightly improved. As a matter of fact, these experiments showed that vision becomes disturbed in the presence of stimuli containing spatial sinusoids of frequency higher than the resolvable maximum. These studies highlighted the importance and adaptive usefulness of having relatively low-quality optics. On the one hand, better optics would not result in better visual performance due to the limitations caused by photoreceptor sampling limits. On the other hand, if the eye optics were of a better quality, our vision would be seriously disturbed by the appearance of flickering moiré patterns due to the undersampling of the finest details of the retinal image. From this point of view, the imperfect optics of the eye would certainly warrant a 'praise of the imperfection'.

Coming to the visual results illustrated in Figure 8.4 we need to say that circuits of the retina and higher structures of the visual system are entirely responsible for the cut-off at low spatial frequency. This is because there is not any similar effect in the optical transfer of low spatial sinusoids across the eye media.

The high-frequency cut-off of the spatial sinusoid detection, with the limit near 60 cycles per degree, occurs only in the ideal conditions for the visibility of such patterns. When the average luminance of the visual sinusoids decreases, the spatial behaviour of the visual system changes substantially. Besides a general decrease of the capability of resolving the spatial pattern at all spatial frequencies, there is an important degradation of the visual performance in the high spatial-frequency range. With very low average luminance the cut-off at high frequencies goes down to values around one cycle per degree. This change is not due to any important extent to a change of the optical quality of the eye or to physical factors and is mainly of a neurophysiological nature. Although, as discussed earlier (see Figure 8.3), in principle the pupillary dilatation consequent on light dimming results in an optical degradation of the retinal image, the effects are observed even in experiments in which the size of the pupil is kept constant. This suggests that the drastic changes of the spatial behaviour of the visual system are due mainly to neurophysiological factors.

The study of retinal function carried out for about 50 years with a variety of experimental approaches (morphological, electrophysiological, biochemical, comparative) has deepened our understanding of the complex mechanisms underlying the transformation of spatial visual performance produced by changes of light intensity on the retina. This phenomenon is called light or dark adaption. As shown in Figure 8.5, going from an intense light to a very dim one our system passes from being able to discern a very fine pattern of sinusoidal stripes to that of hardly discerning a sinusoid whose spatial period is larger than one degree. This might seem a disadvantage inasmuch with such limited performance we could not perform many visual tasks. However, we can imagine the situation in a more positive way if we consider that we can see in moonlight and recognize large objects.

The problems which arise at very dim light come mainly from the quantal nature of light. This emerges particularly when, by dimming the light, the average number of light quanta (or photons) gets very small. In this condition (called 'scotopic' vision) the photoreception task shifts from cones to rods, which are the most sensitive retinal photoreceptors. Rods are extremely sensitive to light and in several animals they come near the maximum possible physical sensitivity, i.e. the capability of detecting a single quantum of light. There are, however, some drawbacks of this extreme sensitivity. One has to do that with the fact that with a certain frequency events similar to that triggered by the absorption of a photon arise spontaneously in a rod even in the absence of any light whatsoever. If one of these events would be able to trigger a physiological response, we would see light in the absence of any external stimulus. Moreover, under very dim illumination the random nature of photon emission would dominate the function of individual rods leading to electrical responses characterized by prominent temporal fluctuations. If every one of these fluctuations were to result into an effective perceptual response, the global visual performance would be seriously disturbed by something like a continuous, fastidious temporal flickering.

Because of these and other problems at very low light levels the retina is organized in such a way that when rods start to be the dominating photoreceptors, the need of having a system capable of high spatial resolution is traded off with the need to have a more sensitive and reliable detection system. This is achieved first through an extensive lateral communication at the level of the rods themselves, due to particular junctions (called gap-junctions) which allow for the diffusion of the electrical signals between neighbouring rods. Moreover, the 'rod pathway', i.e. the pathway by which the electrical signals generated in the rods are conveyed towards the more proximal nerve cells of the retina are characterized by an extensive 'convergence'. In one of the main retinal rod pathway, thousands of rods are connected to a specific subset of the second-order neurons of the retina (the rod-bipolar cells) and further convergence is achieved while these signals proceed towards the ganglion cells through rather complex circuits. Due to this extensive lateral convergence the visual signals become more reliable: the temporal fluctuations due to the random nature of photon absorption are smoothed by a form of spatial averaging, and, moreover, the probability that spontaneous events arising in a photoreceptor result in a fake light response is drastically reduced. This is because isolated events arising in a single rod are diluted within the pool of intercommunicating rods and because of the extensive convergence at the subsequent stages, and thus fail to be transmitted towards the ganglion cells. On the other hand, in the presence on the retina of a light pattern of great extension there is a chance that the electrical events generated in the rods of the pool are correlated and thus sum together and produce a visual response.

The negative consequence of the extensive convergence existing at various levels of the rod pathways is the degradation of the spatial performance of our vision when passing from the high luminance behaviour dominated by cones, to the dim light condition dominated by rods functioning (illustrated by the lowermost graphs of Figure 8.5). As one could expect, rod vision plays an important role in the naked eye observation of the stars. This accounts for the fact that the dimmest stars are not perceived when looking directly at them (when their image would be focused in the rod-free fovea), but are better seen with lateral view (about 20° out of axis, which brings the image on the region of the retina richer in rods).

To conclude, this long digression allows us to understand the complexity of the phenomena involved in the vision of stars and other celestial objects and situate better the discussions on this matter in Galileo's age. In the case of the observation of the nocturnal sky, vision shifts from a condition indicated as mesopic, in which both cones and rods work together (as, for instance, when observing the most luminous stars) to a decidedly scotopic condition (when looking to very faint stars), to a more photopic condition when observing the moon. In general, the pupil is dilated in night vision, which results in an extension of the image of stars due to increased spherical aberration. As the condition of light adaptation moves towards the mesopic phase, the ensuing reduction of light sensitivity contributes to make the image sharper. In the case of the observation of very dim stars the system is extremely sensitive, but because of the faint light reaching the eye, only a part of the image of the star is above the threshold for detection (and the star appears small). In the case of bright stars, the modest decrease of light sensitivity due to the relatively intense light reaching the retina is compensated by the strong effect of contrast which is particularly effective in mesopic condition.

8.3 **The Copernican system, a world of absurdities**

Galileo's concerns about vision had an important cosmological dimension, and this was also in the case of the vision of stars. This particular aspect has to do with one of the most significant objections addressed to the Copernican system. In the *Dialogue* the discussion on this topic is centred mainly on the criticism raised by Simplicio on the basis of the work of Galileo's adversary, Christoph Scheiner. In 1614 Scheiner had published a series of theses defended publicly by a student, Johann Georg Locher, in order to obtain the degree of *Magister artium et philosophiae* from the University of Ingolstadt.[3] Some of the theses were aimed at demonstrating the incongruities and absurdities of the Copernican system based on both theological issues in addition to mathematical and astronomical arguments. The objection expounded in Proposition XIII under the title *Argumentum ex motu et orbe annuo* ('Argument derived from annual motion and orb') was stated in this way:

> According to the opinion of Copernicus and all the Copernicans it is in no way perceptible the proportion that exists between the radius of the Great orb, i.e. the distance of Sun from earth, and the radius of firmament, i.e. the distance from earth of any fixed star whichever; but this is absurd and generates other absurdities as it will appear from what follows. (Scheiner & Locher, 1614, p. 29)

[3] We have mentioned this work in Chapter 4.

Why did Scheiner/Locher say that the proportion between some of the fundamental measures of the cosmos (the radius of the Great orb and the radius of firmament) was in 'no way perceptible'? The traditional model of the cosmos was based on the idea that all stars (with the exception of the sun) are located in a specific crystalline orb or sphere, the eight orbs, also called the sphere of fixed stars. Moreover, on the basis of approximate measurement of the distance from the earth of the various planets, the apparent movement of the various spheres was considered as harmonic, and a measure had been proposed for the diameters of the various orbs, including those of the fixed stars.

For this sphere no direct measurements were possible, other than those depending on logical inferences and philosophical and theoretical mathematical assumptions. This is because the appearance of an orb of fixed stars is based on a perceptual illusion due to the tendency of our visual system to locate all objects at the same distance (see Chapter 2). In the ancient cosmology there was, however, an important limit that constrained the lower figure for the diameter of the eight spheres. This was the absence of any parallax, that is, the absence of any change of the relative position of nearby stars with changes in the relative position of the observer on the earth's surface (see Figure 8.6).

Because of this awareness, old scholars (Archimedes among others) had agreed that the distance of the fixed star should be very large relative to the dimensions of the earth. During the Renaissance a commonly accepted value for the radius of the eighth sphere (or radius of the

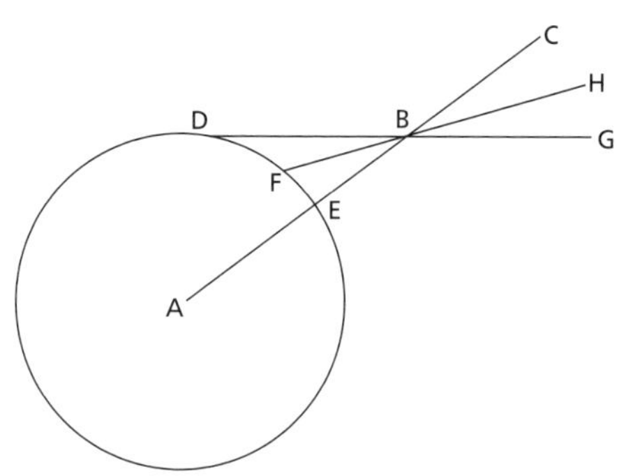

Figure 8.6 Galileo's illustration of parallax, from a dissertation written in 1624 in the form of a letter addressed to Francesco Ingoli. Ingoli was an important catholic prelate and author of a pamphlet entitled *De situ et quiete Terrae contra Copernici systema, Disputatio*. It was written following the condemnation of Copernican theory by the Catholic Church and attempted to demonstrate its untenability on the basis on a variety of arguments, largely derived from the Bible and the ideas of Tycho Brahe. An object in the sky (B) will appear visually at C when viewed from E, but will change its apparent position to H and G when the observer moves to F and D. The more distant the celestial object the smaller is the parallatic change for a given displacement of the observer. Notice that, because of the relative daily rotation of earth's surface relative to the vault of heaven, a parallatic change would occur during the day, even with no real motion of the observer (diurnal parallax). Galileo's example concerns the parallax of a planet, i.e. a celestial globe situated nearer to earth than the fixed star. However, a change would occur also in the relative visual position of nearby fixed stars if they were situated at a relatively short distance from the earth. It is easy to understand this by reference to the figure, by supposing that C, H, and G are three fixed stars of the eighth sphere and noticing that the visual angle separating them would change with the change of the observer's position.

firmament) was that provided by the Persian astronomer al-Ferghani (Alfraganus in Galileo's spelling of the name), i.e. about 20,110 terrestrial radii (amounting to a little more than 128 million km). This distance rendered all possible parallatic changes due to displacements of the observer on the surface of the earth undetectable to the ordinary astronomical tools of the period.

However, the Copernican theory had introduced a much greater motion of the observer relative to the fixed stars, i.e. the movement along the so-called Great orb (*Orbis magnus*), which (as we now know) has a maximum diameter of about 300 million km. To account for the absence of an annual parallax of the fixed stars during such huge revolutions of the earth, Copernicus extended the width of the eighth sphere to values much greater than those previously assumed. The actual values for the distance of fixed stars given by the Polish astronomer cannot be easily rendered in modern terms because they were based on rather inaccurate estimations of some fundamental astronomical parameters (particularly the distance between the earth and sun which was largely underestimated). In modern terms suffice it to say that, assuming an annual revolution of the earth, in order that the parallaxes of the stars might be undetectable with astronomical instruments capable of resolving the angular distance of a minute of arc, the distance of stars needed to be greater than 40 billion km. Taking into account the much shorter distance of the planets, Copernicus's assumption of the immense distance of the fixed stars would have resulted in an almost empty cosmos, with the earth and planets being but extremely small specks within an immense cosmic space. This was one the absurdities addressed by Scheiner and Locher in their *Disputationes* (and also remarked on by other anti-Copernicans). To their eyes (as well as to those of many astronomers of the age) the cosmos of Copernicus appeared therefore to be full of absurdities, mathematically incongruent, and disharmonious.

Some of the absurdities pointed to by Scheiner and Locher were decidedly trivial. One concerned the astrological impossibility of the zodiacal constellations having an influence on earth due to the immense distance of stars. Others were more cogent. The main one had to do with the apparent dimensions of stars, i.e. with the size of the stars calculated on the basis of the immense distances of the fixed stars assumed by Copernicus and the angular size of the stars apparent to an observer. If one accepted the then current measures of these sizes this would imply that the largest stars would have dimensions corresponding to the greatest planetary orbs (Saturn), and the small stars a value corresponding to the dimension of the Great orb. Examples of contemporary measures (those of Tycho Brahe) were 2–3′ for the most luminous and remarkable stars of the sky, like Sirius, Vega, Arcturus, and of 20″ for the barely visible stars of magnitude 6. This was a real absurdity, and one that was not restricted to stubborn anti-Copernicans of Galileo's time, because it implied that the fixed stars were much bigger than our most familiar star, the sun.

8.4 **Great astronomers incapable of seeing**

But let us consider the matter in the way Galileo puts it in the *Dialogue*. It is Simplicio who illustrates the problem with reference to the book of Scheiner and Locher (evidently attributed only to the first author). He does it after having referred to the religious and theological objections raised by the two German scholars:

SIMPLICIO. Let us, then, listen to his other objections, which are more strongly supported. Now here, as you see, he deduces with very precise calculations that if the orbit in which Copernicus makes the earth travel around the sun in a year were scarcely perceptible with respect to the immensity of the stellar sphere, as Copernicus says must be assumed, then one would have to declare and maintain that the fixed stars were at an inconceivable distance from us, and that the smallest of them would be much larger than this whole orbit, while others would be larger than the orbit of Saturn. Yet such bulks are truly too vast, and are incomprehensible and unbelievable. (DIALOGO, p. 350; transl. p. 358)

To which Galileo's alter ego answers:

SALVIATI: I have indeed seen something similar argued against Copernicus by Tycho, so this is not the first time that I have revealed the fallacy—or better, the fallacies—of this argument, built as it is upon completely false hypotheses.

In the following Salviati shows, on the basis of a series of calculations relying on the reasoning of Copernicus, that what is really false in the arguments of the anti-Copernicans is the accepted values of apparent diameters of the stars. The main authority and reference being Tycho Brahe, an astronomer generally noted for the precision of his celestial measurements. According to Salviati (and of course to Galileo) a star of the first magnitude has an apparent diameter of only 5″, and one of the sixth magnitude of 50′″ (one minute third being 1/60 of a second), these values being 240 or 360 times smaller than those of Tycho.

Among Galileo's manuscripts at the Biblioteca Nazionale of Florence there are some loose papers with astronomical observations or annotations, some of which have to do with the apparent diameters of stars and with the distance of the sphere of fixed stars (collected in the *Analecta astronomica* of OG III, pp. 872–880). In some of these annotations Galileo assumes that a star of the first (or, alternatively, of the second) magnitude is as great as the sun. On the basis of the apparent diameter of the star, of the sun, and of the estimated distance between earth and sun, he tries to deduce the distance of the fixed stars. In one case he concludes that this distance is as great as 360 radii of the Great orb. In another case he concludes that the distance of the fixed star is 67,800 times the radius of the sun. The difficulty with these calculations is that the available values of the earth–sun distance and of the diameter of the sun (generally given with reference to the diameter of the earth) were definitely wrong. For instance, in Galileo's time the earth–sun distance was estimated to be about 1000–1200 earth radii (against an average modern value of 23,455). As to the diameter of the sun, in the *Dialogue*, Galileo assumes that it is 11 times the radius of the earth, while modern values are of about 218 earth radii. Using the modern values, Galileo's estimate of the distance of the fixed stars would be above 5 billion km in the first calculation (360 radii of the Great orb), and a little less than 50 billion km for the second calculation (67,800 radii of the sun). Even this last value is a gross underestimation of the distance of the nearest star, Proxima Centauri situated at 4.2 light years (1 light year being 9.4607×10^{12} km). Sirius (referred to as *Canicola*, i.e. the Dog Star) repeatedly mentioned by Galileo is a relatively near star at about the double of the distance of Proxima Centauri.

Galileo was interested in the problem of the apparent size of the stars until the last years of his life as is clear from an unfinished manuscript *Operazioni astronomiche* that he wrote in 1637 (OG VIII, pp. 449–464). He describes in detail the "cord" method for the measurement of the visual angle of luminous stars (and particularly the Dog Star). Moreover, he contrived other methods based on the calculation of the time a star is occulted by an appropriate device, also applicable to the measurement of Sirius. He described them in 1638 to a friend, Niccolò Arrighetti, so that they would not be lost 'in the case he passed away'. These methods, annotated by Arrighetti among his recollections, have been published in the works of Galileo (OG VIII, pp. 464–466). We will discuss them in Chapter 14.

In the *Dialogue* Sagredo invites Salviati to explain the reasons and justifications for the large discrepancies between the commonly accepted values of the angular sizes of the stars and those provided by his reference, a person indicated as 'our Academician', i.e. Galileo himself. Salviati does that by making reference to an argument that we have been considering in the previous chapters with regard to the mountains of the moon, that of the adventitious irradiation emanating from luminous bodies, and of influence in the visibility of small bright objects:

SAGREDO. Then their error consists in their having been very much deceived in taking the apparent diameter of the fixed stars.

SALVIATI. That is the error, but not the only one. And truly I am quite surprised at the number of astronomers, and famous ones too, who have been quite mistaken in their determinations of the sizes of the fixed as well as the moving stars, only the two great luminaries being excepted. Among these men are al-Fergani, al-Battani, Thabit ben Korah, and more recently Tycho, Clavius, and all the predecessors of our Academician. For they did not take care of the adventitious irradiation which deceptively makes the stars look a hundred or more times as large as they are when seen without haloes. Nor can these men be excused for their carelessness; it was within their power to see the bare stars at their pleasure, for it suffices to look at them when they first appear in the evening, or just before they vanish at dawn. And Venus, if nothing else, should have warned them of their mistake, being frequently seen in daytime so small that it takes sharp eyesight to see it, though in the following night it appears like a great torch. I will not believe that they thought the true disc of a torch was as it appears in profound darkness, rather than as it is when perceived in lighted surroundings; for our lights seen from afar at night look large, but from near at hand their true flames are seen to be small and circumscribed. This alone might have sufficed to make them cautious. To speak quite frankly, I thoroughly believe that none of them—not even Tycho himself, accurate as he was in handling astronomical instruments and despite his having built such large astronomical instruments and despite his having built such large and accurate ones without a thought for their enormous expense—ever set himself to determine and measure the apparent diameter of any star except the sun and moon. I think that arbitrarily and, so to speak, by rule of thumb some one among the most ancient astronomers stated that such-and-such was the case, and the later ones without any further experiment adhered to what this first one had declared. For if any of them had applied himself to making any test of the matter, he would doubtless have detected the error. (DIALOGO, p. 353; transl. pp. 360–361)

This passage reveals some of the typical aspects of Galileo's reflection on the tendency of humans, sometimes even of great scholars, to take for granted what is generally considered true, without any critical analysis or personal verification. It contains the essence of his justification that the apparent diameter of small luminous bodies (like stars and the planets with the exception of the moon) is much larger than the effective geometrical angle subtended at the level of the observer's eye. Galileo's argument is based on two main elements: on one side, the comparison of the visual appearances in two different conditions of average illumination and on the other, the correspondence between the observation of a celestial body (Venus) and of a terrestrial light source (the flame of a torch). As we have seen in section 8.2, it is under conditions of high ambient light that the spatial resolution gets better and the perceived size of a small light source is less distorted with relation to its real geometrical dimension. In the case of Galileo, however, there was no reason a priori for assuming that the image of Venus seen in daytime corresponded more accurately to the geometrical image of the planet than the much bigger globe shining in the night sky. The difficulty was, however, rapidly resolved with reference to the terrestrial light source. From afar we overestimate the size of a torch when it is seen under conditions of 'profound darkness' compared to its aspect perceived 'in lighted surroundings'. This is one of the arguments why, in the absence of a specific knowledge of the phenomena and mechanisms of light and dark adaptation, Galileo could conclude that the image of Venus seen in daylight is a better indication of its true size.

8.5 Measuring the stars with a cord

Against the common views of great astronomers, Galileo had other elements for supporting his conclusion that the visibility of stars and planets can be greatly distorted by the subtleties of vision processes. His reasoning was also based on experimental evidence. We will follow how Salviati responds to Sagredo's remark which was intended as an excuse for the doubtful perspicacity of previous astronomers:

SAGREDO. But if they lacked the telescope (for you have already said that our friend came to know the truth of the matter by means of that instrument), they ought to be pardoned, not accused of negligence.

SALVIATI. That would be true if they could not have obtained the result without the telescope. It is true that the telescope, by showing the disc of the star bare and very many times enlarged, renders the operations much easier; but one could carry them on without it, though not with the same accuracy. I have done so, and this is the method I have used. I hung up a light rope in the direction of a star (I made use of Vega[4] which rises between the north and the northeast) and then by approaching and retreating from this cord placed between me and the star, I found the point where its width just hid the star from me. This done, I found the distance of my eye from the cord, which amounts to the same thing as one of the sides which includes the angle formed at my eye and extending over the breadth of the cord. This is similar to, or rather equal to, the angle made in the stellar sphere by the diameter of the star. From the ratio of the thickness of the cord to its distance from my eye, using a table of arcs and chords, I immediately found the size of the angle—taking the customary precaution, used in determining such very acute angles, not to put the intersection of the visual rays at the center of my eye, where they would not go if they were not refracted, but beyond the location of the eye where the actual width of the pupil would permit them to converge.[5] (pp. 353–354; transl. 361–362)

The subsequent objection by Sagredo allows Salviati to stress a fundamental point of Galileo's view of the problem that justifies the basic validity of the method of the cord:

SAGREDO. I understand this precaution, though I somewhat question it; what bothers me most in this operation is that if it is made in the dark of night, it seems to me that one is measuring the diameter of the irradiated disc and not that of the true and naked star.

SALVIATI. Not a bit; for the cord, by covering the bare body of the star, takes away the halo belonging not to it but to our eyes; of this it is deprived the moment the true disc is hidden. In making the observation you will be astonished to see how thin a rope will cover that great torch which seemed incapable of being hidden except by a much larger obstacle. (pp. 354; transl. 362)

This was a fundamental justification for the validity of Galileo's visual experiment (and of all his conceptions about the sizes of small luminous points) which is repeatedly reasserted when he returns to this theme. In his view, the halo, the adventitious rays (which he refers to by different

[4] *Lira* in the original, i.e. Lyra, the constellation of which Vega is the most brilliant star.

[5] The precaution to which Salviati alludes, and that will return in an unfinished treatise written by Galileo in 1637, is not justified in view of the modern knowledge of image formation on the eye. In the framework of modern physiological optics the point from which to calculate the angle subtended by a visual object is the posterior nodal point, which is situated before the centre of the eye (i.e. nearer to the cornea) and not, as implied by Galileo, beyond the eye. As a matter of fact, even in the late years of his life Galileo seemed to have no clear idea of the mechanisms of the image formation in the eye despite the previous studies of Kepler and Scheiner that had clarified the basic process by which the optics of the produce a real image (*pictura*) on the eye's fundus (see Chapters 13 and 14).

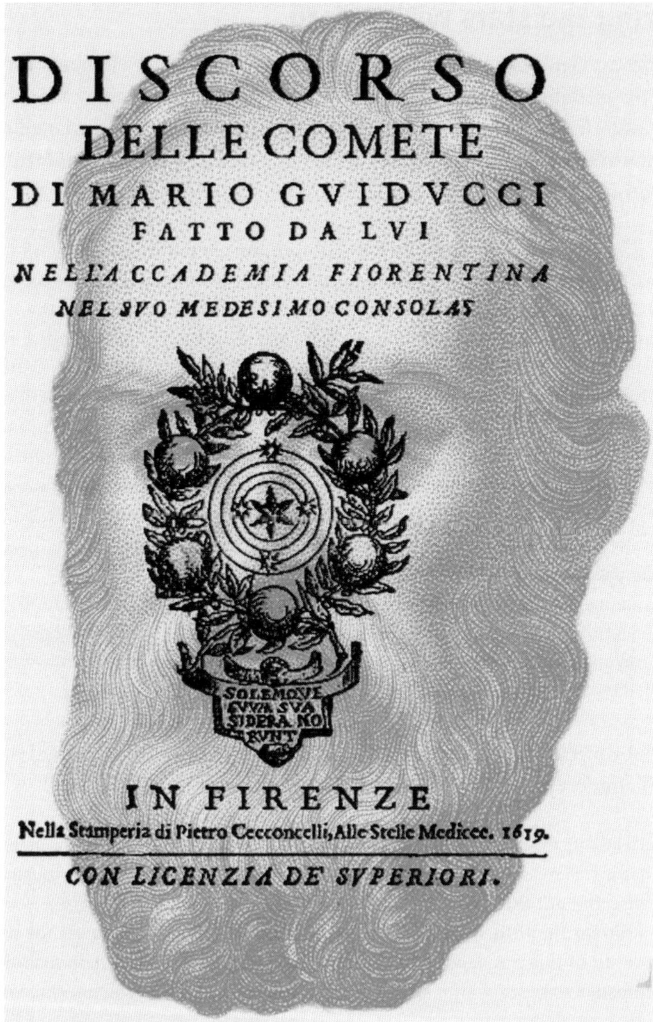

DISCORSO
DELLE COMETE
DI MARIO GVIDVCCI
FATTO DA LVI
NELL'ACCADEMIA FIORENTINA
NEL SVO MEDESIMO CONSOLATO

IN FIRENZE
Nella Stamperia di Pietro Cecconcelli, Alle Stelle Medicee. 1619.

CON LICENZIA DE' SVPERIORI.

Figure 8.7 Galileo's *Discourse*.

terms) are produced mainly within the eye, and are not an objective feature of the luminous object.

The idea is expressed in a particularly clear way in *Discorso delle comete* ('Discourse on the comets') read in 1619 at the Accademia Fiorentina by Galileo's student, Mario Guiducci, and published in the same year under Guiducci's name, but largely due to the pen of Galileo himself (Figure 8.7). In this discourse the problem of the apparent size of star and planets is considered mainly with reference to telescopic observations. Concerning the site of adventitious irradiation this is what we find in this text:

> Here it is necessary first that we upset a false opinion about the nature of this same irradiation, if indeed anyone has put faith in what some philosophers have written to the effect of stars, torches, and all kinds of luminous bodies of all kinds light up and brighten a part of the surrounding air also, which

> in turn at a suitable distance shows its splendor more vividly and more definitely, and that is why the whole torch appears much larger to us. This reasoning is false. The truth is, first, that the air is neither lighted nor brightened; next that this irradiation is not around the luminous object anyway, but is so close to us that if indeed it is not actually within our eyes, it is upon their surfaces; perhaps it is caused by the principal light from the object being refracted in that moisture that is always maintained upon the pupil of the eye by the eyelid. Several things support this. (COMETE, 1619, pp. 31–32: transl. p. 47)

Before continuing the reading of the *Discorso* let us consider the conditions and problem inherent in Galileo's experiment with the cord for measuring the angular size of stars. First, we must be aware the true angular sizes of stars are not only much smaller than those given by Tycho and his followers but are also definitely smaller than those resulting from Galileo's measurements. For instance, Vega, the brightest and apparently largest star of the Lyra constellation, estimated by Galileo to be about 5″ is actually a little less than 1‴ (1 third or 1/60th of 1″), that is, more than 1000 times smaller than the value given by Galileo. This value (precisely 3.28±.06 milliarcseconds as ascertained by modern interferometric techniques) is not only below any possible estimate made by the unaided eye, but was certainly well below the resolution limit of Galileo's telescope. Moreover, as is the case for most of stars, it is also below the diffraction limits of any conventional modern light telescope, and can be measured only with sophisticated techniques (like those based on interferential procedures). In the case of Venus, Jupiter, and Saturn, the existence of a planetary atmosphere made Galileo's telescopic observations even more complex.

In addition to the optical limitations of the telescope (and the physical constraints due to the undulatory nature of light), another measurement problem is the influence of earth's atmosphere. Because of the existence of this atmosphere it is only partially true that the halo or irradiations surrounding the true image of a star is exclusively produced within the eye. A part of it is indeed produced by the atmospheric diffraction of the light rays coming from the star and by atmospheric turbulence. This is, however, a very small portion of the halo visible with unaided eyes and not large enough to influence the outcome of Galileo's cord experiment (in modern astronomy the consequences of atmospheric turbulence can be reduced by using the methods of the so-called 'adaptive optics'). The main difficulty is that, despite Galileo's repeated assertion that the experiment was made in a very precise way, it is nevertheless unrealistic to avoid an important source of error due to the impossibility of keeping the eye totally immobile during the measurement. In addition to possible accidental movements (both of the eye in the orbit and of the head), it is impossible to avoid the rapid involuntary movements of the eyes; microsaccades can span a spatial extent of several minutes of arc, i.e. a value much larger than the apparent visual angle of the stars. The fact that, despite the complexities and intrinsic limits of the method, Galileo was able to reduce by more than 200 times the value of the size of Vega and other stars is further evidence of his extraordinary experimental and logical perspicacity.

Returning to the *Discorso* we can see how the authors justify the idea that the adventitious irradiation issuing from small luminous bodies arises mainly within the eye rather than from the illuminated air surrounding the light source:

> The irradiation appears greater to moist and teary eyes; also if you partially close and compress the eyelids, the rays appear very long, an evident sign that the brilliance is established in the eye and resides there. And what finally shows that it is in the eye is that if we interpose our hand or some other opaque body between the eye and the light, and gently move it as if we wanted to cut out the light, the irradiation is never completely hidden until the actual flame is concealed, but the rays appear quite unaltered between the hand and the eye. This would not occur if the rays were close to the light; that is, between it and the hand. As the hand begins to cut off part of the actual light, parts of the same rays also commence to disappear, namely those which seemed to stem from the opposite part of the light. Thus if

> in raising the hand the lower part of the flame is hidden, those rays will begin to be lost which seem to burst forth from the upper part; and on the contrary, if the hand is placed above the light and is lowered to hide the upper part, then the lower rays will be lost. (COMETE, p. 32; transl. pp. 47–48)[6]

Soon afterwards, another simple experiment is mentioned to support the origin of the adventitious rays emanating from the flame of the candle within the eye:

> The same thing is proven by another most evident experiment. If looking at those rays we lean our head either toward the right or left shoulder—and thus tilt our eyes in the same way, we shall behold the same tilt occurring in the rays, but not in the small flame of the candle, which remain fixed. This is an argument which so much show that those rays are in the eyes, as it demonstrates that the flame is outside and far from them. (COMETE, pp. 32–33; transl. p. 48, modified)

It is worth comparing this passage with that of a modern text of visual science, *The first steps in seeing* by Robert William Rodieck. Interestingly, in order to discuss the image seen when the eye looks at an extremely small light spot, the author considers the vision of a star, and particularly Solaris, the North pole star. In this context he refers to the concept of the point spread function. In order to show that the radiating pattern visible with this type of stimuli originates within the eye and not in the outside world, Rodieck proposes to the reader a simple experiment:

> You can observe point spread function of one of your own eyes whenever you see a radial pattern caused by sunlight reflected from a small bright object. If you tilt your head to the side, the radiate pattern rotates as well, demonstrating that this phenomenon is due to the optics of the eye. Every eye shows these effects, which are due to the arrangements of cells within the lens. But, like fingerprints, every eye differs in the exact patterns. (Rodieck, 1998, p. 82)

There is indeed an amazing correspondence between the writing of a modern retinal physiologist and the words written about four centuries ago by Galileo (and Guiducci) with, perhaps, an element of greater precision in the old text where it is stated that the movement of the rays occur in the same direction of the head movement, and that there is no tilt of the proper image of the small flame.[7]

In many passages of the *Dialogue* Galileo considers the problem of the adventitious irradiation with reference to both stars and terrestrial light sources. Salviati mentions the origin of this irradiation in the context of the experiment of the mirror that we have dealt with in detail in Chapter 5. He tries to explain to Simplicio why a light beam coming out from the surface of a spherical mirror contributes imperceptibly to the ambient light while it appears large and brilliant when looked at directly. He compares its appearance to that of a flame and to the appearance of Sirius:

SALVIATI: First of all, that brilliance which you see so vividly on the mirror, and which seems to you to occupy such a large part of it, is not such a big piece. It is really very tiny, but its extreme brightness causes an adventitious irradiation of your eyes through the reflection made in the moisture at the edges of your eyelids, which extends over the pupil. It is like the little hat that seems to be seen around the flame of a candle at some distance; or you may want to compare it with the apparent rays around a star. For example, if you match the little body of the Dog Star as seen

---

[6] As we shall see in Chapter 14, Galileo was probably inspired from Leonardo in placing the main cause of the irradiation at the level of the eye.

[7] Hermann von Helmholtz is among the scientists who have studied the phenomenon of irradiation from small light sources; he devoted several pages to the phenomenon in the first volume of his *Handbuch der physiologischen Optik* (1867).

in the daytime through the telescope, when it is without irradiations, with the same seen at night by the naked eye, you will perceive beyond all doubt that with its irradiations it appears thousands of times larger than the bare and real starlet. A similar or larger augmentation is made by the image of the sun which you see in that mirror; I say larger, because it is more vivid than that of the star, as it is obvious from one's being able to look at the star with less injury to one's vision than at this reflection in the mirror. (DIALOGO, p. 69; transl. p. 76)

Simplicio replies with an argument based on the visual appearance of a gilded plate struck by the sun, to which Salviati responds by alluding to how the image of a bright light source seen from afar can depend on phenomena taking place in the eye. The observation can be considered as complementary to that of the cord capable of obstructing the vision of an object even when it subtends an angle much smaller than that subtended by the distant light source. In this case, as we shall now see, the attempted obstruction is made around the light source, where the adventitious rays appear. Surprisingly it proves to be largely ineffective in hiding their splendour:

SALVIATI: In order to explain better, let us take a very large gilded plate exposed to the sun; it will show to a distant eye the image of the sun occupying only a part of the plate, that from which the reflection of the incident solar rays comes. It is true that on account of the vividness of the light such an image would appear crowned with a much larger part of the plate than it really did. To verify this, one might note the exact place on the plate from which the reflection came, and likewise figuring how large the shining space appears, cover the major part of this space leaving only the middle revealed; the size of the apparent brilliance would not be a whit diminished, but it would be seen widely spread over the cloth or other material used for the covering. So if anyone, seeing from a distance a little gilded plate shining all over, should imagine that the same phenomenon would have to occur with a plate as large as the moon, he would be as much deceived as if he were to think that the moon is no larger than the bottom of a vine vat. (DIALOGO, p. 71; transl. 78–79, revised)[8]

It should be noted that even though this reasoning is justified for the case of the irradiation issuing from a torch or a candle, it is less so for a star or a planet. This is because in the case of stars and planets part of the irradiation is due to the diffraction of light by the earth's atmosphere, a phenomenon which is amplified by impurities in the air, whereas in the case of a close light source the effect of the interposed layer of air is much less pronounced.

It is to Galileo's great merit that, despite the many possible errors intrinsic to the procedure of his visual experiment, he succeeded in showing how previous measures of the stars (that had been accepted by astronomers of great authority) were greatly overestimated.

8.6 **A telescope-assisted visual experiment**

In the case of *Discorso* (as well as a similar discussion in *Saggiatore*), the central problem regarding adventitious irradiation was concerned mainly with telescopic observations. It is with reference to another telescope experiment that Galileo provided a further piece of evidence pointing to the small size of celestial bodies. The problem raised by Galileo's anonymous adversary (actually Horatio Grassi, the Jesuit who was also his opponent in the debate over *Saggiatore*; see Chapter 1) concerned the reason why the telescope, which was so powerful when magnifying the moon and the sun, seemed much less capable of magnifying the diameter of other planets,

---

[8] As we shall see in Chapter 14, Galileo's experiment correspond to one described by Giovanni Battista della Porta in his *De refractione* published in 1593.

and totally ineffective for the stars. Galileo's explanation was based on the idea that, while the telescope magnified the real external image of the object, it did not magnify the adventitious irradiation because this came mainly from inside the eye. Without entering into the details of his discussion with Grassi, we report here another of Galileo's important experiments supporting his idea that the apparent size of small luminous sources is grossly overestimated by the unaided eye. This experiment described in *Discorso delle comete* involves the phenomenon of light and dark adaptation. Galileo intuitively grasps the fundamental significance of this phenomenon in his astronomical observations, despite having no explicit and clear knowledge about it. The new experiments involve the most brilliant star in the sky, Sirius, referred to by Galileo/Guiducci as *Cane* and three of the most visible planets of the sun, Venus, Jupiter, and Saturn:

> In confirmation of what I am saying, let the telescope be fixed upon the Dog Star, for example, before dawn: it will not appear much larger than if seen without the telescope. Now let us follow it until the sun rises. We shall see it remain the same size through the telescope, but to the unaided eye it will seem gradually to diminish in such a way as to be seen smaller than the least visible of the night stars. And finally the sun rises, it will be made infinitely smaller and it will be completely lost; yet it will still be seen very well through the telescope, looking always the same. Venus, Jupiter and in sum all the stars observed though the instrument appear to us no larger by night than by day, yet the same stars seen with the naked eye are very large in the dark and very small in the lighted sky. This is a sure argument that that which is seen through the instrument is the pure object robbed of its alien rays. The same is deduced from its perfect and sharp figure, sometimes horned [*falcata*] in Venus, oval in Saturn, and circular in the other stars. (COMETE, pp. 28–29; transl. pp. 44–45)

With reference to a passage of the *Dialogue* on the different shape and size of Venus in daytime and at night, Galileo had more faith in observations made in daylight. This was based on the comparison with what happened with the shape and size of a flame seen at different distances and in different conditions of illumination. A similar type of argument is made in *Discorso delle comete* where the visibility of terrestrial light sources is invoked on several occasions to support arguments about celestial bodies.

As discussed in sections 8.1 and 8.2, among the relevant factors are the various optical aberrations of the eye (chromatic, spherical, astigmatic, and those due to the imperfect transparency of ocular media). These aberrations play a progressive role as the pupil size increases in response to the dimming of ambient light. As a consequence, the blur of the retinal image increases as the optical point spread function becomes broader, with a relative increase in peripheral light intensity. The increased light sensitivity due to the shift from cones to rods of the predominantly active photoreceptors (as well as other functional adaptations of the neural circuits of the retina) make the eye sensitive not only to the light of the central lobe corresponding to the main image of a luminous point, but also to the surrounding zones. This results in a substantial increase of the size of the perceived image. The actual dimensions of the perceived image depends on the luminance of the source, because the lateral spread of the light would produce an excitation of photoreceptors only if its intensity is sufficiently high for their activation. One of the consequences of the blur would be loss of detail of the shape of the luminous body (in the case of Venus it would appear spherical even when it is falciform due to its phases).

As the ambient light increases with the rising sun, the pupil diameter decreases, thereby reducing the effects of optical aberrations. Consequently, the image of a luminous point on the retina would become more precise, with a narrowing of its lateral extension. The shift from rods to cones would result in only the more central parts of the light distribution being effective in triggering a visual response. The consequence is a substantial reduction of the perceived size of a point source; in Galileo's case it can be assumed to be Sirius, whose true angular size is less the 6/1000 of a second of arc, a value largely below the resolution limit of both the naked eye and the telescope. With a larger, non-spherical luminous body, there would also be a better correspondence between the apparent and physical size.[9]

Telescopic observations would be less affected by the factors considered here. This is because of the larger size on the retina of the image of the point source and also because of the light capturing properties of the instrument (resulting in more light adaptation). The actual size and shape of the image on the retina would depend on the magnification of the telescope and the quality of its optics and also on the quantity of light that the telescope could capture. The physical aperture of the telescope is larger than that of the human pupil. As remarked in the *Discorso*, in the case of the telescopes used by Galileo the interplay of these factors resulted in a perceived size of a luminous point source only slightly larger than that seen with the naked eye. Moreover, because of the light collecting property of the telescope, the visibility of a very bright star like Sirius (indeed the brightest star in the sky with an astronomical magnitude now estimated to about −1.4, i.e. more than four times brighter than Vega) is likely to be due to light adaptation of the eye, irrespectively of the changes in the ambient illumination. This is probably the reason why the Dog Star was 'seen very well through the telescope, looking always the same' when observed both in the night and day.

In *Saggiatore* Galileo mentions an experiment similar to that on the Dog Star made by observing Jupiter during the night and day with both the naked eye and a powerful telescope. He writes:

> With the telescope, its disc will be seen as always of the same size, but as seen by the naked eye it will progressively shrink as the dawn brightens. Near sunrise Jupiter—which in the dark surpasses all the stars of the fifth magnitude—is reduced to a smaller appearance than a star of the fifth or sixth magnitude, and finally at sunrise it is reduced to an indivisible point and becomes completely lost. Yet after that it has disappeared to the naked eye, it continues to be seen through the telescope large and round all the day. (SAGGIATORE, pp. 219–220; transl. p. 326)

The telescope used in observing Jupiter was one capable of magnifying the surface of the object seen by about 600 or 1000 times (i.e. one having approximately 20 or 30 times linear magnification) and—according to Galileo—it caused the planet 'to swallow up its coiffure of rays, and makes it similar to the full moon'. With a comparable telescope this is what happened to the appearance of Sirius:

> But the very tiny disc of the Dog Star, though enlarged a thousand times by the telescope, cannot equal its irradiation size as to appear completely shorn. Yet since the rays near the outer edges are somewhat weak and separated, the disk is very easily seen amid the discontinuity of the rays. The more the telescope enlarges this, the more distinct and the less irradiated it appears. (p. 218; transl. p. 325)

It seems as if, with more powerful and improved telescopes, in 1623 Galileo was near to separating, in the case of Sirius, the central images of the stars from the surrounding annular illumination due to light diffraction and optical aberrations. It would seem that for Galileo there was nothing definitely peculiar about the stars as stars but simply the fact that they were tiny luminous

9 In exceptional circumstances, and particularly with a very clear atmosphere, people with extremely acute eyesight can almost see the falciform shape of the crescent of Venus. This is because the phase of thin crescent subtends a visual angle of about 60″, a value not very far from the resolution limits of particularly good eyes.

visual objects. As he remarks in *Saggiatore*, essentially similar visual phenomena would occur with any terrestrial object seen under conditions making it appear as a minute shining body:

> For candles shine, and blazing torches seen from distance, and any small pebbles, and bit of wood or other small bodies [*qualunque sassetto, legnuzzo o altro piccolo corpicello*], and even the leaves of plants or drops of dew struck by the sun; and from certain viewpoints these are irradiated as much as the most refulgent star, and when seen through the telescope they show the same type of enlargement [*tenore*] that stars do. (p. 86; transl. pp. 230–231)

8.7 Driving a car in the night with Galileo's thoughts

If Galileo were to live in modern times, it could easily be surmised that he would find other examples, besides candle flames, as analogies to the problem of the visual appearance of stars. Suppose, for instance, that we are driving during the night on a relatively solitary country road and Galileo is seated by us. All is dark until a car approaches with its headlights appearing initially as small light sources shining. Surely our companion would direct our attention to the appearance of the light, and especially to the adventitious rays spreading in all directions from the light bulbs, and varying in their extension and directions as we move our eyes and/or the car approaches. Perhaps he will ask us to stop for just a little, while the car is still distant and take a pencil or a small screwdriver to show how completely that broad brilliance is obliterated when the object hides the head lights. Perhaps he would also remark that our pupil is wide when looking at the distant headlights.[10] As the car approaches the brightness of the headlight increases and can even become somewhat disturbing, until it is at few tens of metres from us. If we, and the other driver, do not proceed at fast speed, we will have the time to notice a rather unexpected phenomenon.

Rather suddenly, at the moment we can see the headlights distinctly we will realize that the irradiation appears to decrease substantially. Galileo would remark then that we would still see a glare around the headlamps, but this is clearly less luminous than the light issuing directly from the bulbs, and that it is clearly distinguishable from the image of the main light sources. Perhaps he would also tell us that our pupils became narrower while looking at the headlights while nearer to them. If we doubted him he would ask us to stop the car and demonstrate what happens if we look at the headlamps of our car by alternatively turning the lights on and off.

Surely he would use particularly colourful expressions to describe the phenomenon by which, when seen from near, lights are stripped of their adventitious rays, or are sheared of their luminous covers as luminous lambs, or swallow their shining coiffure. And surely he would tell us, somewhat proudly, that he can do the same with the stars and planets, simply by looking at them with the new glass that he invented (or at least considerably improved) 'some years ago'.

The problem of irradiation surrounding a light source is amply discussed by Galileo in *Saggiatore* with reference to both celestial bodies and terrestrial lights. In particular, in chapter 49 he differentiates between a fainter and ampler irradiation belonging to the illumination of the air surrounding light sources (and easy to distinguish perceptually from the main light source, even with the unaided eye), and a more intense and more restricted luminosity, indistinguishable from

[10] The phenomenon of the constriction and dilatation of the pupil with changes of ambient light is considered by Salviati and Sagredo in the *Dialogue* in the context of the discussion of the visibility of stars (DIALOGO, p. 355; transl. p. 363). Galileo was well aware of it because it had been thoroughly studied in the circle of his friend Paolo Sarpi, and by Fabricius ab Aquapendente, his colleague at the University of Padua, and also his physician. (See Chapter 13.)

the light source when this is viewed from a distance. The telescope could help in separating visually this second irradiation from the main image of the light source, an effect that Galileo denotes metaphorically as 'to undress', 'to strip out', 'to shear'.

It is, of course, a fiction to place Galileo in a modern automobile but it is not very far from truth, inasmuch as every moment of ordinary life provided the opportunity for Galileo to exercise his 'acute' vision. Indeed the experience of the car headlights at night presents us with a way to appreciate how Galileo succeeded in reducing the estimated size of stars and thus strongly contributed to make more plausible the universe of Copernicus.

8.8 New Jesuit assaults and the disruption of the eighth orb

The importance of the discussion on the apparent size of the fixed stars with reference to the cosmological and mathematical plausibility of the Copernican system has been remarked upon. With relatively simple visual experiments, Galileo had succeeded in demonstrating that the angular size of the stars was much smaller than previously supposed. This enabled him to defend the heliocentric system from criticisms of the conservative cultural milieu, and from Jesuits who had fully endorsed the anti-Copernican politics of the Vatican authorities, especially after the official censure of Copernicus by the Holy Office in 1616.

The pro-Copernican aspect of the new-found dimensions of the stars, derived from the cord experiment, is clearly expressed in the *Dialogue* through the words of Salviati, in refuting the anti-Copernican arguments of Scheiner and Locher. It is also asserted in others texts by Galileo dealing with the relationship between the size of the Great orb and of the sphere of the fixed stars (as, for instance, a long letter addressed in 1624 to Francesco Ingoli: OG VI, pp. 502–561; see also the legend to Figure 8.5).

As noted in Chapter 7, the Catholic Church was obliged to abandon the traditional cosmology of Ptolemy and was inclined to endorse the system of Tycho Brahe against that of Copernicus. After the death of Galileo, this project was pursued by Giovanni Riccioli with his *Almagestum novum*, published in 1651, i.e. less than 10 years after Galileo died. The importance of the angular sizes of stars as support for Copernicus makes it little wonder that in his monumental work Riccioli questioned the validity of Galileo's method in measuring the size of stars. Indeed the basis of his own measurements, the Jesuit proposed substantially larger values than those of the Tuscan scholar (although not as large as those of Tycho Brahe and his followers). For instance, Riccioli concluded that Sirius had a diameter of 18″ and Arcturus a little less than 17″, based on his observations, made in collaboration with Grimaldi and some other brothers. The method used by Riccioli and Grimaldi was a telescopic comparison of the apparent diameter of the star with those of other celestial bodies (like Saturn and Jupiter). Unlike Galileo's method, it did not involve a procedure of occultation. Because of that, it suffered from the errors that Galileo had pointed out repeatedly. The values found by Riccioli and Grimaldi were smaller than those of Tycho only because of the use of a telescope (and one surely improved with respect to that of Galileo). Due to these smaller estimates, Riccioli was obliged to assume a value of the radius of the sphere of the fixed star much greater than those accepted by previous authors (210,000 times the radius of the earth instead than the 20,110 of al-Ferghani and that of 14,000 of Brahe). This made the Copernican hypothesis a little less absurd than Scheiner's and Locher's assertions about it 40 years earlier.

Despite Galileo's experimental and logical efforts to account for the presumed absurdities of the Copernican system with respect to the distance of the fixed stars, he was far from trusting the existence of the sphere of fixed stars. In other words, he did not believe that the stars were all at approximately the same distance from earth. This emerges in the letter addressed in 1624 to Francesco Ingoli, a stubborn adversary of the Copernican system. In the well-established astronomical tradition, Ingoli had asserted (in 1616) the necessity of locating the earth at the centre of the universe, i.e. at the centre of the eighth sphere or firmament. This was also because during their supposed revolution around the earth, the stars always appear the same size, which would be impossible if they were not moving together along a circular orbit centred on the earth. This is Galileo's refutation of Ingoli's argument:

> Let us come to the second [argument] by which you pretend, together with Sacrobosco, to be capable of demonstrating that the earth is at the centre of the firmament, because the fixed stars, situated in whatever part of the sky, always appear to us the same size. I tell you that it lacks not only one, but all the conditions needed for a correct conclusion. First, you suppose that the stars of the firmament are all in the same orb: *this is so doubtful to be known, that neither you nor others would ever be capable of demonstrating it.* (OG VI, p. 523, our emphasis)

In another passage, Galileo deals with the orbits of the satellites of Jupiter that he had discovered with his telescope. The existence of satellites which rotate around a globe different from the earth made less cogent one of the fundamental assumptions of the Ptolemaic system—the need to have an absolute centre of the universe. This centre was both the site around which all satellites and stars rotated and also an absolute reference point. In this context Galileo remarked:

> If it would then be necessary to assign to the totality of the stars an inferior site, that is a centre, and superior one, that is toward the external parts, this is doubtful to determine; in the [existing] ambiguity it seems to me more reasonable to assume that it is no rather than yes, because (as I have already said) *I do not believe that the stars are placed all on a spherical surface, such that they would be equally distant from a given point.* (p. 536, our emphasis)

These two passages make clear that Galileo did not trust the existence of a sphere of the fixed stars, nor that those stars (either fixed, or freely moving), were at one and the same distance from the earth. A criticism of the fixed-stars orb conception is developed in the Second Day of the *Dialogue* in the context of a general censure of the Ptolemaic system. Galileo, was not, however, too explicit in such type of assertions.[11] This was likely because it implied the possibility of an infinite universe, with a plurality of worlds and without an absolute centre. Such statements had physical and religious dimensions and were considered heretical by the Catholic Church. A similar conception had been one of the imputations addressed to Giordano Bruno and a justification for his condemnation by the tribunal directed by Cardinal Roberto Bellarmino which was followed by his execution by burning at the stake in Rome in 1600.

In Galileo's age, the idea of the existence of an eighth orb, although strongly asserted by the conservative milieu and by Jesuits, was already being questioned, particularly after the various observations that had made the idea of the existence in the sky of solid orbs problematic. Independently of Bruno, criticism of the existence of the eight spheres was particularly strong among British Copernicans. The first cosmological image of a universe with stars spreading outwards, towards a potentially infinite space was published in an English text by Thomas Digges; he was an important astronomer and mathematician, the son of Leonard Digges who was also an astronomer (and astrologer). This image was inserted by Thomas Digges as an appendix to an astrological work by his father, having an impressively long title beginning with *A Prognostication euerlasting of right good effect....* Thomas's appendix, also with a long title and a strong Elizabethan style, *A Perfit*

[11] A short and somewhat ironical allusion to the problem of the infinity of Universe is contained in a letter addressed by Galileo to Fortunio Liceti on 20 September 1639 (OG XVIII, pp. 106–107).

Description of the Cœlestiall Orbes according to the most aunciente doctrine of the Phythagoreans, latelye reuiued by Copernicus and by Geometricall Demonstrations approued, appeared starting from the 1576 edition of Leonard's *Prognostication*. Interestingly, as seen in the text referring to the disrupted sphere of 'starres fixed' written by Thomas, and reported in the legend to Figure 8.8, the modernity

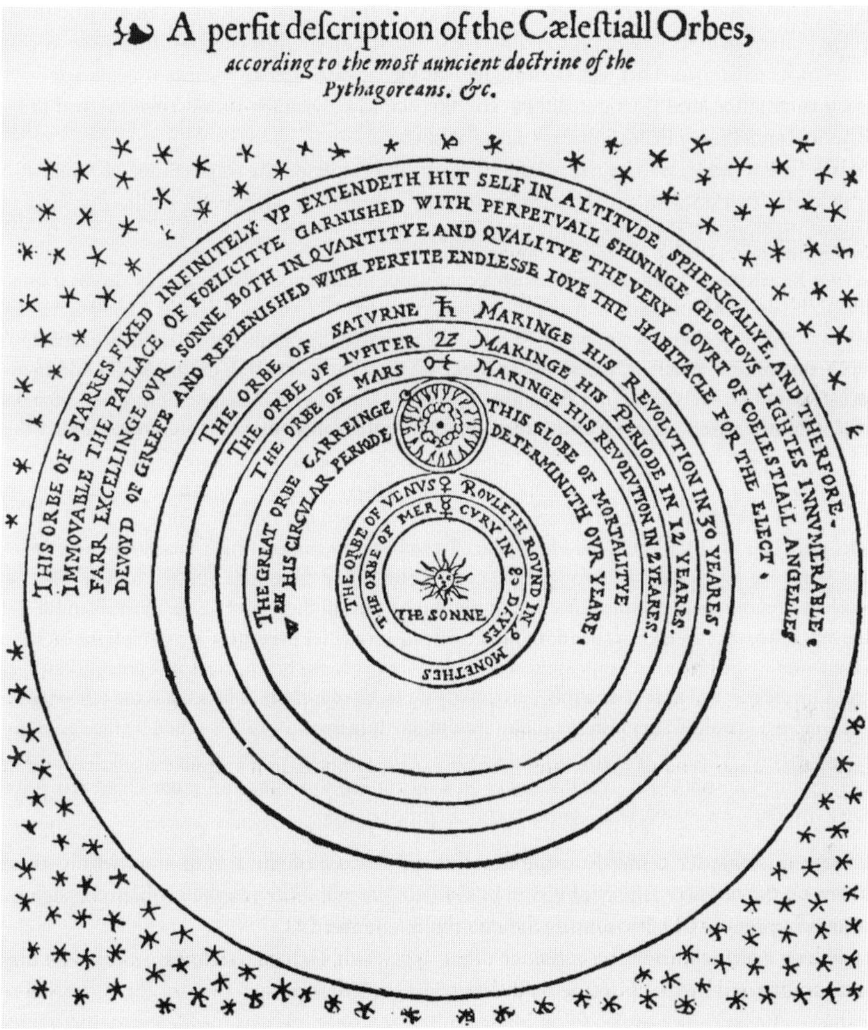

Figure 8.8 The first published image with a representation of the Copernican system based on the idea that stars spread in the far regions of the cosmos at variable distances from the sun, without being inserted in a specific orb. The text referring to the stars reads as follows: 'This orbe of starres fixed infinitely up extendeth hit self in altitvde sphericallye, and therefore immovable the pallace of foelicitye garnished with the perpetvall shininge gloriovs lightes innvmerable farr excellinge ovr sonne both in qvantitye and qvalitye the very covrt of coelestiall angelles devoyd of greefe and replenished with perfite endlesse ioye the habitacle for the elect'. Reproduced from Digges, L. and Digges, T., *A prognostication euerlasting of right good effect fruitfully augmented by the auctor, contayning plaine, brief, pleasaunt, chosen rules to iudge the weather by the sunne, moone, starres, cometes, rainebow, thunder, cloudes*, 1576, Aldbrough, St John Publications.

of Digges's ideas went along with a religious attitude with strong implications of an esoteric and astronomical character.

8.9 The monkey and the mirror

Galileo did not believe that there were sound physical and logical arguments to assume the existence of a sphere of fixed stars. Nor did he trust his sensory impressions sufficiently to provide evidence of its existence. This was because he was well aware that all remote objects appear to be at the same distance, and thus the stars in the sky would be visually located on one and the same hypothetical sphere, regardless of their actual distance.

Horatio Grassi (addressed by the pseudonym of Sarsi) stressed the importance of visual appearances in order to establish the physical nature of comets. In *Saggiatore*, Galileo replied to his adversary (through Virginio Cesarini) in this way:

> As your Excellency will note, Sarsi has such a confidence in the sense of sight that he deems it impossible to be deceived any time that a spurious object may be set aside a real one. I confess that I do not have such a perfect discriminatory faculty, but resemble the monkey that firmly believed he saw another monkey in a mirror, and so live and real did the image seem to him that he did not discover his error until he had run behind the mirror four or six times to catch her. Assuming that what Sarsi sees in his own mirror are not true and real men at all, but are mere images [*vani simulacra*] like those the rest of us see in ours, I should like to know what those visual differences are by which he so readily distinguishes the true from the spurious. For my part, I have countless times been in one room with closed shutters and have seen on the opposite wall the reflection of sunlight coming through some tiny hole, and as far as vision could tell I have judged it to be a star, no less bright than Venus and the Dog Star. When we walk over a field toward the sun, in how many thousands of straw and pebbles, little polished or moistened, will the reflection of the sun be seen in the aspect of the most splendid stars? Sarsi has but to spit upon the ground, and undoubtedly he will see the aspect of a natural star from that point toward which the sun's rays are reflected. Furthermore, any body placed at a great distance and struck by the sun will appear as a star, particularly if placed so high as to be seen as the other stars are seen. And who could distinguish the moon seen in daytime from a cloud touched by the sun? Surely, no one. Finally, if simple appearances can determine the essence of a thing, Sarsi must grant that the suns, moons, and stars seen in still water or in a mirror are true suns, real moons, and actual stars. (SAGGIATORE, pp. 89–90; transl. pp. 232–233, slightly revised)

We close this chapter centred on the illusory appearance of the size of stars with this strong statement on the possible fallacy of vision by Galileo. We will return to the problem of seeing stars in the last chapters of our book, and particularly in Chapter 14.

In Chapter 9 we will move to consider other aspects of Galileo's reflection on visual appearances, characterized by more decidedly geometrical considerations.

Chapter 9

Heavens sensed

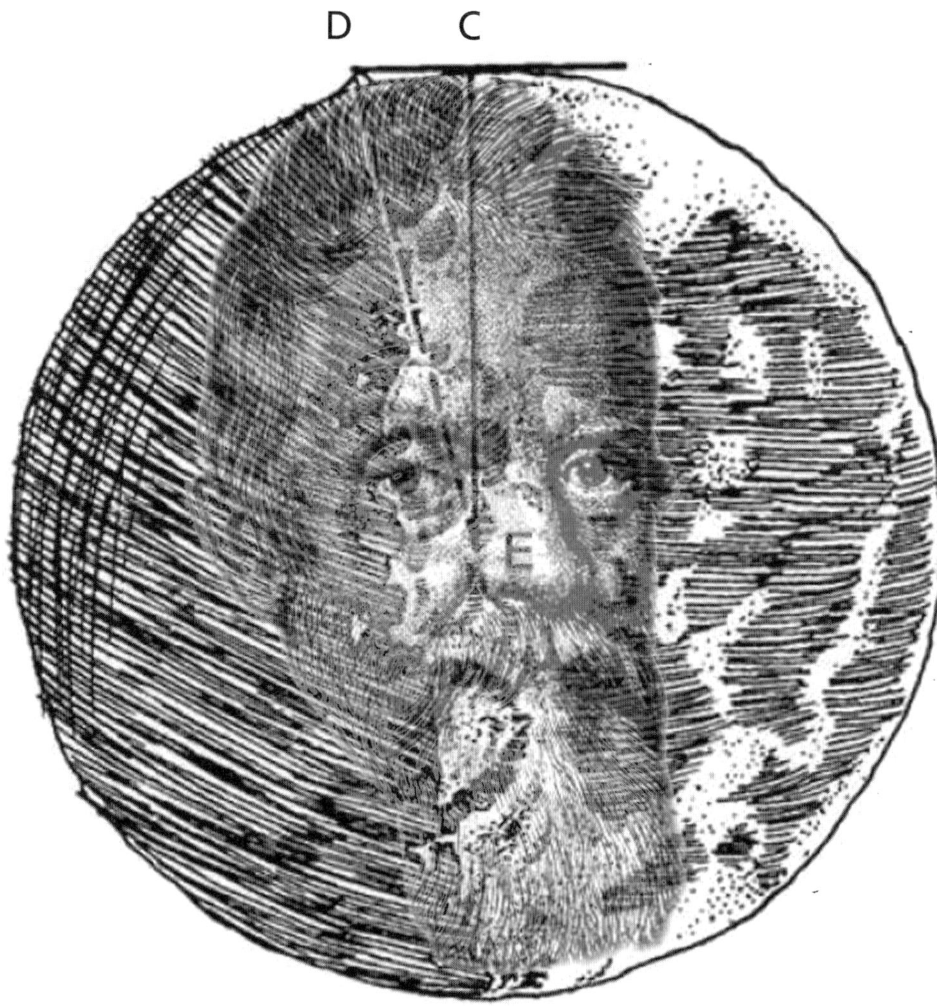

Figure IX *Measuring the lunar mountains* by Nicholas Wade. The height of the peaks of the moon could be estimated by Galileo (shown in a portrait derived from an engraving by Ottavio Leoni) following the scheme described in *Sidereus nuncius*.

In the previous chapters we have addressed Galileo's great interest in the senses (particularly vision) and have remarked on his emphasis on their possible unreliability (or decided fallacies). This is encountered in many passages in *Sidereus nuncius*, *Saggiatore*, and the *Dialogue* as well as in his letters on sunspots, the *Discorso delle comete*, and a number of booklets and private letters. To examine all these materials in an exhaustive way would require many more pages of our book, and we prefer to leave the interested reader to examine these texts in order to verify personally the importance of Galileo's concern with vision in the framework of his global scientific and intellectual approach.

9.1 Surveyors of the skies

In our analysis of Galileo's writings on the senses we have emphasized phenomena that would be considered as belonging to visual psychophysiology or psychophysics. Examples include spatial contrast, chiaroscuro and shadowing, the visual appearance of luminous spots, and the mechanisms of light reflection.

Much less attention has been paid to another important facet of Galileo's interests in vision—one involving geometry and perspective. The main reason for our choice is that this second aspect engages approaches that were more common in the research of astronomers and mathematicians of his age, and thus its presence in Galileo's work does not connote it in a specifically visual way. Moreover, it would have obliged us to expound several geometrical and astronomical technicalities that we considered beyond the scope and especially the style of our book. Among Galileo's writings there are texts like the letters on sunspots where the geometrical-perspective reasoning has a fundamental relevance, being at the heart of Galileo's attempt to show that the spots seen with the telescope are on the surface of the sun or very close to it, and not—as maintained by Scheiner—in the cosmic space surrounding the sun. Despite the acuteness and precision of Galileo's observations and conclusions in this context, and notwithstanding the remote location of the heavenly targets, in this respect the localization of sunspots belongs to a somewhat ordinary surveyor approach. One similar to that of military engineer or surveyor charged with measuring the distance and the position of an unreachable enemy fortress.

This said, there are at least two aspects of Galileo's use of geometrical perspective that are worth considering here. One concerns a particular facet of the discussion dealing with the trajectory of comets (and also of the apparent movement of new stars) in which Galileo was involved, particularly after the publication by Horatio Grassi of a pamphlet on the three comets which appeared in 1618 (Figure 9.1). Another is evident in the discussion on the mountainous nature of the moon (although—as seen in Chapter 6—this was dominated by visual considerations like those concerning the play of shadows and light and the adventitious rays). In this context, Galileo's method for measuring the height of lunar mountains drew upon geometrical perspective. Although, as in the case of localizing sunspots, the technique was based on methods of trigonometry similar to those used by surveyors, nevertheless, it is worth considering it in some detail. This is because of the remarkable effectiveness of the method: the measurement of the height of lunar mountains turned out to be considerably more precise than that for mountains on earth. It is also because of its historical importance in adding a new note to the process by which humans were determining aspects of celestial bodies, thereby making them progressively more similar to earth.

Before considering these two particular instances of Galileo's geometrical perspective, a problem already mentioned in Chapter 2 should be noted. That is, the presumed asymmetry of the vault of the heavens invoked by Jacopo Mazzoni against the Copernican doctrine. Galileo addressed

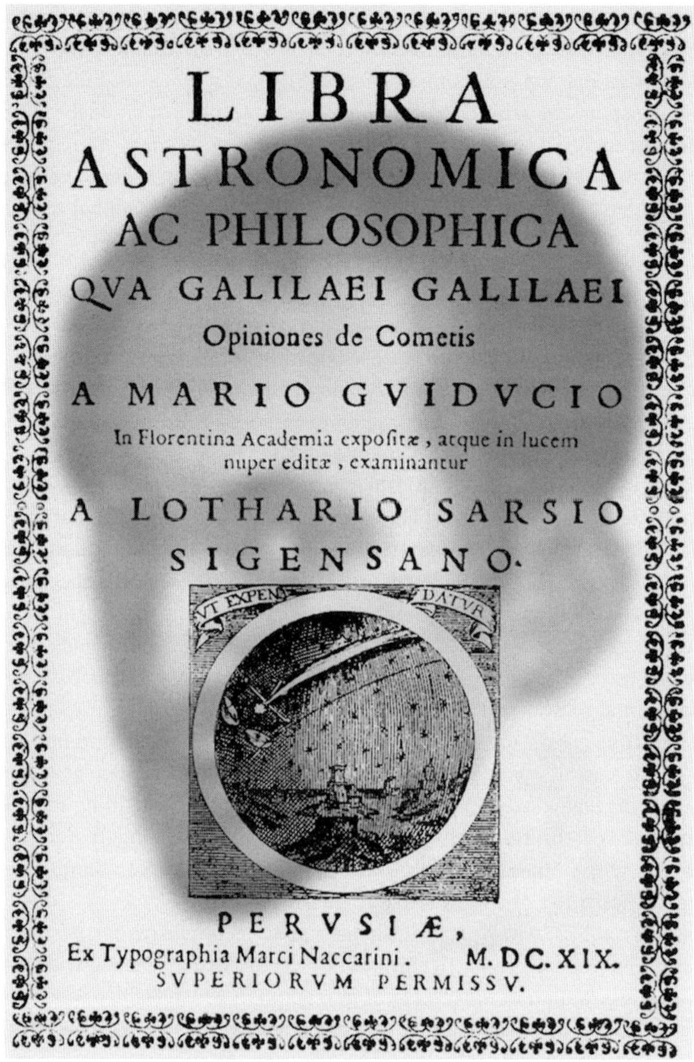

Figure 9.1 *Horatio Sarsi!* by Nicholas Wade. The shadowy presence of Horatio Grassi hovers behind the title page of *Libra Astronomica* written under the pseudonym Lothario Sarsi.

this problem in his 1597 letter to his former teacher; this seems to be Galileo's first writing dealing with vision in a geometrical manner.

9.2 **Ascending comets and straight lines through the skies**

Galileo's interest in comets was stimulated by a text published in 1619 by Horatio Grassi. It appeared in print in the anonymous form of a *Disputatio* on the three comets of the year 1618 held in the Roman College by 'one of the fathers' of the Society of Jesus (*De tribus cometis anni M.DC.XVIII.: Disputatio astronomica publice habita in Collegio romano Societatis Iesu ab uno ex Patribus eiusdem Societatis*). Grassi's authorship was, however, easily identifiable (Grassi, 1619b).

Stimulated by members of his intellectual entourage, Galileo replied to Grassi with the *Discorso delle comete*, written in collaboration with his pupil Mario Guiducci (see Figure 8.7) and delivered by Guiducci at the Accademia Fiorentina in May 1619.[1] The *Discorso* was at the origin of the controversy on comets between Galileo and Grassi which would last for several years and would include, on Galileo's side, one of his most important works, *Saggiatore*. In the previous chapters, we have already mentioned several passages from both *Discorso* and *Saggiatore* that are of particular visual relevance, and both texts can be considered as treatises on vision applied to astronomical observations. They contain discussions on some of Galileo's most typical visual themes, and particularly those on diffuse reflection and the visual appearances of stars and planets. They also feature some of Galileo's real or virtual experiments on vision. As already mentioned in Chapter 1 with reference to the reflection of sunlight on the sea at sunset, the theme of the mechanism of visual reflections is particularly well developed in *Saggiatore*. This is mainly because Galileo attributed most of the appearance of comets to a particular type of diffuse reflection—that occurring when sun light shines over a vaporous mass.

The theory to account for the aspect and trajectory of the comets of 1618 expounded in *Discorso* and *Saggiatore* has an important liaison with his interest in the new star of 1604. As already mentioned in Chapter 2, this extraordinary phenomenon represented the first occasion for Galileo's involvement in a public debate on astronomical issues. This occurred during three lectures held at the University of Padua, of which we have a few fragments containing some important observations and annotations. The new star was also at the origin of two pseudonymous Galilean texts published in 1605 and 1606, the already mentioned *Cecco de Ronchitti* and *Alimberto Mauri* (Figure 9.2). In the case of the discussion on the new star, one of the visual problems considered was concerned with geometrical perspective. It is not by chance that the peasant Cecco de Ronchitti, the protagonist of the homonymous work written in *pavano*, the dialect of Padua, was a land surveyor. Speaking with his friend Natale about mathematicians, he says: 'It's the Mathematicians you've got to believe. They are surveyors of empty air, just like I survey fields and can rightly tell you how long they are, and how wide. Just so can they' (RONCHITTI, F4v; transl. p. 38).[2]

In the case of the new star the absence of detectable parallax pointed to its location high in the vault of the heavens, a feature in disagreement with the Aristotelian conception of the immutability of the skies. Galileo's interpretation of the phenomenon was that it was not a true star, but a terrestrial exhalation ascending towards the skies along a rectilinear trajectory perpendicular to the earth's surface which had reached a considerable distance from the earth. Even though in evident contrast with the Aristotelian theory of the impenetrability of the skies, this conception was in line with the astronomical novelties that, starting mainly from the second half of the previous century, had pointed to a fluidity of cosmic matter. This had emerged particularly after parallax was being customarily applied to the observation of comets and other celestial novelties, starting particularly from the careful study of the new star of 1572 carried out by Tycho Brahe. Due to their unconventional trajectories, and because of their high location in the skies, comets would have broken the orbs of heavens in their celestial movement, were these orbs made of a

---

1 Although in the Bibliographic Abbreviations and References we mention both Galileo and Guiducci as author of the text, for the purpose of narration we assume Galileo's exclusive authorship of the *Discorso delle comete*; this assumption is amply justified by the available manuscripts.

2 *El bisogna credere a gi smetamatichi, que gi è pertegaore de l'aire, secondo, che an mi a pertego le campagne, e si a posso dire, a rason, quanto le xè longhe, e larghe, e così an iggi.*

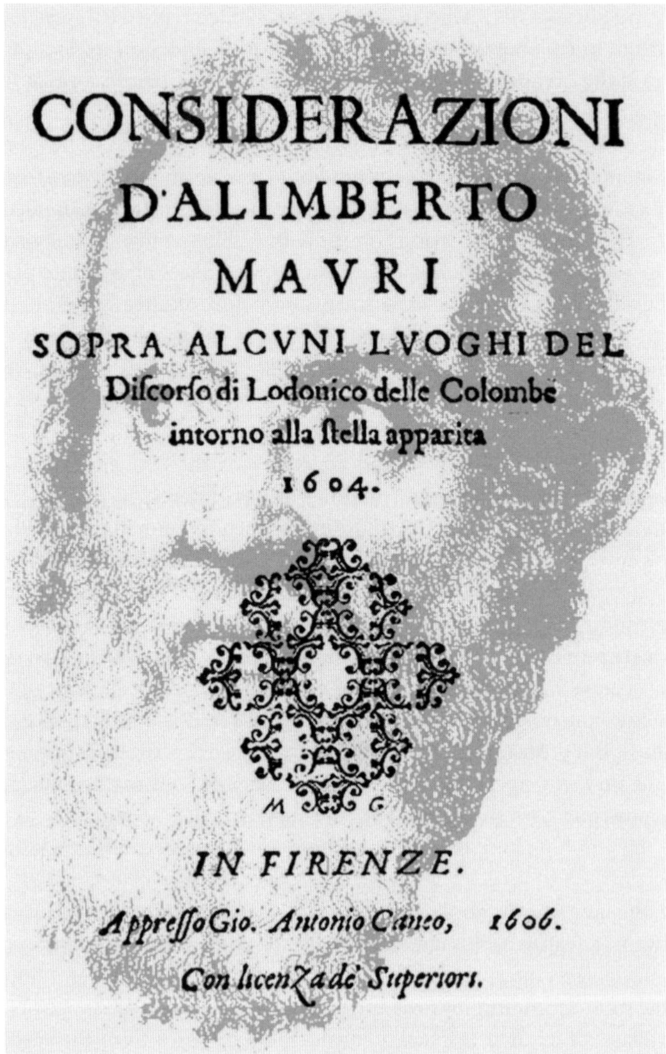

Figure 9.2 *Galileo-Mauri* by Nicholas Wade. Galileo's portrait is derived from an engraving in Bethune (1829) and is shown hiding behind the title page of *Considerazioni d'Alimberto Mauri* (1606).

solid matter. Moreover, since the middle of the sixteenth century, the study of the effect of optical refraction on the appearance of the celestial bodies initiated by Peter Ramus (Pierre de la Ramée) and Jean Pena greatly contributed to undermine the faith in the existence of crystalline orbs.

Within the framework of the new conception of fluid skies, the idea that planets were moving freely in the cosmic spaces 'like birds in the sky, or fish in the sea' was being substituted to that of their movement with their respective solid sphere 'like knots in a wooden board'. As we shall see in Chapter 10, the idea of continuity of universe was also congenial to Galileo's general atomistic conception of matter which led him to assume that the various terrestrial and celestial spheres corresponded simply to different degrees of expansion of the same primordial particles.

It is within this cosmological context that Galileo formulated his theory of a terrestrial exhalation ascending perpendicularly towards the sky in order to account for the appearance of the new star of 1604. Because of its high location in the heavens, this exhalation would be capable of reflecting sunrays and shine even in the middle of the night, in contrast to what happened for more ordinary terrestrial exaltations like clouds, fog, rainbows, or smoke. This idea had a very long ancestry being rooted in the conceptions expounded in the fifth century BC by the Greek philosopher Xenophanes of Colophon. In the more recent past, the idea of terrestrial exhalations had been invoked by various scholars to account for the appearance of comets and the new star of 1572. Among them were John Dee and Thomas Digges in England, Cornelius Gemma in Belgium, and Elias Camerarius in Germany.

Many years later, in the *Discorso delle comete*, Galileo would return to his theory of ascending terrestrial exhalations in order to account for the visibility and motion of the three impressive comets that appeared between August and December 1618. This was to refute the theory of comets expounded by Horatio Grassi in his *Disputatio*. Following Tycho Brahe, whose cosmological conception was endorsed by the Society of Jesus after the condemnation of Copernicus by the Vatican authorities, Grassi aimed at demonstrating that the 1618 comets moved in the sky along circular orbits like planets. To this purpose he made reference to a method of cartographic representation of the sky on a planar surface endorsed by Grienberger in 1612 in his Catalogue of old and new stars (see Chapter 6). This was the so-called gnomonic projection largely based on the studies of Clavius; both Clavius and Grienberger had been Grassi's predecessors as mathematicians at the Roman College. In the astronomic usage of the gnomonic projection, the centre of the world is assumed as projection centre of the cartographic representation, and the position of stars and planets are projected on a planar surface tangentially to the sky sphere on the specifically selected point. In this way the great circles of the celestial sphere passing through that point are displayed on the projection surface as straight lines. This is because the orthogonal intersection between two planar surfaces is always a straight line (Figure 9.3).

In the gnomonic projection, deformations are minimal around the tangent point of the sphere with the projection plane, and become progressively more important as the distance from this point increases. The utility of the method in astronomy is also due to the fact that the gnomonic representation corresponds to the perceptual data for an observer located at the centre of the sky's sphere. This is because there is an absolute identity between the lines of sight of the observer and the lines used for the projection of the sphere onto the projection surface. Since there is nothing in physical reality corresponding closely to a sky sphere (which is exclusively based on a perceptual phenomenon), any observer looking to the vault of the heavens would always feel to be at its very centre, irrespective of his actual location (see Chapter 2).

The importance attributed by Grassi and the Jesuits of the College to this type of projection was emphasized by the magnificent plate used in the *Disputatio* to illustrate the motion of the comet according to this method of projection (Figure 9.4).

In the study of the 1618 comet Grassi looked for evidence supporting the cosmological theory of Tycho Brahe, as a better option to Copernicanism which had been condemned by the Catholic Church in 1616. Following the Danish astronomer who had proposed that, similar to planets, the comet of 1577 moved along a great circle of the sky vault, Grassi wished to demonstrate that the comets also followed a similar path in the skies. He was convinced that he could conclude this if he was able to demonstrate that the gnomonic projection of the 1618 comet trajectory corresponded to a straight line. This was indeed what appeared from the plate attached to the *Disputatio* (Figure 9.4) and it seemed thus unavoidable to conclude that the trajectory of the comet followed the predictions of the Tychonic system.

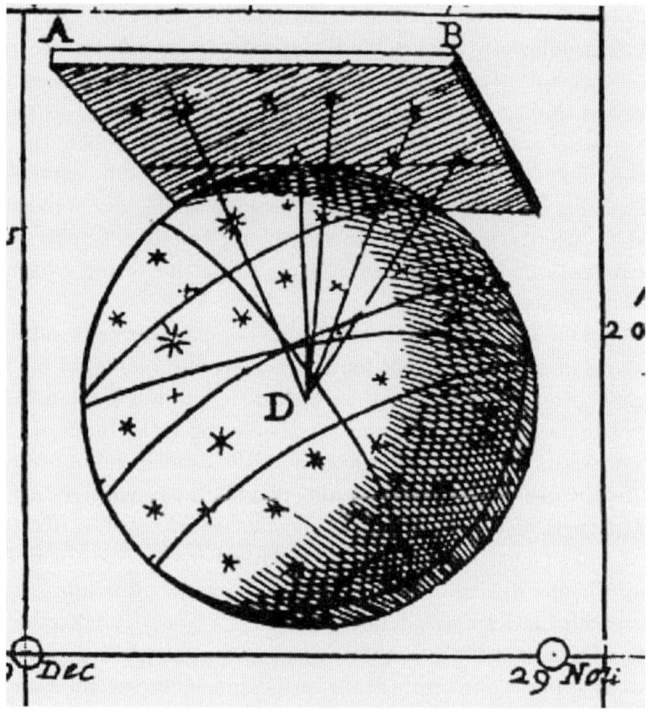

Figure 9.3 The image used by Grassi in his *Disputatio* to illustrate the technique of gnomonic projection. The celestial meridian passing through the point of contact of the projection plane and the sphere of the sky appear as a straight line on the gnomonic representation.

Grassi's conclusion seemed perhaps unavoidable but certainly lacked caution. While it is true that the gnomonic projection of great circles of the celestial sphere always results in straight lines, the reciprocal is not necessarily correct. In the *Discorso* Galileo pointed out the fact that Grassi's reasoning could be justified if the only distinction to be made was between great circles and other circles of the sky sphere, as for instance the celestial parallels (the only minor circles actually considered by the Jesuit as possible alternative to the great circles). If, however, one admitted the possibility that the comet would move in the three-dimensional space in a more free way, outside the strict limits assigned by Grassi, then the equation 'straight projection = trajectory along a great circle' did not hold.

After having objected that in the conditions considered by Grassi 'to the observer, two sorts of motion appear straight: those which really are straight, and those circular motions which are made along great circles', the author of the *Discorso* remarked:

> When I am saying this I am speaking only of simple motions; speaking generally, all movements made within a given plane would appear to be along a straight line to an eye situated in the same plane. Thus, whoever wanted to prove faultlessly that the movement of a comet was along a great circle would be under the necessity of proving first that it was not really and inherently along a straight line, which has not been done and which would perhaps not be easy to do. (COMETE, p. 36; transl. pp. 50–51)

The argument by which Galileo refuted the conclusion of the Jesuit on the motion of comets has to do with the intrinsic ambiguity of representing a three-dimensional element on a

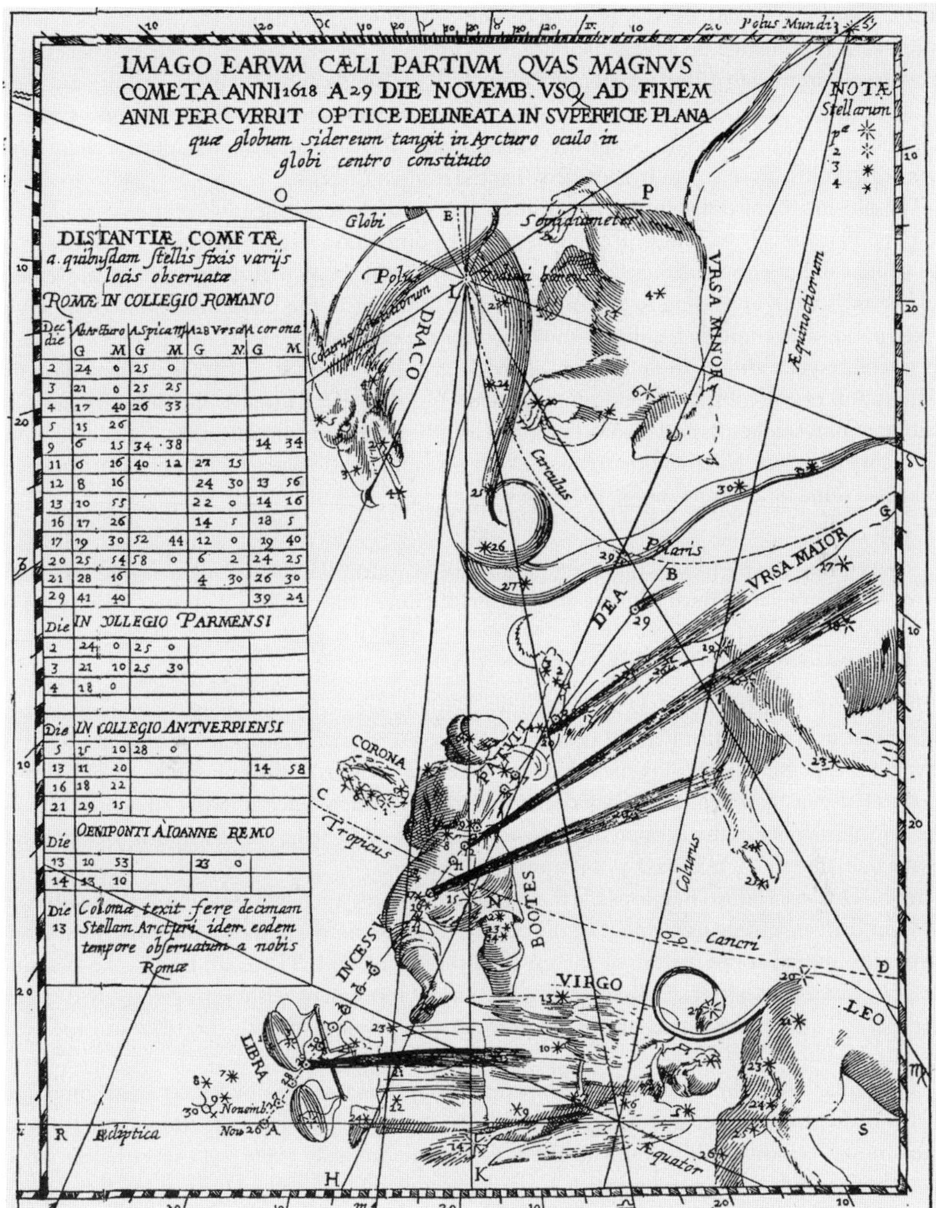

Figure 9.4 A detail of the plate from Grassi's *Disputatio* featuring the trajectory of one of the 1618 comets. The trajectory is represented by the straight line going from *H* towards the *Polus Mundi* (the north pole of the sky sphere). In the baroque allegory of Grassi's language, the trajectory bears the inscription, derived from Virgil, '*incessu patuit Dea*' (in her gait the Goddess reveals herself).

two-dimensional planar surface. If, given certain conditions, a particular three-dimensional feature can be represented on a planar surface in an unequivocal way, the opposite is not necessarily true. In an unrestricted three-dimensional space, a multitude (potentially an infinite number) of shapes could correspond to a given two-dimensional representation. In the *Discorso* Grassi is accused of 'an imperfect logic' because he has not taken into account that possibility. A charge that was indeed difficult to accept by a professor at the Roman College!

The allusion to the possibility that rectilinear movement seen on the vault of the sky could correspond to genuinely rectilinear trajectories in three-dimensional space is used to introduce what we could call the *pars construens* of the *Discorso*. That is the idea that the rectilinear movement on the sky's vault appearing to the observer, and recorded in the gnomonic projection, might correspond to a genuinely rectilinear movement of the comet in space. This hypothesis, which is in several respects similar to that proposed by Galileo for the new star of 1604, was based on the assumption of a rectilinear ascending movement, from the earth towards the sidereal spaces, of 'sublimations, smokes, vapors, exhalations, and all other thin and light materials'. Galileo develops his theory of comets with relation to the idea of a substantial homogeneity between earth and sky, as he had done for the new star of 1604. He writes:

> Never having given any place in my thoughts to that vain distinction (or rather contradiction) between the elements[3] and the heavens, there is for me no qualm or difficulty about the idea that the material of which a comet is formed having sometimes invaded these nether regions of ours, and being sublimated here, having surmounted the air or whatever else it is that it is diffused throughout the immense reaches of the universe. (COMETE, p. 39; transl. p. 53)

As happened for the new star of 1604, it was with an explicitly anti-Aristotelian (and cryptically pro-Copernican) attitude that Galileo alluded to the idea of homogeneity between earth and sky and to a possible ascending movement of terrestrial matter. In the opinion he would express in the *Dialogue*, these materials 'may rise as they please without encountering any obstacle from the impenetrability of the Peripatetic heavens, which I hold to be far more tenuous, yielding, and subtle than our air' (DIALOGO, p. 44; transl. p. 52).

In the *Discorso* Galileo develops his theory on the basis of a scheme showing that a rectilinear and uniform ascending movement of the comets ('a most simple and equable movement along a straight line from the surface of the earth to the sky': COMETE, p. 40; transl. p. 54) would be perceived by a terrestrial observer as a rectilinear movement with a progressively decreasing speed. This corresponded nicely to the observational data of both the 1577 and the 1618 comets.

This explanation, similar to that developed at about the same time by Kepler (and some time earlier by Kepler's teacher in Tubingen, Maestlin), although attractive in its simplicity, is—as we know now—erroneous. It belongs to the series of intellectually acute, but nevertheless incorrect, theories by Galileo among which is particularly notable his hypothesis of sea tides amply expounded in the *Dialogue*.

9.3 **Copernican ambiguities**

Towards the conclusion of the *Discorso delle comete* Galileo develops a consideration pointing to his Copernican option, although he does it in the veiled manner to which he was obliged after the

---

[3] Meaning the sublunary world which, as we know, was supposed to be made of the four elements (earth, water, fire, and air) as opposed to the composition of the heavens based on the ether or quintessence.

condemnation of Copernicanism. This represents a fundamental passage of the *Discorso*, which is at the heart of the argument around which all the text is built. Galileo says:

> I shall not pretend here to dissimulate that I know that if the material in which the comet takes form has only a movement straight and perpendicular to the earth surface (that is, from the center toward the sky), the comet should appear to be directed exactly toward the zenith; yet it did not appear so, but declined toward the north. This forces us either to change what has been said until now or else to retain that, but to add some other cause for this apparent deviation. I cannot do the one, nor I should dare to do the other. (COMETE, p. 44; transl. p. 57, revised)

Galileo's reference to the comet having 'declined toward the north' concerns the fact—noticed by many astronomers and illustrated in the plate of Grassi's *Disputatio*—that the comet had changed its direction pointing towards the celestial north pole: starting from the constellation of the Libra it had passed across Boötes, reached afterwards the tail of Ursa Major, and eventually disappeared before reaching the polar constellations (see Figure 9.4). According to the scheme of the *Discorso* an object ascending towards the sky along a purely rectilinear path perpendicular to the earth's surface should have tended progressively towards the zenith of the observer, without any systematic deviation, this conflicting with the displacement towards the celestial north pole that had characterized the apparent movement of the real 1618 comet on the vault of the heavens (Figure 9.5). How can this deviation be accounted for within the framework of the hypothesis of a pure rectilinear movement of ascension?

The way Galileo introduces a possible explanation of this apparent incongruity is an indication of the rhetoric strategy by which he attempts to propose his Copernican option. Although hidden behind the veil of hesitant wording, his message was easy to understand by his ideal reader, i.e. the

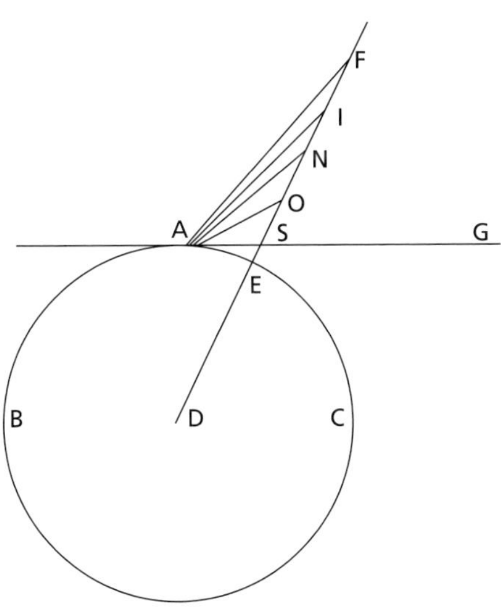

Figure 9.5 The drawing which in the *Discorso delle comete* illustrates the idea that an object ascending vertically from the surface of the earth towards the sky would be seen by a terrestrial observer located in a different region of the earth as progressively approaching the zenith of the observer (while at the same time diminishing its speed of ascension). E–F is the rectilinear trajectory of the object, A the position of the observer. Reproduced from Galileo–Guiducci, *Discorso delle comete di Mario Guiducci*, 1619, Cecconcelli.

reader who, starting from *Mauri*, qualified as *discretto e intendente* (discreet and understanding), to whom—as he wrote 'I submit my every work and labour'.

The attentive reader was warned of the importance of what he was going to read by the indirect and cautious form by which Galileo introduced the argument ('I shall not pretend here to dissimulate that I know'). Two alternatives were considered and, for different reasons, excluded. The second (the one the author dared not to consider) was particularly significant because, as was the custom in the dissimulation rhetoric of the age, it was left undeclared and was entrusted to the exclusive understanding of the reader. Galileo alluded to the fact that the north declination of the comet could be accounted for, not by a movement of the celestial object, but by a movement of the observer, and particularly by one due the motion of the earth in its annual revolution around the sun. Even if Galileo did not explicitly say how this could happen, the mere admission of such a possibility was, of course, to put himself within a decidedly Copernican perspective.

Galileo's view corresponded to Kepler's theory of comets. In 1604, in a short appendix added to chapter 10 of *Astronomiae pars optica* ('Optical part of astronomy') the German astronomer had surmised that the apparent movement of comets (like that observed by Regiomontanus in 1472, and the more recent comet of 1577 studied by Brahe) could be explained by assuming a rectilinear ascending movement combined with the movement of the observer due to the revolution of the earth around the sun (OPTICA, p. 334; transl. pp. 345–6).

In the same year, during the preparation of his lectures on the new star, Galileo had alluded to a similar explanation when commenting on the hypothesis proposed by Elias Camerarius in 1572 (and strongly criticized by Brahe). Like other mathematicians of the epoch, Camerarius supported the idea that the phenomenon of the new star could be accounted by a rectilinear ascending movement. As with the 1618 comet, the astronomical observation showed that a luminous body deviated from the zenith while decreasing in its apparent size. In his annotation, Galileo explicitly wrote that 'Camerarius's observation could be true'; in his view, this was due to the star increasing its distance from the zenith because of the annual motion of the earth, which 'at that time aimed toward the southern regions' (*quae tunc ad austrum tendebat*). A movement of the observer towards the southern direction of the cosmic sphere, while the luminous body continued its rectilinear ascension towards the vault of the skies, could account for an apparent displacement towards the celestial north pole.

In the *Discorso delle comete*, soon after implying his Copernican explanation for the singular movement of the 1618 comet, Galileo mentioned a cosmological reflection of the Roman philosopher Seneca:

> Seneca recognized and wrote how important it was for the sure determination of these matters to have a firm and unquestionable knowledge of the order, arrangement, locations, and movements of the parts of the universe. In our age we still lack this; hence we must be content with what little we may conjecture here among the shadows, until there shall be given to us the true constitution of the parts of the universe—inasmuch that which Tycho promised us still remain imperfect. (COMETE, p. 44; transl. p. 57)

By noting the imperfection of the constitution of the world proposed by Tycho (that he would not consider worthy of being placed among 'the chief systems of the world' in his 1632 *Dialogue*), Galileo aimed to make explicit to Grassi that he had understood the anti-Copernican attitude underlying the latter's endorsement of Brahe's world system. Moreover, the allusion to Seneca was itself cryptically pro-Copernican. This was because in book VII of Seneca's *Quaestiones naturales* there was an important passage alluding to the possible revolution of the earth around the sun (a hypothesis supported in antiquity by Aristarchus of Samos and some followers of Pythagoras):

> It will also be relevant to this question if we learn whether the earth revolves while the earth stands still, or the universe revolves while the earth stands still. There have been people who said that we are unknowingly carried about by the natural world; and that sun risings and settings are not due to a movement of heavens, but rather that we are rising and setting. The subject is worthy of examination to know in what condition we are; whether our lot was the most sluggish or the most rapid of abodes; whether God moves all things around us, or us around them. (OG II, p. 283; transl. from Reeves, 1997, revised)

Galileo had transcribed this quotation in his notes on the new star of 1604, this suggesting that he had mentioned it in his public lectures at the University of Padua. He did not report it, however, in *Discorso delle comete*, nor in *Saggiatore*. Nevertheless, the 'discreet and understanding reader' of his age knew Seneca and his cosmological reflections expounded in the *Quaestiones naturales*. He was therefore ready to grasp the pro-Copernican valence of the reference to the Roman philosopher. In the rhetoric of the dissimulation to which Galileo was obliged after the condemnation of Copernicus, alluding to an opinion without expressing it overtly, could have a stronger communicative force than a direct and explicit statement.

9.4 The height of lunar mountains: a (rather) precise surveying of remote regions

We end now with our considerations about how Galileo dealt with comets (and new stars), in texts where the ambiguity had both visual and rhetorical implications, and come to the other aspect of his scientific enterprise, that of the height of lunar mountains. We introduce this theme by first referring to a remark expressed by Galileo in his third letter on sunspots made when commenting on what Scheiner had written about the difficulty of measuring extremely distant phenomena. Galileo considers the possibility of deriving the properties of natural matter in a different way:

> But if we want to limit ourselves to learning certain properties, it does not seem to me that we need despair of grasping these in the most remote bodies any more than in the closest ones. At times, indeed, such knowledge will be more exact in the former than in the latter. And who does not know the periods of the motions of the planets better than he does that of the waters of sundry seas? Who does not know that the spherical figure of the Moon was recognized much earlier and more quickly than that of the Earth? And is there not still a controversy over whether the Earth itself remains immobile or wanders, while [at the same time] we are quite certain of the motions of not a few stars.
>
> I want to conclude from this that although one would attempt the investigation of the substance of the solar spots in vain, this does not mean that certain of their properties [*affezioni*]—their location, motion, shape, size, opacity, mutability, appearance, and disappearance—cannot be learned by us and then serve as our means better to speculate upon other more controversial conditions of natural substances. (ISTORIA, pp. 101–102; transl. pp. 254–255)

Galileo's measurement of lunar mountains might appear as a clear illustration of the possibility of understanding the properties of distant as well as near bodies. This is because Galileo's error in this measurement was relatively modest compared to the more or less current values of the mountains of the earth. The matter requires, however, some qualification. The interesting point about the mountains on the moon is that, given the assistance of the telescope, the conditions of the observation were more favourable than those for terrestrial mountains.

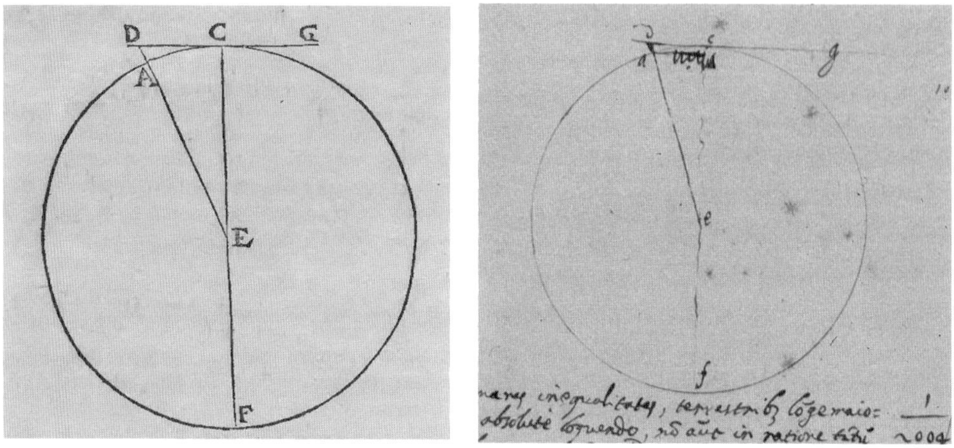

Figure 9.6 The scheme used by Galileo in *Sidereus nuncius* to illustrate his method of calculating the height of a lunar mountain. The figure at the left is from the printed copy of the work, that at the right from the Galilean manuscripts at the National Library of Florence (BNF GAL 48, F16r; © Biblioteca Nazionale of Florence, Italy).

To follow Galileo's reasoning we will refer to the image published in the *Sidereus* and to that in Galileo's hand among the manuscripts of National Library of Florence (Fig. 9.6).

Having determined a luminous point in the dark zone of the moon (D, in the two images), not far from the terminator (i.e. the line separating the dark and light boundary), Galileo assumes that it corresponded to the peak of a mountain just illuminated at sunset. The point chosen (relative to a particularly high lunar mountain) was found to be at the distance of about 1/20 from the moon diameter. On the basis of the known diameter of the moon (that Galileo considers to be 2/7 of the diameter of the earth assumed to be 7000 Italian miles, i.e. about 10,346 km (1 Italian mile corresponding to about 1478 m, which would result in a value of the moon diameter of 2956 km)), he calculates the length of CD, i.e. the distance of the luminous point from the terminator (147.8 km in modern units). Galileo assumes further that, because of the great distance of the moon from earth, the sunrays arrive at the moon surface parallel to the line of sight, which means that the triangle CDE is a right triangle. By applying Pythagoras' theorem to this triangle, he can calculate the length of EB (the hypotenuse of the triangle) and then, by subtracting, from the value obtained, the segment EA (i.e. the value of the moon radius) he arrives at the conclusion that the particular mountain measured is 'more than 4 Italian miles' (i.e. more than 5912 metres).

This achievement is noteworthy, but we need to consider the concluding statement of the relatively short section of *Sidereus* dealing with the height of lunar mountains:

> But on the Earth there no mountains exist that reach a perpendicular height of 1 mile high. It is evidence therefore that lunar prominences are loftier than the terrestrial ones. (SIDEREUS, p. 14; transl. pp. 52–53)

This statement is surely wrong if we consider that the tallest mountain in the visible part of the moon, Mons Huygens, has a height of about 5400 metres, and thus well below that of Mount Everest on the earth. Using Galileo's values for the diameter of the moon, his calculation would amount actually to about 7380 metres, which would represent an overestimation by about 30 per cent of the real altitude (the error would be a little greater if we use the modern value for the moon's diameter). However, the calculation was extraordinarily exact if compared to the available measurements of mountains on earth. Nevertheless, Galileo's claim that 'on the Earth there are no mountains reaching a perpendicular height of even 1 mile high' appears surprising. It is true that the measurement of the height of mountains on earth made by classical authors was in the order indicated by him. For example, Eratosthenes of Cyrene (the famous geographer who provided a celebrated and rather accurate measurement of earth's circumference) and other scholars of Greek antiquity give values of the mountains they measured in the range of less than 3000 metres which correspond to the actual mountains they measured with an error similar to that made by Galileo with the mountains of the moon (assuming that he was actually measuring Mons Huygens).

It is very likely that Galileo was considering exclusively the values of terrestrial mountains calculated by the classical scholars when he claimed that the mountains on the moon are much higher than those on earth. In his era, the error of calculations or estimations of the terrestrial mountains was much more impressive. This is clear if we compare values at the time of Galileo with the modern measurements. We will take as an example the altitude of the Pico del Teide in Tenerife (Canary Islands) which attracted the interest of sailors and voyagers because of its impressive appearance from sea. Against a contemporary value of 3718 metres, in the Renaissance Joseph Justus Scaliger gave 90,000 metres, Francesco Patrizi 105,000 metres, up to the impressive 463,000 metres estimated by Cardanus (Gerolamo Cardano). Some time after *Sidereus*, in 1616, the Dutch astronomer Willebrord Snel (Snellius or Snell) arrived at the more reasonable value of 8,230, while, after Galileo's death, the German geographer Bernhardus Varenius (Bernhard Varen) increased this value to 11,800 metres (Cajory, 1929; Adams, 1932).

Despite the relatively good precision of Galileo's measurements, some more remarks are required. One is that the illustration from *Sidereus* might suggest that Galileo was measuring the height of the mountains situated at that border of the moon where, according to his repeated and justified assertions, no mountain could be seen with his telescope. In a letter addressed to the German physician and astronomer Johann Georg Brengger on 8 November 1610, Galileo makes clear that it was just for the purpose of geometrical calculation that he drew the scheme used in his measurement of the height of lunar mountains in this way (OG X, pp. 466–473; see Figure 9.7). As he wrote, the actual mountain that he measured was located near the central part of the moon. Brengger, an acquaintance of Marcus Welser, had raised several objections to the method used in the measurement of lunar mountains in a text that Welser had forwarded to Galileo on 20 October 1610 (OG X, pp. 460–464).

We know from the letter to Brengger that Galileo chose to measure a particularly high mountain, situated where the terminator was smooth (this indicating that no other mountains in the line of sight might occlude the passage of sunrays and thus lead to a false estimate of the height of the peak to be measured). Moreover, he states explicitly that he measured the angular distance from the terminator of the luminous peak with the telescope. This was preferred to another method, suggested by Brengger as a better one, based on the time needed by the luminous peak to merge into the illuminated part of the moon, because this was more prone to errors.

In conclusion if we compare the remarkable inconsistencies in the values for a terrestrial mountain (Pico del Teide) current in Galileo's time, with that resulting from his own measurement reported in *Sidereus*, it is difficult not to share his opinion that we need not despair of grasping the properties of natural objects 'in the most remote bodies any more than in the closest ones'. Bear in mind that even though Pico del Teide was on a remote and exotic island, it could be seen and

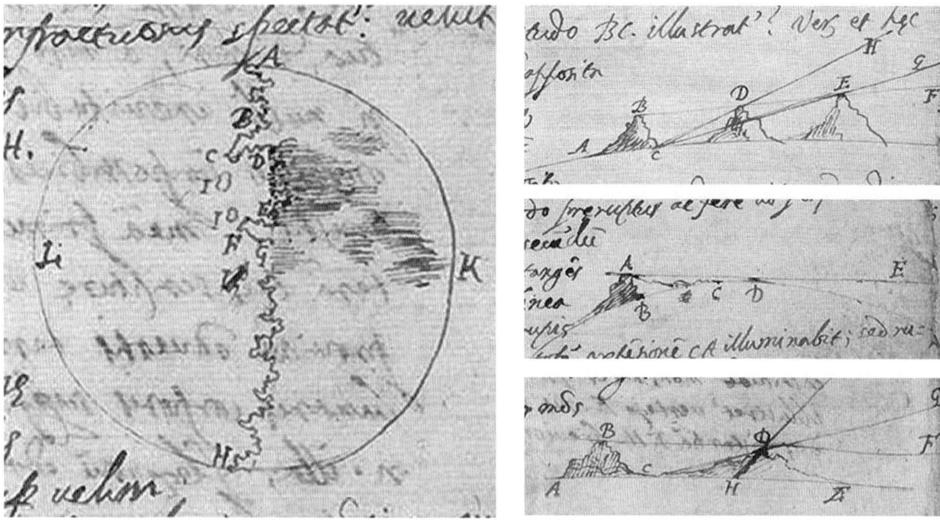

Figure 9.7 Some of the drawings accompanying a letter to Brengger by which Galileo illustrates his method for calculating the height of a mountain on the moon and the reasons for the possible inconsistency of the method suggested by the German scholar (BNF GAL 53, F34r and 36v; © Biblioteca Nazionale of Florence, Italy).

even climbed. The method used by Galileo was indeed conceptually simpler than a triangulation method applicable to the measurement of a mountain on the earth.

On another point, we are inclined to endorse the opinion of Aleixandre Koyré who said that, with Galileo, we passed from a world of approximation to a universe of precision. As in many other aspects of Galileo's work, this was not only the consequence of better methods of measuring and calculating, but also of a singular ability to see and to interpret visual appearances correctly.

Chapter 10

Galileo's sensory philosophy

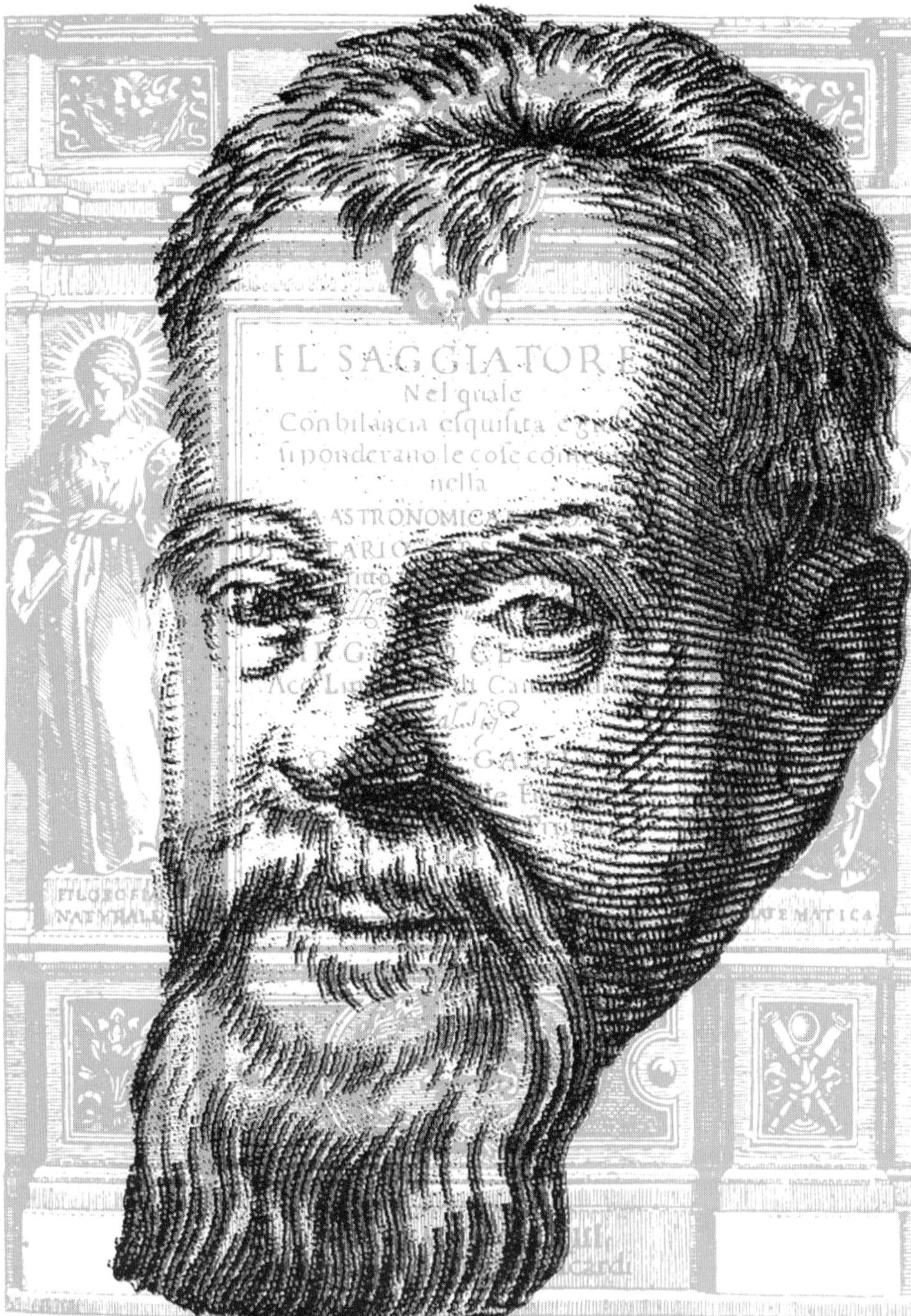

Figure X *Galileo's Saggiatore* by Nicholas Wade. Galileo's portrait is derived from a painting by Francesco Villamena and is framed by the frontispiece of *Il Saggiatore*.

Credit: Frontispiece of 'The Assayer' by Galileo Galilei, 1623 (engraving), Villamena, Francesco (1566–1624) / Private Collection / Photo © Christie's Images / The Bridgeman Art Library.

Galileo's interest in vision has been considered in the previous chapters and it is now time to analyse the philosophical foundations underlying his conception of senses. This is in the context of his considerations of the unreliability (and possible fallacy) of the senses. Galileo's attitude contrasts with his insistence on the need for 'sensible experiences' in order to arrive at correct conclusions in the various fields of scientific investigation, and in order to achieve a trustworthy knowledge of the world.

This can be addressed through some rather well-known pages in chapter 48 of *Saggiatore*, in which Galileo discusses two different qualities of physical bodies that were later referred to as 'primary' and 'secondary' qualities.[1] These pages are generally discussed on a purely philosophical basis, outside the context of Galileo's general approach to science and reality, and with no reference to his understanding of the mechanisms underlying the psychological and physiological dimensions of sensory processes.

10.1 **Tastes, odours, colours, and so forth are no more than mere names**

Galileo develops the properties and causes of sensations within the framework of a discussion on the nature of heat and of its relation to motion. Addressing (His Excellency) Virginio Cesarini, to whom *Saggiatore* is dedicated, Galileo writes:

> It now remains, in accordance with the promise made above to your Excellency, for me to tell you some of my thoughts about the proposition, 'Motion is the cause of heat,' and to show in what sense this may be true in my opinion. But first I must give some consideration to what we call 'heat,' for I much suspect that in general people have a conception of this which is very remote from the truth, believing heat to be a real attribute, property, and quality which actually resides in the material by which we feel ourselves warmed.
>
> Therefore I say that upon conceiving of a material or corporeal substance, I immediately feel the need to conceive simultaneously that it is bounded and has this or that shape; that it is in this place or that at any given time; that it moves or stays still; that it does or does not touch another body; and that it is one, few, or many. I cannot separate it from these conditions by any stretch of my imagination. But that it must be white or red, bitter or sweet, noisy or silent, of sweet or foul odor, my mind feels no compulsion to understand as necessary accompaniments. Indeed, without the senses to guide us, reason or imagination alone would perhaps never arrive at such qualities. For that reason I think that tastes, odors, colors, and so forth are no more than mere names [*puri nomi*] so far as pertains to the subject wherein they appear to reside, and that they have their habitation only in the sensitive body. Thus, if the living creature [*l'animal vivente*] were removed, all these qualities would be removed and annihilated. Yet since we have imposed upon them particular names which differ from the names of those other previous real attributes, we wish to believe that they should also be truly and really different from the latter. (SAGGIATORE, pp. 196–197; transl. pp. 309–310)

After examining the sense of hearing (by negating expressly the existence of 'sonorous or transonorous qualities'), he writes:

> I do not believe that for exciting in us tastes, odors, and sounds there are required in external bodies anything but sizes, shapes, numbers, and slow or fast movements; and I think that if ears, tongues,

[1] Although in the context of post-Galilean science the expressions 'primary' and 'secondary qualities' were introduced by Locke, they existed in the Scholastic philosophy, although with a different meaning. In particular for most of the scholastic philosophers, primary qualities corresponded to the elementary qualities of the Aristotelian philosophy, i.e. hot, cold, wet, and dry.

> and noses were taken away, shapes and numbers and motions would remain but not odors or tastes or sounds. These, I believe, are nothing but names, apart from the living animal just as tickling and titillation are nothing but names when armpits and the skin around the nose are absent. And as the four senses considered here are related to the four elements, I believe that vision, the sense which is eminent above all others, is related to light, but in that ratio of excellence which exists between the finite and the infinite, the temporal and the indivisible; between darkness and light. Of this sense and of the matters pertaining to it, I pretend to understand but a trifle, and since a long time would still not suffice to explain that trifle—or even to hint at its explanation in writing—I pass this over in silence. (pp. 199–200; transl. pp. 311–312)

These statements have generally been considered indicating a purely subjective conception of knowledge, with reference to the phrase 'mere names' attributed by Galileo to 'tastes, odors, and sounds', which would suggest that the sensations would be without any substantiality and consistence outside the subject capable of perceiving them (denoted by 'the subject wherein they appear to reside' or 'the sensitive body' or 'living creature'). Historically, only the so-called primary qualities have been considered as a proper object of investigation according to the paradigm of the (supposedly) Galilean science. This contributes to explaining why the research in the field of sensations has lagged behind that of physics by about two centuries.

In the pages of *Saggiatore* the discourse on sensations as 'mere names' seems to intrude as an extraneous body into the polemics on the nature of comets that continues that initiated with the *Discorso delle comete*. Nonetheless, it represents a vital aspect of Galileo's conception of the world that had been building up since his youth. Far from being simply a facet of his theory of sensation and knowledge, it is connected to all the dimensions of his scientific endeavour (studies on motion, mechanics, hydraulics, floating bodies, astronomy) and also to his philosophical and metaphysical conception of reality.

10.2 **A moving hand, a statue, and a living man**

In the conclusion to his first letter on sunspots, where he deals with visual themes (see Chapter 2), after mentioning the difficulty encountered in dealing with the new and intricate matters of astronomical observation, Galileo writes:

> I do not want on this account to despair and to abandon the enterprise; on the contrary, I would hope that these novelties might serve me wonderfully to tune up a few pipes of this grand [but] discordant organ of our philosophy, which, in my view, many organists labor in vain to tune to perfection [*accordare al perfetto temperamento*]. And this is because they go about leaving and preserving three or four of the principal pipes out of tune, such that it is impossible for the others to respond in complete harmony. (ISTORIA, p. 28; transl. p. 7)

In Galileo's view there is little doubt that among the 'three or four of the principal pipes' that make the organ of natural philosophy discordant, there is also that of a theory of sensations, and that this theory must be in complete harmony with the entire structure of the grand organ of natural philosophy (i.e. science at large).

The example that Galileo develops in *Saggiatore* in order to clarify his conception of senses is particularly efficacious. It concerns the nature of the tickling sensation:

> I believe I can explain my idea better by means of some examples. I move my hand first over a marble statue and then over a living man. Now as to the action derived from my hand, this is the same with respect to both subjects so far as the hand is concerned; it consists of the primary phenomena of motion and touch which we have not designated by any other names. But the animate body which

> receives these operations feels diverse sensations according to the various parts which are touched. Being touched on the soles of the feet, for example, or upon the knee or under the armpit, it feels in addition to the general sense of touch another sensation upon which we have conferred a special name, calling it tickling; this sensation belongs entirely to us and not to the hand in any way. It seems to me that anyone would seriously err who might wish to say that the hand had within itself, in addition to the properties of moving and touching, another faculty different from these; that of tickling as if the tickling were an attribute which resided in the hand. A piece of paper or a feather drawn lightly over any part of our bodies performs what are inherently quite the same operations of moving and touching; by touching the eye, the nose, or the upper lip it excites in us an almost intolerable titillation while in other regions it is scarcely felt. Now this titillation belongs entirely to us and not to the feather; if the animate and sensitive body were removed, it would remain no more than a mere name. And I believe that many qualities which we come to attribute to natural bodies, such as tastes, odors, colors, and other things, may be of similar and no more solid existence. (SAGGIATORE, p. 199; transl. pp. 309–310)

The meaning of this passage, which recalls and develops a similar example from *Discorso delle comete*, is rather evident. Outside the individual capable of perceiving, sensations have an undoubted physical reality (easy to individuate in the case of tickling although a little less so in the case of other sensations, especially the sensation of light). In his mechanistic and atomistic conception of the world Galileo tends to identify this reality with the motion of matter; the properties of matter are considered to be corpuscular, but he refuses to attribute it to a specific sensory dimension. A specific sensory quality is acquired only with regard to a specific sensory apparatus. Nothing in the world exists outside us that is specifically 'colour', 'odour', 'taste', 'sound', 'tickling', or 'warmth'. The sensorial connotation is the consequence of an action exerted by the external agencies on specific structures of the sensitive individual (animal or human), where it activates specific sensory processes. With reference to the old theory of the 'four elements', Galileo establishes a relation similar (but not identical) to that adopted by Aristotle, between—respectively—the elements of earth, water, air, fire on one side, and the tactile, gustatory, acoustical, and olfactory sensations on the other side (and also between vision and light, of which he seems to suggest the analogy with the ether or quintessence). However, he did not believe, as Aristotle did, that specific sensory qualities existed in external reality, outside the sensitive individual.

10.3 **Aristotle and his real sensibles**

For Aristotle (Figure 10.1) colour, taste, odour, sound, touch (or the tangible quality) were the proper objects of sensation (i.e. *aisthēta*, i.e. sensibles; or *aisthētai poiotētes* i.e. sensible qualities), i.e. specific qualities of external reality having an autonomous existence, independent from the existence of individuals capable of perceiving them, and finalized to produce a specific sensory modality. They belonged to the category called 'proper sensibles' (*idia aisthēta*) being expressions of a specific quality of the external object potentially interacting with a particular sense (of which it was the 'proper' object). Colour[2] (like the other proper sensibles) was therefore considered as existing in the real world, independently of its action on the specific sensory mechanism of the perceiving individual, even though their existence *in actu* required interaction with the correspondent sense. The physical reality of proper sensibles is asserted by Aristotle in various passages. For example, in *De anima* ('On the soul') when speaking of earlier conceptions (and particularly of those

[2] The Greek term for colour, *chrōma*, had a somewhat wider meaning than colour nowadays and also included black and white. In Aristotle's conception, the different hues resulted from a mixing in different degrees of black and white.

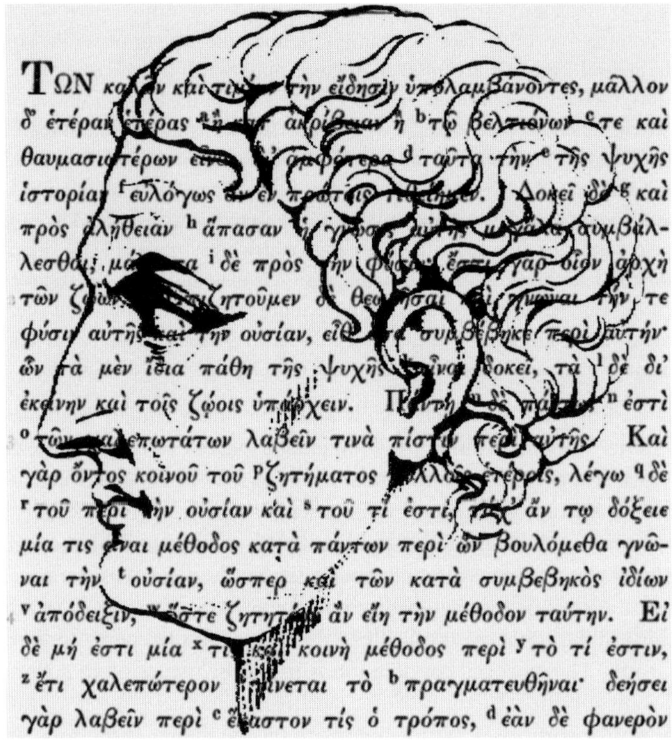

Figure 10.1 *Aristotle's De Anima* by Nicholas Wade. A portrait of Aristotle (derived from an engraving in *The historic gallery of portraits and paintings*, 1810) is combined with Greek text from *De Anima*.

expounded by atomists) he wrote: 'This relation of the object to the subject of sensation was not rightly comprehended by the early natural philosophers [*próteron physiologoi*]. They thought that there was nothing white or black apart from vision, and no flavour independently of taste' (transl. Wallace, 1882, p. 137).

For Aristotle, touch, requiring contact in order to experience it, was often taken as the most important sense, and the one relative to which others could be related: 'The primary form of sense is touch, which belongs to all animals' (Ross, 1931, p. 413b). It is perhaps for this reason that Aristotle maintained that touch is a single sense, that the number of senses is restricted to five, and that: 'there cannot be a special sense-organ for the common sensibles either' (p. 425a). Touch presents more problems because its sensitivity is not localized to a particular sense organ, and the experiences derived from the skin are many and varied. Aristotle confronted these aspects of anatomy and experience and reached similar conclusions:

> In dealing with each of the senses we shall have first to speak of the objects which are perceptible by each.... I call by the name of special object of this or that sense that which cannot be perceived by any other sense than that one and in respect of which no error is possible; in this sense colour is the special object of sight, sound of hearing, flavour of taste. Touch, indeed, discriminates more than one set of different qualities. Each sense has one kind of object which it discerns, and never errs in reporting that what is before it is colour or sound (though it may err as to what it is that is coloured or where that is, or what is sounding or where that is). Such objects are what we propose to call special objects of this or

> that sense. 'Common sensibles' are movement, rest, number, figure, magnitude; these are not peculiar to any one sense, but are common to all. (Ross, 1931, p. 418b)

Later in *De anima* Aristotle distinguished between experience and organ: 'By a "sense" is meant what has the power of receiving into itself the sensible forms of things without the matter.... By "an organ of sense" is meant that in which ultimately such a power is seated' (p. 424a). This, again, provided problems for the experience of touch, because there was no specific organ associated with it. Once more, the issue was voiced by Aristotle: 'If touch is not a single sense but a group of senses, there must be several kinds of what is tangible. It is a problem whether touch is a single sense or a group of senses. It is also a problem, what is the organ of touch' (p. 422b).

Aristotle distinguished the proper from the common sensibles (*koina aisthēta*), these being those properties of objects that we can apprehend through the work of various senses (most frequently touch and vision): 'motion, rest, shape, size, number, unity', with the addition of the broad categories of time and space. Another important distinction he made concerned the so-called 'sensibles *per accidens*' (or 'incidental sensibles': *aisthēta kata sunbebēkos*), which are those qualities that can be accidentally associated to a proper sensible, but are not an essential constitutive element of it.

One of the important distinctions between the different sensibles of Aristotle's theory of sensations concerned the possible occurrence of errors. For him errors arise more commonly in the case of incidental sensibles, and they might also happen in the case of common sensibles, whereas no error can occur in the case of proper sensibles. Concerning these last ones, the impossibility of errors seems to belong to their very definition:

> The so-called object of sense-perception may mean three different things, of which two are said to be perceived directly in themselves, the third incidentally and with regard to its concomitants. Of the two first- mentioned, one is proper and confined to each one of the senses separately, the other is common to them all. By the proper is to be understood that which it is impossible to perceive by any other sense than that appropriated to it and with respect to which that sense cannot be deceived. So it is that colour stands to sight, sound to hearing, flavour to taste: touch, however, it must be added, deals with a number of different qualities. Each single sense in fact discerns these different qualities, and is subject to no delusion as to whether it be a colour or whether it be a sound that it perceives: its only doubt is what it is that is coloured or where it is, or what or where is the body that is sounding. Such are the objects of perception which are said to be peculiar to each separate sense. The common sensibles are movement, rest, number, figure, magnitude such properties being peculiar to no one single sense but shared in common by them all. Movement for instance is perceived at once by touch and by sight. (Aristotle, *De Anima*, II, 5; transl. Wallace, p. 93, revised)

A deception can arise in the case of incidental sensibles, when, for example—as Aristotle puts it—by seeing from afar a person dressed in white one says that he is 'the son of Diares', because normally the son of Diares is dressed in white. There is no possibility of error in the perception of the white colour (a proper sensible), but the error is possible in the association of this sensation with the idea of the 'son of Diares', an association which is purely incidental and contingent. By examining the various circumstances in which there could be errors or fallacies of the senses, one gets the impression that this never occurs at the very moment of sensation (considered to be always trustworthy), but in a somewhat later phase which implies a more or less explicit act of judgement. This may occur in associating a particular sensation with another one belonging to a different sense (this happens with common sensibles) or with a memory or concept (as it happens with incidental sensibles). In this context it is appropriate to mention that Aristotle's confidence in senses is repeatedly asserted in the *Dialogue* by his spokesman Simplicio as when he says that for the Greek philosopher the data of senses must be preferred to any logical argument:

> SIMPLICIO: Aristotle would not give assurance from his reasoning of more than was proper, despite his great genius. He held in his philosophizing that sensible experiments were to be preferred above any discourse built by human ingenuity, and he said that those who would contradict the evidence of any sense deserved to be punished by the loss of that sense. (DIALOGO, p. 24; transl. p. 32)

Aristotle's survey of the senses was more extensive than those of his predecessors (see Beare, 1906). Most of the knowledge we have of the earlier Greek commentators derives from the writing of his pupil, Theophrastus (*c.* 370–286 BC). Without his work *On the Senses* our understanding of early theories of the senses would be even more meagre. Theophrastus categorized writers on the senses into two groups: those who considered that the senses were stimulated by similarities or by opposites. Thus, taste and touch could be treated as similar, since both involve contact. The means of sensing by sight, hearing, smell, and taste was speculated upon by most writers, but less was said about touch. For example, with regard to Alcmaeon of Croton (*fl.* 500 BC), Theophrastus wrote: 'All the senses are connected in some way with the brain; consequently they are incapable of action if [the brain] is disturbed or shifts its position, for [this organ] stops up the passages through which the senses act. Of touch he tells us neither the manner nor the means of its operation' (Stratton, 1917, pp. 89–91).

Alcmaeon located the centre of sensation in the brain, although Aristotle did not adopt this view, referring the processes of perception to the heart. In the context of touch, Anaxagoras (*c.*500–438 BC) discussed sensing warmth and cold, and Democritus contrasted heavy with light, and hard with soft. Plato wrote that touch distinguished between hot and cold, hard and soft, heavy and light, as well as rough and smooth. Theophrastus himself said relatively little about touch. His theory of the senses in general involved some intermediary between the object and the sense organ; for vision, hearing, and smell this could be more readily maintained than for touch.

The approach by Galen (Figure 10.2) to the senses displayed the advantages of anatomical dissection. He berated Aristotle for denying that all the senses do not have connections with the brain: 'Hence all the instruments of the senses—if we are to believe our eyes that see and our hands that touch them—communicate with the encephalon' (May, 1968, p. 391). Galen's theory of the senses was physiological, and it was based on the concept of pneuma advocated by Empedocles: 'Unless the alteration in each sense instrument comes from the encephalon and returns to it, the animal will still remain without sense perception' (May, 1968, p. 403). Galen restricted his discussion to the 'four sense instruments in the head, namely, the eyes, ears, nose, and tongue, all of which take the source of their sensation from the encephalon' (p. 400).

The situation remained relatively unchanged through the medieval period: 'Aristotle's account of sensation and perception was held in great esteem in the Middle Ages, and his systematic approach and many of his specific doctrines were widely copied' (Kemp, 1990, p. 35). Attention was directed principally at interpretations of vision, with much less heed paid to the other senses. Developments did occur in fusing Aristotle's account of the senses with Galen's pneumatic physiology, and the medical tradition of describing diseases of the senses became more refined.

10.4 The sensibility of a modern peripatetic

In Galileo's day, the theme of the different sensibles of the Aristotelian tradition, and of the causes or deceptions in sensory appearances, was reconsidered in 1612 by Giulio Cesare Lagalla (or La Galla), professor at the University of Rome, in a small book entitled *De Phoenomenis in orbe lunae*

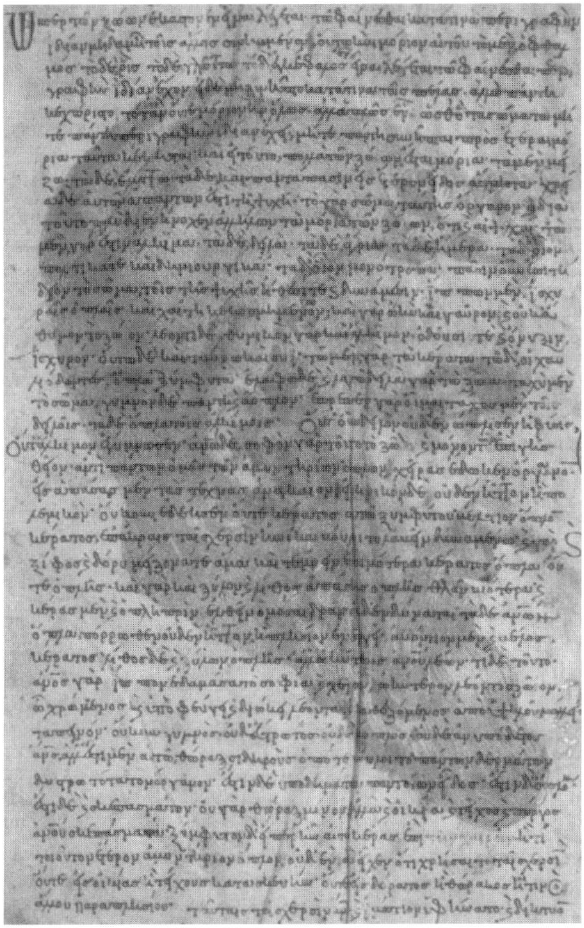

Figure 10.2 *Galen's usefulness* by Nicholas Wade. A profile portrait of Galen is combined with a page of Greek text from his *On the usefulness of the parts of the body.*

('On the phenomena in the orb of the moon'). It critically discussed the observations of the moon made by Galileo with his telescope (and various related scientific novelties). In this book Lagalla asserted the infallibility of sensations in the case of the proper sensibles, considered as specific properties (*passiones*) of the object, and, in accordance with the Aristotelian doctrine, he admitted the possibility of error only in the case of common sensibles and sensibles *per accidens.* For the common sensibles he invoked a classical example, that of the rod (or a stick) partially immersed in water, which appears to be bent. For the sensibles *per accidens* he uses the example of somebody who thinks they have met Socrates when they happen to encounter a man resembling him because of a flat nose and frizzy hairs.

In the marginal annotations that he writes in his personal copy of Lagalla's work, Galileo counteracts the arguments of the peripatetic philosopher with incisiveness and wit by evidencing the intrinsic inconsistency of his adversary's reasoning. As for instance when, with a pungent irony, he writes:

> If sense is deceitful with common sensibles, then when one sees a bird flying or a horse running, this is false. (OG III, p. 399)

Or when, speaking about the rod of Lagalla's example, he says:

> If sight is deceitful in judging the rod, half-immersed in water, as broken, because the figure is a common sensible, then it should also be deceitful when it is out of the water, where the figure is still a common sensible: to what purpose then to introduce the water? (p. 394)

Or when, in the same context, he says:

> Is he [Lagalla] not aware of the fact that, when he says that sight is deceitful when it judges, on the basis of colour, the wood to be straight or broken, he is placing the deception in the proper sensible, and not in the common one. (p. 397)

Within the framework of peripatetic philosophy to which he adhered, in his *De Phenomenis in orbe lunae*, Lagalla, despite recognizing the importance of Galileo's achievements with the telescope,[3] attacked almost all his interpretations of the astronomical novelties and also many other aspects of the new science that was undermining the foundations of Aristotelian philosophy. In particular he rejected the Copernican idea of the mobility of earth and of the centrality of sun, he was against the mountainous nature of the moon's surface, he also opposed Galileo's interpretation of the causes of the lunar candour, and he retained the idea of the immutability of skies against the evidence of new stars. He also criticized Galileo's idea of the applicability of mathematical reasoning to the study of natural phenomena. As a matter of fact all Lagalla's discussion on the possible fallacies of common sensibles aimed at undermining the importance of experimental evidence as a means to arrive at reliable scientific conclusions.

One of the points addressed by Lagalla concerned the infinity of the cosmos and the plurality of worlds. These he imputed mainly to the philosophy of Democritus, which was revived in his era particularly by 'an author of a condemned name' (that, although not mentioned, was easily identifiable as Giordano Bruno). Despite his lack of scientific penetration, Lagalla was able to understand that many of Galileo's astronomical discoveries were indeed fitting with the idea of a cosmos less limited and geocentric than that of the traditional Aristotelian and Ptolemaic conceptions and more akin to the idea of an infinity of worlds advocated by Bruno. Among Galileo's relevant observations were the discoveries of the four satellites of Jupiter (which made clear that the world could accommodate more than a planetary system) and the great number of stars revealed by the telescope and the starry nature of the galaxies. These pointed to a potentially infinite number of celestial bodies among which the earth might lose its cosmological and anthropological centrality.

10.5 Atomistic condensations and expansions

Atomism was central to Galileo's conception of the world and it invested many facets of his scientific and intellectual vision of natural phenomena. It was also central to his conception of senses, which was closely related to his global conception of reality and to his effort to supplant the traditional philosophy of Aristotle with an entirely new philosophy. This was implied in the metaphor of the 'discordant grand organ' in need of re-tuning, which bore an obvious reference to Aristotle's *Organon* of philosophy. Galileo invoked the metaphor of the organ in various writings in addition

[3] Lagalla was one of the members of the Roman intelligentsia who benefitted from the telescopic demonstration given by Galileo during his visit in Rome in the springtime of 1611. Besides confirming the reality of telescopic appearances, in his book Lagalla narrates the episode in which the Tuscan scholar, with use of his instrument, made distinctly visible the inscriptions on a monument at a distance of 'not less than 2 miles' from the observation place (OG III, p. 330; on the episode see another testimony in OG XI, p. 117).

to the first letter on sunspots. A reference to the atomism of Democritus is developed in the writings of Galileo and of his student Benedetto Castelli. This particularly concerned his analysis of floating bodies (in 1611) in opposition to some members of the Florentine conservative intelligentsia (and particular his old adversary Lodovico Delle Colombe), and in the *Discorso intorno alle cose che stanno in su l'acqua o in quella si muovono* ('Discourse on the matters that float on or move inside the water') published in 1612. Atomism, in both its physical and mathematical dimensions is also central to the first day of the dialogue in the *Discorsi e dimostrazioni matematiche intorno a due nuove scienze*, the last great work of Galileo published in 1638, four years before his death.

In addition to these works, atomism was also a fundamental reference in many of Galileo's other texts from the early research on gravity which had been largely inspired by the physics of Archimedes. Galileo rejected the explanation based on the Aristotelian idea of absolute gravity and levity (as specific attributes of the various elements, with the element of earth being the heaviest and the element of fire being the lightest). Galileo developed instead the conception of 'gravity in species' (i.e. specific gravity) which would result from the different states of condensation and rarefaction of matter composed of minute corpuscles interspersed by vacuum. In one of his first texts which referred to atomism (the manuscripts dealing with motion known as *De motu antiquiora*)[4] the concept of condensation and rarefaction is considered within the framework of a Platonic myth of creation. Having created the world, the Divine Maker (*divinus Opifex*) concentrated the by-products of the creation of the very vast celestial sphere (*vastissimae caelestis excrementa spherae*) at its centre, in order to avoid offending the sight of the most blessed immortal spirits of the heavens. Afterwards, however, in order not to leave empty an immense cosmic space (and also with the aim of attenuating the extreme physical gravity of the concentrated matter), the Maker expanded the primordial matter such as to locate it progressively in zones corresponding to the traditional four spheres of elements (i.e. the concentric spheres of earth, water, air, and fire). Within the framework of this allegorical representation (that anticipates the myths of creation present in the *Dialogue* and in the *Discorsi*), Galileo could undermine Aristotle's explanation of natural motion in the terrestrial world (based on the concept of absolute gravity and levity). He could also connect one of the basic aspects of traditional cosmology (the four spheres of the terrestrial world) to the physical concepts of condensation and rarefaction, capable of accounting for the specific gravity hypothesis invoked to explain his own experiments on motion and floating bodies. The four elements belonging properly to the four spheres were nothing other than four differently condensed aggregations of the same small particles. As to the matter of the heavens this would represent the ultimate level of rarefaction of the primordial matter and it would be akin to light. A resonance of this conception linking the constitution of the world to a terrestrial physics of strong Archimedean and atomistic inspiration is indeed present in the earlier considered pages of *Saggiatore* dealing with senses, where Galileo establishes a relationship between the various sensations on one side, and the four elements on the other side, and adumbrates a correlation between vision and light.

Within the framework of atomism, the different qualities of objects cannot be accounted for by the Aristotelian categories of matter and form, and need to be explained on the basis of the different states of configuration and movement of the minute bodies from which the matter of universe is made. This is what Galileo tries to do in *Saggiatore* by elaborating the sensorial conceptions of

[4] See OG I, pp. 243–417. An excellent discussion of the importance of atomism in Galileo's work is found in Galluzzi, 2011.

the classic atomists and inserting them within the framework of his global epistemological and ontological vision of the world, based on a concept of order and necessity, and strongly averse to any trivial anthropomorphic finalism.

10.6 The silence of Nature

By saying that tastes, smells, colours, etc. would have no existence in the absence of the individuals endowed with sensory capabilities, Galileo is not simply asserting the intrinsic subjectivity of sensations nor is he putting sensations outside the realm of scientific investigation. In marked contrast to the dominant Aristotelian tradition, he is saying that nature does not contain specific signals for the purpose of sensory communication with living beings. Put in other terms, there is no specific language through which nature talks to living beings (and especially to humans) by signs especially adapted to their sensory processes. For Galileo, sensations are the results of actions exerted on the sentient individual (*corpo sensitivo*) by purely objective elements, lacking any definite sensory attribute. These elements (or agencies) are identified with matter in movement of diverse rarefaction or subtlety: on the one hand the dense and tough matter involved in tactile sensation and, on the other, the extremely rare 'ultimate and deepest level of resolution' of the matter which might possibly account for light and, through it, vision.

If we take aside the more mechanistic aspects, this is the epistemological conception which underlies modern sensory physiology. In the external world there are no flavours, no odours, no colours, no sounds, but only molecules, mechanical or electro- magnetic waves (or other types of energies) which are a part of the universe. All this exists independently, and has no definite and constitutive relation with sentient individuals. Throughout evolution, sensory systems have arisen and become adapted to exploit these moving molecules or energies in order to gather information about the external (or internal) world. By themselves, however, molecules have neither taste nor smell, mechanical vibrations are not intrinsically sonorous, and electromagnetic waves are not coloured. Sensory qualifications arise from the interaction between the objective environmental elements with specific biological systems of varying complexity, but all evolved in such a way as to interact effectively with them. Not only the characteristics but also the very existence of these qualifications depends on the characteristics and existence of those biological systems. If they were removed, sensory qualities would lack any definite reality.

In Galileo's own words:

> I think that tastes, odors, colors, and so forth are no more than mere names so far as pertains to the subject wherein they appear to reside, and that they have their habitation only in the sensitive body. Thus, if the living creature were removed, all these qualities would be removed and annihilated. (SAGGIATORE, p. 196; transl. p. 309)

To evaluate the modernity of Galileo's conception of sensation we could compare these words with two short passages from modern books dealing with sense physiology. In the chapter entitled 'Coding of sensory information' written by Esther P. Gardner and John H. Martin in a contemporary textbook of neuroscience, the authors write:

> Colors, tones, smells, and tastes are mental constructions created by the brain out of sensory experience. They do not exist, as such, outside of the brain. Thus, we can answer the traditional question raised by philosophers: Does a sound exist when a tree falls in the forest, if no one is near enough to hear it? We now believe that the fall causes vibration in the air but not sound. Sound only occurs when pressure waves from the falling tree reach and are perceived by a living being. (Gardner & Martin, 2000, p. 412)

In *Eye and Brain*, a very popular volume on visual physiology and psychology, Richard Gregory pointed out some of the basic principles of visual perception in contemporary science with these words:

> We should realize quite clearly that without life there would be no brightness and no colour. Before life came, especially higher forms of life, all was invisible and silent though the sun shone and the mountains toppled. (Gregory, 2005, p. 85)

10.7 **Chromatic ambiguities**

Colour vision provides an apposite example to illustrate these modern views of sensory science. Similar to some of the most evolved monkeys, humans perceive colours through the interaction of electromagnetic oscillations of wavelengths between 400 and 700 nanometres with a photoreceptive system based on three types of retinal cones. These cones are sensitive to a rather wide band of wavelengths, with peaks of sensitivity around, respectively, 430, 550, and 570 nanometres loosely named as blue, green, and red cones. In ordinary conditions, stimulation with long wavelength waves tend to induce a sensation of red, while the stimulation with intermediate or short wavelengths produces, respectively, the sensation of green or blue. Because of this we tend to speak of red, green, and blue lights, in the tacit assumption that colours are objective and unequivocal attributes of specific forms of light.

Isaac Newton's prism experiment (Figure 10.3) represented an advance in colour science, by changing the origin of chromatic sensations from intrinsic qualities of the objects (as Aristotle maintained) to specific properties of light radiations. In the famous article on the *Philosophical Transactions* in which he communicated his discovery, after linking the various colours of light to their different degree of refraction through the prism, he wrote:

> Colours are not *Qualifications of Light*, derived from Refractions, or Reflections of natural bodies (as 'tis generally believed,) but *Original* and *connate properties*, which in divers Rays are divers. Some Rays

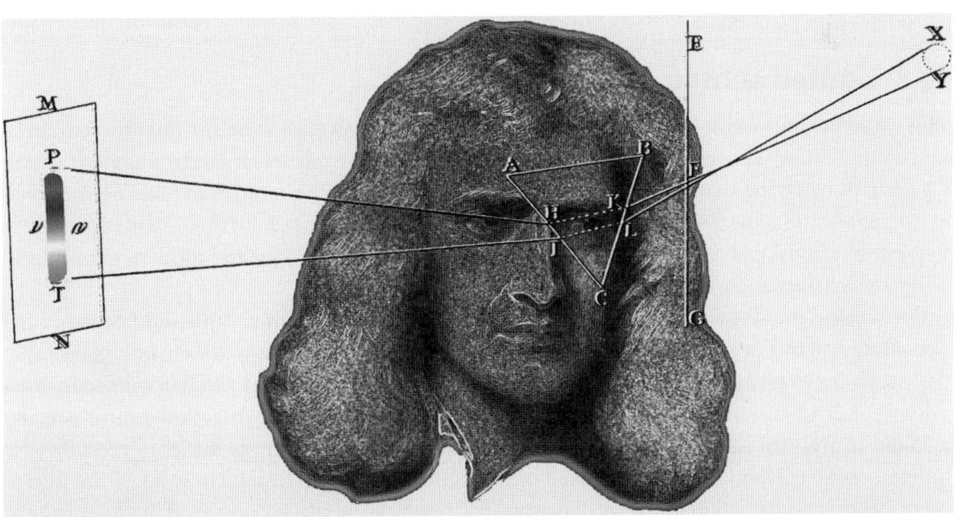

Figure 10.3 *Newton's spectrum* by Nicholas Wade. The portrait of Isaac Newton (derived from an illustration in Wood, 1885) is combined with his diagram of a beam of sunlight passing through a prism and forming an elongated spectrum (from his *Opticks*, published in 1704).

> are disposed to exhibit a red colour and no other; some a yellow and no other, some a green and no other, and so of the rest. Nor are there only Rays proper and particular to the more eminent colours, but even to all their intermediate gradations. (Newton, 1671/1672, p. 3081: original emphasis)

Despite great progress in the physics of light promoted by Newton's prism experiment, the close relationship he established between luminous rays 'which differ in degrees of Refrangibility' and colours, has been somewhat misleading from the point of view of the physiology of colour sensations. This is because of the inherent ambiguity resulting from the mechanisms of colour vision, based on the differential stimulation of three types of broad-band retinal receptors. A person can have exactly the same chromatic sensation, for instance of yellow, either in the presence of electromagnetic oscillations of about 600 nanometres wavelength, or in the presence of an appropriate combination of two waves, one in the longer and the other in the shorter region of the spectrum (for instance, 630 and 550 nanometres). This would happen when the two wavelengths of the combination are capable of stimulating the red and green sensitive cones exactly in the same way as the single 600 wavelength oscillation does. This means that, starting from the perception of a given chromatic hue (yellow in this case), we cannot infer in an univocal and straightforward way the characteristics of the stimulating light.

But there is more. The experiment in which exactly the same yellow sensation is perceived with different types of light is valid only for an individual possessing a particular type of system of three type of cones with those determined bands of sensibility. A person (or an animal) looking at those same lights might have a different sensation originating from the single-wavelength light and from the composition of two different wavelengths. For humans this could happen in the case of anomalies of colour vision. Most animals have a different system of colour vision from ours: for instance, one based on only two type of cones (as is the case for most mammals), or four types of photoreceptors (as in honeybees), or three cones, but different from primates (as in some fishes, reptiles, and birds). To further complicate the matter, exactly the same light (or combination of lights) irradiating from an object can appear of different colours to the same individual, depending on the characteristic of the light in the background surrounding the object and on the condition of light adaptation.

10.8 **Limited senses**

This could be summarized by saying that electromagnetic waves exist in nature but there would be no colour if there were no individuals capable detecting those particular electromagnetic waves. Or perhaps by saying that 'tastes, odors, colors, and so forth are no more than mere names so far as pertains to the subject wherein they appear to reside, and that they have their habitation only in the sensitive body', as Galileo wrote a little less than four centuries ago (and modern neurophysiology straightforwardly confirms).

Concerning the sensation of sound present in the quotation from Gardner and Martin (and also alluded to by Gregory), we have here another opportunity to point to the elusive relationship that exists between external agencies and sensations. In the presence of mechanical oscillations, a living individual endowed with an appropriate system of acoustic detection would perceive a sound if pressure waves of a certain intensity and frequency reach the auditory receptors (in humans some particular types of ciliated cells situated in the inner ear). However, if the instrument producing the oscillations (a diapason, for example) is placed on the skin (for instance, on the palmar surface of the finger or near some joints) an entirely different sensation would result: a kind of swarming or numbing sensation that we normally call vibration because usually we associate it with a vibrating body. This means that a given mechanical stimulus can produce two entirely different sensations with reference to the specific sensory apparatus it is capable of stimulating. In other words, there are mechanical oscillations in the real world but it would be impossible to say what is a sound and what is a vibrating sensation without the presence of a living and perceiving individual.

With reference to mechanical stimulation the discourse could be broadened by taking into consideration the action exerted on the body surface by strong pressure. In response to this type of stimulation, a normal individual would perceive pain in addition to the tactile sensation.

There are, however, particular neurological conditions in which a person might be deprived of the pain sensation. This may happen, for instance, in syphilitic myelopathy (*tabes dorsalis*) and also in a very rare syndrome of congenital insensitivity to pain (congenital analgesia). In these circumstances, in the presence of a violent mechanical stimulus, the person would still perceive only pressure sensation, but would not feel pain.

The discussion could be broadened further by considering less conventional senses, some of which were unknown in Galileo's age. Among them are the electric sense of many fishes, the echolocation system of bats, the magnetic sense which contributes to the migratory orientation of birds, and the capability of detecting the angle of light polarization present in some fishes, reptiles, and birds. Within an Aristotelian perspective, one would be obliged to assume the existence of other proper sensibles, in addition to the physical entities constitutive of the universe (corpuscles, forces, energies) for any new sensory modality.

10.9 **A closed world**

The investigation of sensory organs was particularly vibrant in Galileo's era, particularly their gross anatomy, and it involved some of his former colleagues in Padua (like Fabricius ab Aquapendente—his personal physician—and Giulio Casseri; see Chapter 1). On the basis of his knowledge, Galileo could not anticipate the development of modern sensory science. However, being an accurate observer (and a 'true philosopher' as he declared to be) he was aware that Aristotle's proper sensibles would have implied an unjustified, and potentially unlimited, multiplication of the '*entia*' of the external world (in the form of 'qualities', 'affections', or 'virtues'). This would have occurred as a consequence of the multiplication of the possible relational targets on which the external object might possibly interact in the sensory process (the sensitive man or the insensitive statue in the case of the tickling sensation in his expressive example). According to an Aristotelian view, any new dimension of sensitivity would require a new proper sensible. The number and characteristics of these proper sensibles thus would depend on the number and characteristics of the sentient individuals, a position that Galileo considered to be unjustified. This difficulty was one of the reasons why the Aristotelian tradition tended to keep a fixed number of senses (five) and refuted, by ad hoc hypotheses, the possibility of new sensations. A particularly serious consequence of this has been the obstacle to accepting the existence of other senses like vestibular sense and other forms of proprioception in humans (Wade, 2003) and, moreover, electroreception and electrolocation, the complex sensory organization by which many fishes can detect the presence of other organisms and swim avoiding obstacle even in the most complete darkness (Moller, 1995; Finger & Piccolino, 2011).

10.10 **Of an inexorable nature, of books, plants, and brains**

The idea of a world characterized by definite sensory qualities specifically adapted to senses (particularly to human senses) was diametrically opposed to Galileo's basic principles regarding the nature of the universe. Although the universe can be known to humans according to Galileo's famous aphorism of the 'book of universe', it was not specifically constructed to be comprehensible for them. The metaphor of nature or universe as a book, which is present in many of Galileo's writings, is (as already mentioned in our Chapter 1), particularly well developed in *Saggiatore*:

> Philosophy is written in this grand book, I mean the universe, which stands continually open to our gaze. But it cannot be understood unless one first learns to comprehend the language and comprehend the characters in which it is written. It is written in the language of mathematics, and its characters are triangles, circles, and other geometric figures, without which it is humanly impossible to understand a single word of it; without these one is wandering about in a dark labyrinth. (SAGGIATORE, p. 25; transl. pp. 184–185)

The allusion to the language of mathematics and to its abstract characters (triangles, circles, and other geometric figures) serves to highlight the difficulty rather than the ease of deciphering it. Galileo says that nature is regulated by well-defined laws, and its therefore knowable, but these laws are difficult to investigate and require considerable effort to be understood, being written in a language that is not directly suited to human comprehension. In Galileo's view, the book of nature or of the universe is not meant for communicating a specific message to humans. In this sense, despite the similarity of terminology, the book of the universe implied by Galileo's words is opposite to 'the book of the world' of medieval and Renaissance scholars. According to these different views, endorsed, for instance, by Giordano Bruno and Tommaso Campanella, the world was the book by which God communicated to human beings his deep messages, often in a somewhat mysterious way, according to a language rich in symbolism of religious, and often astrological and alchemical dimensions.

Galileo frequently develops the theme of nature characterized by inexorable laws, not necessarily accessible to the human understanding. This theme is evident in the discussion on the relationship between the language of the Bible and that of nature. This is what he wrote in his letter to Castelli on 21 December 1613:

> The Holy Scripture and nature both equally proceed from the divine Word, the former as the dictation of the Holy Spirit and the latter as the most observant executrix of God's orders; moreover, in order to adapt itself to the understanding of all people, it was appropriate for Scripture to say many things which are different from absolute truth in appearance and in regard to the meaning of the words; on the other hand nature is inexorable and immutable, and she does not care at all whether or not her recondite reasons and modes of operations are revealed to human understanding, and so she never transgresses the terms of the laws imposed on her. (OG V, p. 282; transl. Finocchiaro, 1989, p. 50).

Galileo expressed himself in similar terms in his 1615 letter to the Grand Duchess of Tuscany, Christina of Lorena. In this important text, when speaking of 'the open book of the heavens', he stresses the difficulty of investigating the secrets of nature:

> Nor should anyone think that the reading of the very lofty words written on those pages is completed by merely seeing the sun and the stars give off light, rise, and set, which is as far as the eyes of animals and of common people reach; on the contrary, those pages contain such profound mysteries and such sublime concepts that the vigils, labors, and studies of hundreds of the sharpest minds in uninterrupted investigations for thousands of years have not yet completely fathomed them. (OG V, p. 329; transl. Finocchiaro, 1989, p. 103).

In another letter addressed on 21 May 1611 to Msgr. Piero Dini, a Vatican prelate and one of his colleagues at the Accademia Fiorentina, Galileo discussed the theme of the language of nature and of its independence with respect to the possible understanding that humans can have of it.

This discussion is inserted within the context of his discovery of the satellites of Jupiter and the incredulity by which this observation had been received by the conservative intelligentsia of the time. There are many atomistic allusions in the text, signifying Galileo's general intellectual approach:

> It would appear boldness, or even temerity, on my side if I attempted to circumscribe within the narrow limits of my understanding the understanding and operating of nature. In the past few days, when I was in the house of my lord, the Most Illustrious and Excellent Marquis Cesi, I saw the pictures of 500 Indian plants, and I had to declare that, either they were a fiction, denying that such plants are to be found in the world, or, if they did exist, they were vain and superfluous, since neither I nor any of those present knew their qualities, properties and effects. Certainly I do not believe that in the most ancient and coarse centuries, nature abstained from producing the immense variety of animals, gems, metals and other minerals, from providing those animals with any of their members, muscle, articulation; and that, moreover, it failed to move the celestial spheres, and, in sum, to produce and operate its effects; and that happened because those people, unaware of the properties of plants, stones and fossils, did not know the function of all parts of animals, and did not penetrate the courses of the stars. And indeed it would appear to me ridiculous to assume that the things of nature start to exist, when we start to discover and understand them. (OG XI, p. 107)

On the one hand, nature does communicate with humans through a language specifically adapted to their senses. On the other hand, nature does not receive any ontological justification from the knowledge that humans can have of its production and of its ways of operating.

In the *Dialogue* the theme of the inexorability of nature, and of the possibility that its ways of operating could exceed human imagination, recurs many times. An aspect of the relationship between nature and the possible understanding of it by humans emerges in a passage in which Sagredo points to the absurdity of the conceptions of the Aristotelian philosopher Scipione Chiaramonti. In the context of his criticism of the astronomical novelties, Chiaramonti stated that one of the absurdities implied in the Copernican conception had to do with fact that it attributed the same motions to 'things of very different nature'. In his opinion this could not happen because:

> Observation teaches us that the operations and motions of matters of different nature are diverse. And reason confirms this, for otherwise we should have no way of comprehending and distinguishing their nature, if they did not have their special motions and operations capable of guiding us to the cognition of their substances. (DIALOGO, p. 264, revised)[5]

To the Aristotelian principle invoked by the peripatetic philosopher, Sagredo wittily replied:

> Two or three times in this author's argument I have noticed that in order to prove that matters stand in such-and-such way, he makes use of the remark that in just this way they accommodate themselves to our comprehension, and that otherwise we should have no knowledge of this or that detail; or that the criterion of philosophy would be ruined; as if nature had been made the brain of man, and then arranged everything to conform, to the capacity of his intellect. But I should think rather that nature first made things in her own way, and then made human reason skilful enough to be able to understand, but only by hard work, some part of her secrets. (DIALOGO, p. 258; transl. pp. 264–265)

For Aristotle, and for his followers of the Middle Ages and Renaissance, things existed only in the function of mankind for whom their existence is justified. This ontological finalism had also

[5] The readers acquainted with Dante's *Divina commedia* (Divine comedy) may perhaps remember that a similar principle (different causes should produce different appearances and vice versa) is invoked by Beatrice in the II *Canto* of the *Paradiso* in order to rebut one of the possible explanations for the spotted aspect of the moon face.

a gnoseological implication. The existence of a thing is justified by its being knowledgeable. The geocentric conception in cosmology was just an aspect of this fundamental anthropocentric view based on the idea that the sun, planets, and stars were there just to make life on earth possible and to exert a variety of influences on mankind. Genuinely new discoveries posed problems because it was difficult to conceive that something, created or existing specifically for humans, might have existed for millennia without humans having knowledge of it. Besides being centred on mankind, the old universe was thus closed not only physically but also because all had been created for ever, and nothing really new could arise and develop in it.

In the cognitive sphere, an earth at the centre of the universe (and a human microcosm at the centre of the macrocosm) corresponded with humans capable of knowledge because they could interpret the signals that nature was continuously sending to their senses. The removal of mankind from this privileged, central situation had far-reaching implications for Galileo's conception of senses. If there is nothing essentially sensorial in the external world, nor specifically adapted to interact with the senses, then the senses should adapt themselves to objects so that information about them could be gathered. Sensory qualities are the consequence of such interactions which are oriented to objects rather than to mankind. This means that objects, but not sensory qualities, can exist without humans having knowledge of them. Since this interaction is not inscribed within a providential organization of the world, it does guard against the possibility of errors which can arise in various ways and are expressions of the limitation of our sensory capability. However, in spite of sensory limits, and notwithstanding the complexity of 'nature's way of operating', humans can obtain proper knowledge of reality if they are aware of the limits of their senses and submit the sensory appearances to the scrutiny of reason ('the eyes of mind').

The Copernican heliocentric conception removed man from his privileged position in the universe and the new science promoted by Galileo deprived humans of their privileged access to the special language of nature. As would later happen for other revolutionary phases of scientific progress, this was a price that human arrogance had to pay in order to extend man's inquisitive power to the world and on its laws. It also provided the conditions for novel avenues for investigating sensory physiology. So new that only after about four centuries are we starting to appreciate the importance and novelty of the reflection on the theme of senses in the work of Galileo.

10.11 **The long path from Galileo's sensory science to modern sensory physiology**

The particular nature of Galileo's interest in the senses, and especially in vision, may explain why his reflections had initially more impact on philosophical thinking than on the progress of sensory science. His elaboration of the two classes of sensory attributes of objects became the basis of Locke's (1690) distinction between 'primary' and 'secondary' sensory qualities expounded in the *Essay Concerning Human Understanding*. Galileo's general reflections on the senses had an important echo on the debate concerning the cognitive relation with reality. It involved various philosophers like Descartes, Gassendi, and Malebranche in France; Hobbes, Locke, Berkeley, and Hume in Britain; and Leibniz in Germany. They developed different views of the ontological and epistemological status of the primary and secondary qualities.

It was via a philosophical route that Galileo's sensory science resurfaced in the nineteenth century, to lay the foundations of modern sensory physiology. In a footnote at the end of section 1 of the first volume of the 1787 edition of his *Kritik der reinen Vernunft* ('Critique of pure reason'),

Kant, who was familiar with Galileo's work, expressed a conception of sensations somewhat similar that of *Saggiatore*:

> The taste of a wine does not belong to the objective determinations of the wine, not even if by the wine as an object we mean the wine as appearance, but to the special constitution of sense in the subject that tastes it. Colours are not properties of the bodies to the intuition of which they are attached, but only modifications of the sense of sight, which is affected in a certain manner by light. (Kant, 1787, p. 77)

In contrast to Galileo (and Locke and Descartes), Kant (Figure 10.4) placed the notion of space in the mind of the perceiver, as a form of necessary 'a priori intuition'. He distinguished it, however, on epistemic and ontological bases, from colours, tastes, etc. to which he assigned the more subjective status of sensations (i.e. pure alterations of the perceiving subject) rather than

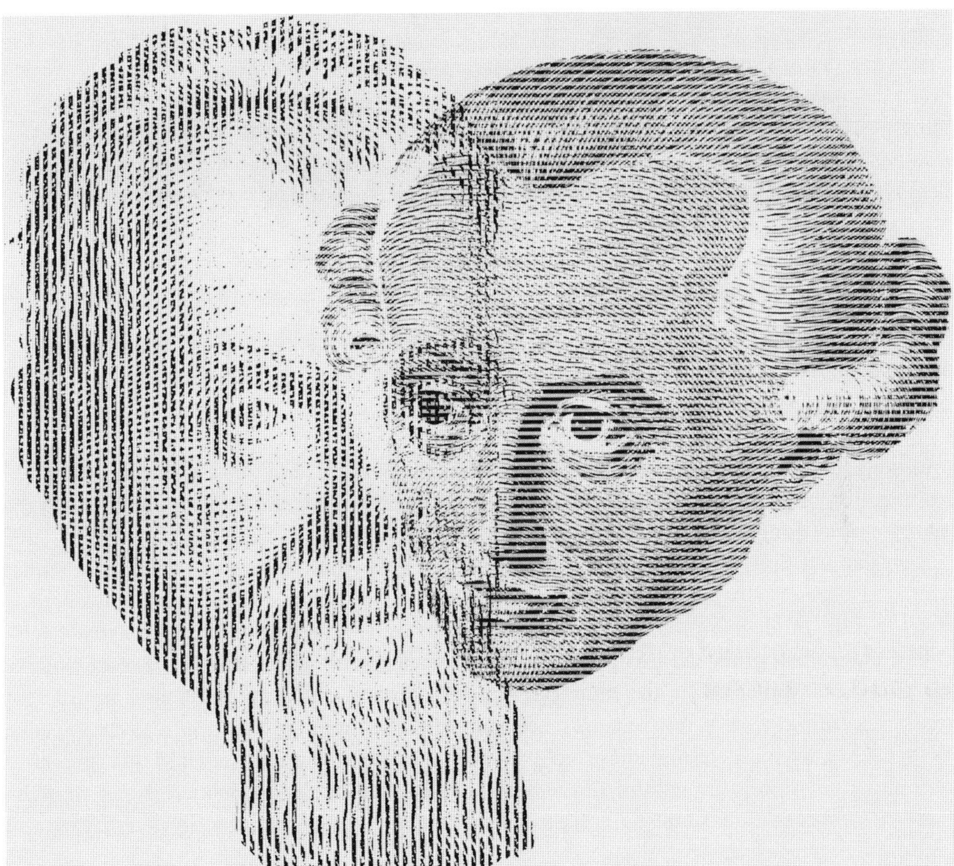

Figure 10.4 *Galileo Galileo and Kant seeing eye to eye* by Nicholas Wade. Galileo's portrait is based upon Leoni's engraving and that of Immanuel Kant is derived from an engraving in Hartenstein (1853). Kant developed a transcendental theory of mind which drew upon both rationalism and empiricism without being allied to either. Rather than accounting for ideas in terms of experience, Kant adopted the opposite strategy of accounting for experience in terms of conceptual categories. That is, our conscious, phenomenal world is a cognitive construction. He accepted that all knowledge arises from the senses, but it is not treated in a passive way.

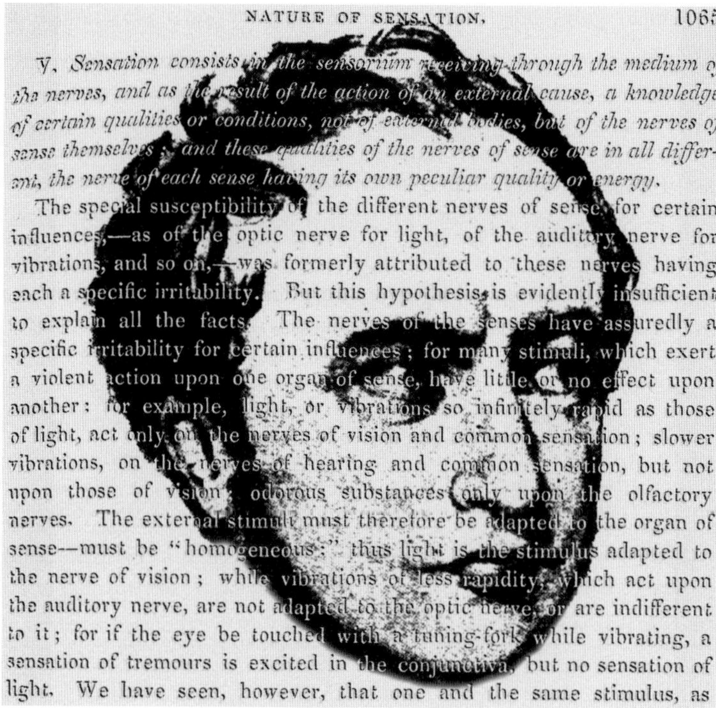
NATURE OF SENSATION. 1065
V. Sensation consists in the sensorium receiving through the medium of the nerves, and as the result of the action of an external cause, a knowledge of certain qualities or conditions, not of external bodies, but of the nerves of sense themselves; and these qualities of the nerves of sense are in all different, the nerve of each sense having its own peculiar quality or energy.
The special susceptibility of the different nerves of sense for certain influences,—as of the optic nerve for light, of the auditory nerve for vibrations, and so on,—was formerly attributed to these nerves having each a specific irritability. But this hypothesis is evidently insufficient to explain all the facts. The nerves of the senses have assuredly a specific irritability for certain influences; for many stimuli, which exert a violent action upon one organ of sense, have little or no effect upon another: for example, light, or vibrations so infinitely rapid as those of light, act only on the nerves of vision and common sensation; slower vibrations, on the nerves of hearing and common sensation, but not upon those of vision; odorous substances only upon the olfactory nerves. The external stimuli must therefore be adapted to the organ of sense—must be "homogeneous:" thus light is the stimulus adapted to the nerve of vision; while vibrations of less rapidity, which act upon the auditory nerve, are not adapted to the optic nerve, or are indifferent to it; for if the eye be touched with a tuning-fork while vibrating, a sensation of tremours is excited in the conjunctiva, but no sensation of light. We have seen, however, that one and the same stimulus, as

Figure 10.5 *Müller's doctrine* by Nicholas Wade. The portrait of Johannes Müller is based on an illustration in Hirsch (1929). It is combined with text from Müller describing an aspect of his doctrine of specific nerve energies.

intuitions (these being more universally valid). The view of space (and time) as intuitions derived from the impossibility, within the framework of Kant's transcendental idealism, of knowing the '*Ding an sich*' (thing in itself).[6]

Kant's conceptions became a philosophical reference for the German physiologist Johannes Müller (Figure 10.5) when formulating his doctrine of 'specific nerve energies'. This doctrine states that the modality of the sensations produced by different stimuli on a given nerve is relatively independent of the nature of the stimulus, but is a specific expression of the sensory nerve stimulated. As Müller put it 'the same external cause excites different impressions in different senses, according to the nature of each sense, namely the sensation of the specific nerve' (Müller, 1840, p. 251). Even if determined normally by external causes, sensations are always expressions of internal 'conditions or qualities' of the nerves. The action of external stimuli is only to excite these internal conditions of the nerves, also referred to as 'energies' from the Greek term ενεργεια (action, vigour) used by Aristotle.

[6] As shown in a recent essay by Gary Hatfield, Kant's conception of primary and secondary qualities changed considerably since his first writings (as, for instance, *Physical Monadology* of 1756) up to his more developed formulations of his mature works. Another important aspect of Kant's (and Helmholtz's) treatment of primary and secondary qualities remarked by Hatfield is the reference to the Newtonian conception of force as primordial to the categories of space and time (Hatfield, 2011).

Müller, who criticized contemporary philosophers for ignoring the biological constraints imposed by the specificities of sensory mechanisms in their theories of knowledge, provided many examples of the subjective and internal nature of sensations, and of its specific dependence on the characteristics of the sensory apparatus. For instance: 'the same number of vibrations in a tuning-fork, which imparts its sensations to the auditory nerve, will be perceived as tickle in the nerves of touch. Something completely different to vibrations must be produced if it should be experienced as sound, and this requirement lies in the auditory nerve' (Müller 1840, p. 256). As Müller warned afterwards, with words which resound with the passage from *Saggiatore*:

> there is no sound in the world without a living ear, but only vibrations; without a living eye there would be no light, no colour, no darkness in the world, but only the imponderable oscillations that correspond to light and its matter, or their absence. (Müller, 1840, p. 261)

In elaborating his general views of sensory physiology, Müller was summarizing and extending observations and conceptions developed before him by several scientists, but the philosophical grounds of his doctrine were undoubtedly inspired by Kant, as is also clear in the work of Müller's student, Hermann Helmholtz (Figure 10.6). In his monumental volumes on physiological optics and hearing, and in other texts as well, Helmholtz elaborated Müller's views of the senses on both a physiological and a philosophical basis, and thus laid the theoretical framework for the subsequent development of modern sensory neuroscience (see Cahan, 1994; Finger & Wade, 2002a, 2002b).

Like Müller, Helmholtz rejected any close correspondence between the sensations on one side and the reality they represent on the other. The process whereby sensations are produced involved both the external objects and the sentient individual: the way they interacted was somewhat similar to a chemical reaction. The outcome depended on the nature of both reacting elements and the laws of the process can only be specified with relation to the properties of the two elements. For Helmholtz, sensations were 'signs', 'tokens', or 'representations', which, in order to provide us with knowledge of reality, need to be 'interpreted' or 'deciphered' by our mind; they need not be similar to the external things they represent:

> The sensations of the senses are tokens for our consciousness, it being left to our intelligence to learn how to comprehend their meaning. Evidently, any other sensations, not only of sight but of other senses also, produced by a visible object when we move our eyes or our body so as to look at the object from different sides or to touch it, etc., may be learned by experience. The content of all these possible sensations united in a total idea forms our idea of the body; and we call it perception when it is reinforced by actual sensations. The only psychic activity required for this purpose is the regularly recurrent association between two ideas which have often been connected before. (Helmholtz, 1925, pp. 533–534)

In spite of this, and of the consequent impossibility of knowing the ultimate nature of the world (Kant's 'thing in itself'), the representations derived from senses are of fundamental significance, the consistency of the law of causality assuring the validity of the inferences based on sensory data:

> It is in this way that the representations of the outer world are images of the regular flow of natural events, and if they are formed correctly following the laws of thought, and if by our actions we can interpret them correctly in reality, then these interpretations are the only true ones; all others are false. (Helmholtz, 1867, pp. 446– 447)

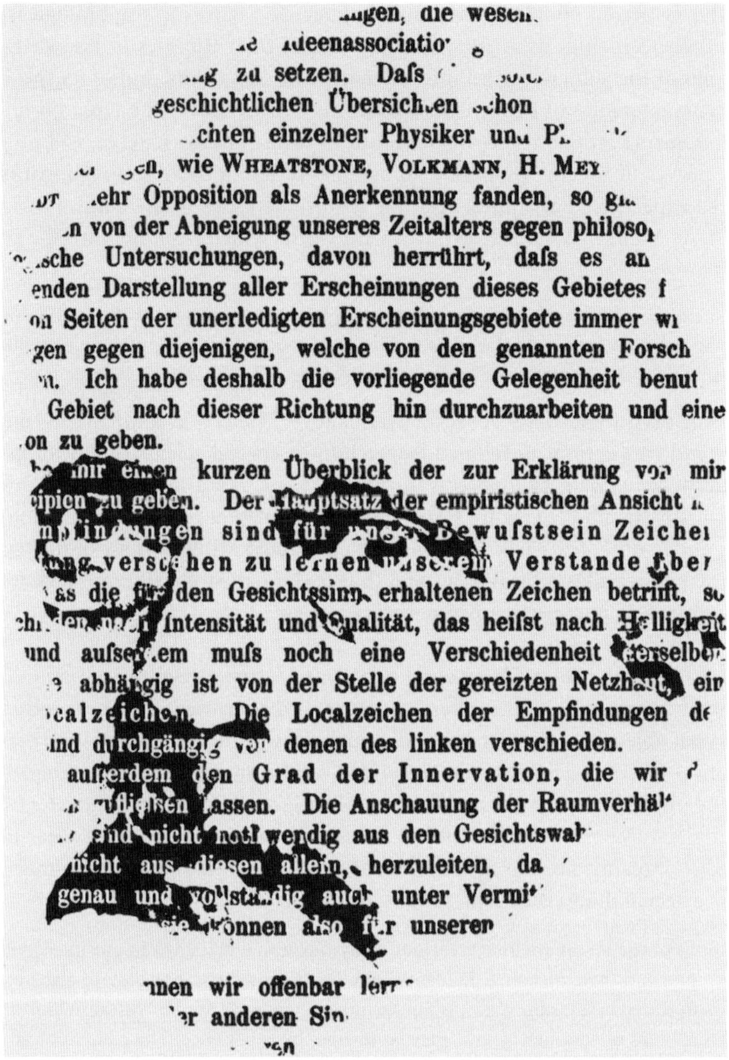

Figure 10.6 *Tokens of sensation* by Nicholas Wade. A portrait of Hermann Helmholtz (derived from a frontispiece in Helmholtz, 1924) can be seen in German text from Helmholtz (1896) describing the intelligence of perception. He adopted the concept of unconscious inference to account for the way in which we learn to see and how common perceptions can arise from varied patterns of stimulation.

In 1868, in a famous lecture on 'The New progresses of the theory of vision' (*Die neueren Fortschritte in der Theorie des Sehen*) Helmholtz wrote:

> Similar light produces under like conditions a like sensation of colour. Light which under like conditions excites unlike sensation of colour is dissimilar. (Helmholtz, 1895, p. 226)

For Helmholtz, the regularity of the production of a given sensation in a given sentient individual, 'under like conditions', ensures that the subjective and apparent character of sensations is not by itself deceitful as it could happen for pure illusions devoid of any usefulness in the path of human knowledge.

To exemplify the deception to which we are prone by assuming a close correspondence between the external world and sensations, he referred to the long-held supposition of the existence, in the rays of the sun, of a heating agent distinct from light, by which the sun might produce a heating effect and a sensation of warmth, in addition to that of light (an agent long referred to as 'caloric fluid'):

> As long as humans did not reflect on the nature of sensations, they were inclined to report immediately on the quality of sensations of external things, and to assume two agents corresponding to two sensations. (Helmholtz, 1867, p. 195)

Helmholtz was a contemporary of Charles Darwin. An important aspect of the new conception of the senses that emerged from his own work (and from that of Müller) is that it removed the obstacles that, in the Aristotelian tradition, prevented sensory science from becoming a part of the Darwinian paradigm. In the course of evolution, living organisms could develop new senses, better adapted to their evolving lifestyle and to their habitat; in order for this to be possible, the existence in the external world of proper sensibles, specific for any new sense, need not be invoked. The new vista on sensory science which emerged with Müller and his students was indeed open to new senses (and thus potentially Darwinian). This emerges in a passage in which, after having remarked that light does not suffice to make objects manifest, Müller wrote:

> Many other agents would similarly play the same role; if there were for electricity, as for light, a delicate organic reagent, electricity would also have, as light does, the property of revealing the existence of a material world. (Müller, 1840, p. 258)[7]

By 1840, when the second edition of Müller's *Handbuch der Physiologie des Menschen* was published, the idea of a possible electric sense was nothing more than a theoretical possibility. It was indeed four years later that James Stark, a Scottish surgeon, discovered in the tail of the skate the existence of a small organ similar to the big organs by which electric fishes (torpedoes, electric eels, and Nile catfishes) produce their powerful shocks (Stark, 1844). It was many years later that the French microscopist, Charles-Philippe Robin, and the Russian physiologist, Aleksandr Ivanovich Babukhin (or Babuchin), showed that these small organs produced a weak electricity (Robin, 1865; Babuchin, 1877). It was more than a century before electroreception and electrolocation (the mechanisms that allow several fish species to detect the presence of other animals and navigate in the complete darkness) were discovered in Cambridge by the (German) zoologist Hans Werner Lissmann (Lissmann, 1951, 1958; Lissmann & Machin, 1958). In this context Müller's remark might appear somewhat prophetic, but it should be considered that the new sensory physiology that he was promoting was dynamically open to new senses. This was because senses were conceived as adaptations developed by animal

[7] In another respect, electricity played an important role in both defining the senses and providing evidence for the doctrine of specific nerve energies. Indeed this relationship was appreciated many years before Müller in the physiological enquiries of Charles Bell: 'If light, pressure, galvanism, or electricity produce vision, we must conclude that the idea in the mind is the result of an action excited in the eye or in the brain, not any thing received, though caused by an impression from without. The operations of the mind are confined not by the limited nature of things created, but by the limited number of our organs of sense' (Bell, 1811/2000, p. 12). Before Bell, Alessandro Volta had come near the doctrine of specific nervous energies in his studies on animal electricity (see Piccolino, 2003; Piccolino & Bresadola, 2003/2013).

and humans to a universe where there exists nothing specifically 'sensible', but only matter in movement, oscillations, and energies.

This was what Müller and Helmholtz argued in the nineteenth century and Galileo with extraordinary astuteness foresaw more than two centuries earlier, in the pages of *Saggiatore* which have been the heart of the argument in this chapter.

Chapter 11

The problem of Galileo's predecessors

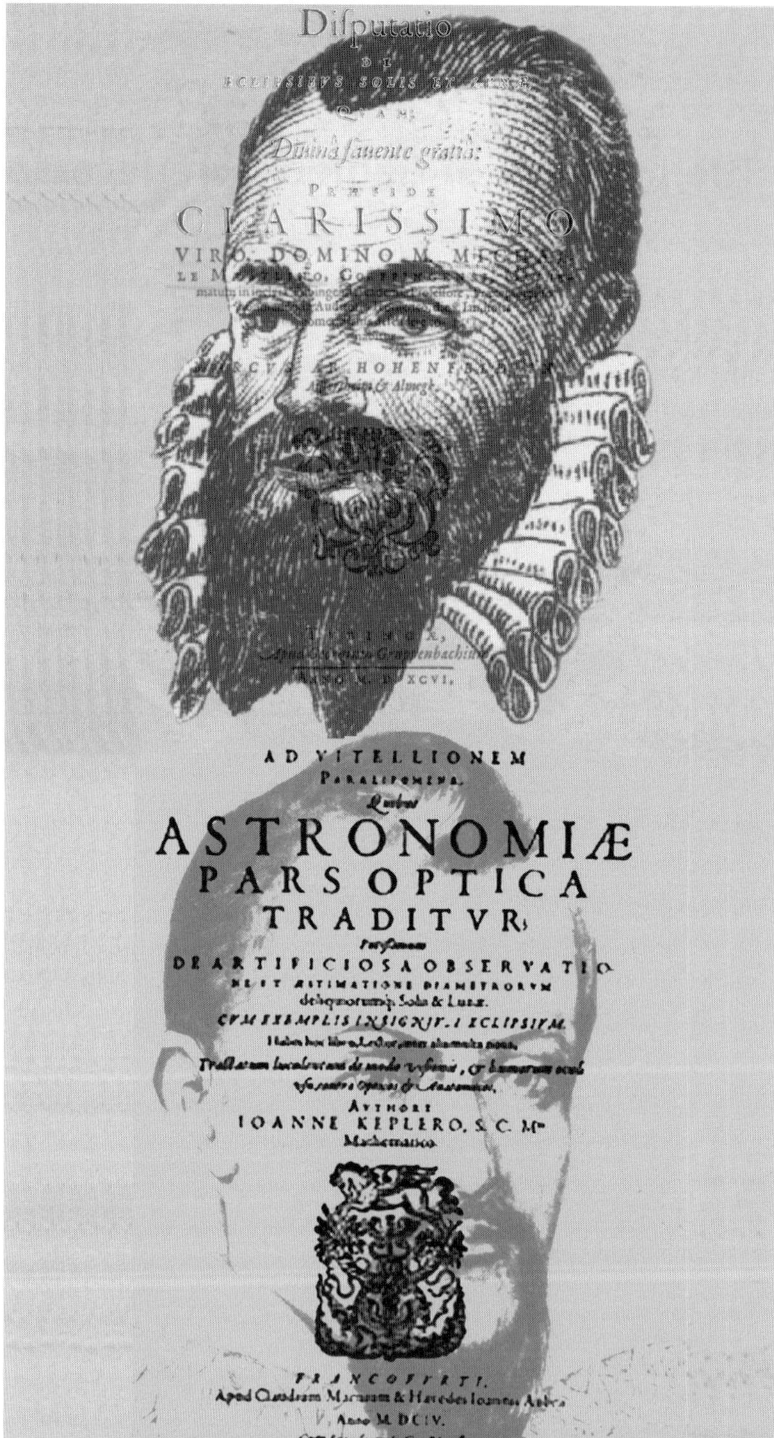

Figure XI *Maestlin's disputes and Kepler's optics* by Nicholas Wade. Michael Maestlin is shown together with the title page of his *Disputatio*. Kepler (shown with the title page of his *Optica*) initially studied under Maestlin.

In most of the previous chapters we have let Galileo express his interest in visual appearances in his own words. Our interpretations of the texts have been rather limited and directed mainly at clarifying what Galileo was saying, and to place his reflections and discussions within particular scientific and logical contexts. Our choice has been dictated by our desire to put together Galileo's words on vision, which are dispersed in many of his writings; some of these are not easy to access (particularly for those unacquainted with Italian or Latin languages). In doing so we have opted for a narrative style which often reflected that found in Galileo's texts. Although not in a proper and defined way, our effort has aimed at reconstituting the treatise on vision and colours *De visu et coloribus* that Galileo announced on 7 May 1610 to Belisario Vinta (the secretary of Tuscany Grand Duke) but never completed (OG XI, p. 352). Our choice has generally obliged us to limit the comments and to avoid any comprehensive doxography aimed at placing Galileo within an historical and scientific context.

We have occasionally mentioned that some of Galileo's conclusions developed from hypotheses formulated by previous scholars. Nevertheless, we are aware that the view of Galileo emerging from our book is possibly that of a solitary inventor of new vistas in the field of vision (as in other scientific and intellectual domains). This impression is indeed largely distorted and inappropriate because many of the themes were certainly not invented by Galileo. Even the telescope, the instrument with which his name is connected, was not his genuine invention, being derived from the instruments produced in Holland about 1608, and which arrived at Padua and Venice in 1609 (the *occhiali in canna* to which we have alluded in Chapter 1).

As the famous Hungarian physiologist Georg von Bekesy remarked in his Nobel lecture delivered in 1961, invention is indeed a subtle and difficult art and people have difficulty even simply imagining really new things. Normally every invention is based on previous elements that are assembled together in a more or less original way. These prior elements generally have a complex history and it is especially arduous to pinpoint precisely when some particularly novel aspect of this history has emerged.

This has undoubtedly occurred with many of Galileo's ideas and achievements in the particular domain of visual science. This notwithstanding, there is hardly a single aspect in which his way of dealing with the matter can be considered a simple repetition of previous ideas or arguments. What is more, Galileo's visual (and sensory) science is inserted within the framework of a vigorous effort aimed at reforming the scientific and intellectual approach to the knowledge of reality. This is perhaps the most significant aspect of Galileo's intellectual enterprise, a feature that has made the Pisan scholar a kind of cornerstone in Western cultural history. A person, or better a 'hero', who is still intensively studied more than four centuries after publication of his first telescopic observations and he remains the subject of heated controversies and passions.

11.1 **Plucking the crow of Aesop**

Nevertheless, in *Sidereus* (and to a large extent in subsequent works, too) Galileo himself was sparing in presenting and discussing his sources and references (as was the practice then[1]). When he did, it was usually for reasons of polemics or in order to deliberately attenuate the revolutionary character of his assertions or theories. The latter was done in the hope of avoiding possible criticisms and condemnations from ecclesiastic authorities, by showing that he was simply re-stating

[1] A rather striking example of this behaviour is the *Dioptrique* of Descartes in which the French philosopher pays no tribute to the optical work of his predecessors (and particularly Kepler and Scheiner) from whom he derived some fundamental conceptions (see Chapter 13).

old opinions. For instance, he was able to attribute the Copernican opinion of the movement of the earth around the sun to Aristarchus, Pythagoras and his followers (and sometimes also to Plato and other scholars).

In Galileo's day, this aspect of *Sidereus* was remarked upon in a more or less pungent way. In a letter sent to Kepler on 16 April 1610 (about one month after the publication of *Sidereus*) Georg Fugger, the ambassador in Venice of the Emperor Rudolph II, wrote: 'That man [Galileo] can, and is used to, gather up the feathers of others, so that he can adorn himself with them like the crow in Aesop' (OG X, p. 316). On his side, three days later, Kepler in a long letter addressed to Galileo (and printed on 3 May with the title of *Dissertatio cum nuncio sidereo*), although expressing his admiration for the brilliant findings announced in the landmark text of his Italian colleague, nevertheless highlighted Galileo's astronomical predecessors, largely by making reference to his own (i.e. Kepler's) observations and opinions (OG X, pp. 319–340; Kepler, 1610).

Michael Maestlin, Kepler's teacher in Tubingen, in commenting on the *Dissertatio* of his former student (probably being aware of the Aesopian metaphor applied to Galileo in Fugger's letter) wrote to his former student on 7 September 1610:

> In your essay (the copy of which you sent me is very pleasant to read; of this I give to you very great thanks) you did the exceedingly good job of plucking that Galileo of his feathers. He is not the first inventor of the telescope, nor is he the first person to notice the rough surface of the moon, nor the first to tell the world there are many more stars in the sky than those recorded until now in old texts. And also for the rest. (I also render you my thanks again for the very honourable mention you did of me in your Dissertation, not the thanks that I owe you, but the greatest that I can make.) (OG X, p. 428)

Kepler's *Dissertatio* touched on most of the themes that we have considered in our book. It is perhaps interesting to follow his reasoning, and particularly his reference to Galileo's possible predecessors, in order to highlight the extent to which Galileo was simply pursuing previous ideas and to what measure he was original in his scientific theories. In addition to Kepler's text we would also take into account another work which was a reference for him (and also for Galileo) in their considerations of the aspects of the moon. This is Plutarch's text generally known by the Latin title, *De facie quae in orbe lunae apparet* (Figure 11.1); it has already been mentioned in Chapter 6, when dealing with the lunar mountains. The reason for our choice is because Plutarch and Kepler can be considered the authors who best represent the knowledge on the moon appearances in classical antiquity and in Galileo's time.

With regard to the parenthetic allusion at the end of Maestlin's letter, we consider first a particularly important point in Kepler's expressed appreciation for the achievements of his teacher. These mainly concern Maestlin's observations and opinions on the appearance of the moon. Among these was his correct interpretation of the cause of the weak light in the dark zone of the moon (the ash light, secondary lumen or lunar candour of Galileo's texts). In that respect Kepler invited Galileo to consider Maestlin's opinion that he 'had fully transcribed in the Optical part of Astronomy, Ch. 6, n° 10, page 252' (Kepler was thus referring to the important work he published in 1604 with a long title, generally known as either *Astronomiae pars optica* or *Ad Vitellionem paralipomena*: see Chapter 13).

In this work, after critically reviewing several opinions of recent authors on the nature and origin of the phenomena, Kepler wrote:

> On the other hand, my first teacher, Maestlin, to my knowledge discovered the true cause, and taught it to me and to all attending his lectures 12 years ago, and publicly explained it in 1596 in theses 21, 22, and 23 of his Disputation on Eclipses. (OPTICA, p. 254; transl. p. 266)

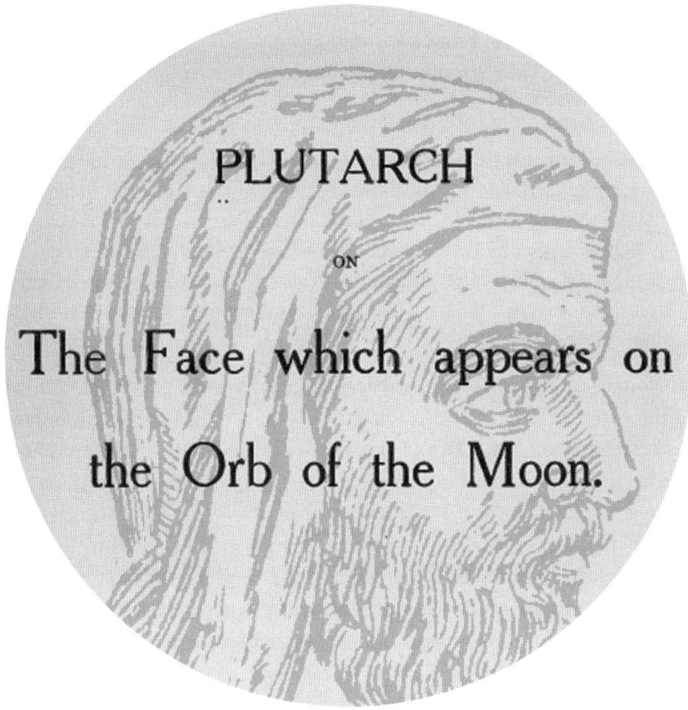

Figure 11.1 *Plutarch's face in the moon* by Nicholas Wade. Plutarch's profile is presented together with the title page of a translation of his book (Prickard, 1911).

Afterwards Kepler reported a long citation from the *Disputatio de eclipsibus solis et lunae* of his teacher where Maestlin expounds his interpretation of the phenomenon:

> On the light which is seen in the horned moon near the horns, diffused through the whole body, it is agreed by those who see it that it is not overshadowed by the brightness of the daylight, which either remains in the evening after the setting of the sun, before twilight (that is, while it is still bright day), or in the morning, with the dawn, precedes the rising of the sun. On the other hand, it is agreed that this same light is weakened on the rest of the days farther removed from new moon, so much so that about quadrature, when the moon is a long way above the horizon in the dead of night, nothing, or very little, of it is seen to remain [and that only by people with the sharpest vision]. Therefore, from this light's being separable, it is concluded that it is not, as certain people wish (among whom is Reinhold), born along with the moon and proper to it, but, just like that great monthly light, is similarly foreign and borrowed. For unless this were so, it would assuredly be seen much more brightly in the dead of night than in the illuminated air of daylight. Moreover, the derivation of this light upon the moon is shown by its position with respect to the earth. For in the new moon, the moon, placed between the sun and the earth, sees that face of the earth which the sun illuminates, placed directly beneath it. But we acknowledge that the strength and brilliance of the sun's rays reflected individually on the single parts of the earth is such that in sunny places it dulls the sharpness of the eyes; and furthermore, that it fills with light the inner recesses of buildings, wherever it is allowed to enter even through a little crack. Who will deny this same thing of the whole of the light itself, gathered and reflected from the whole earth together with the water? We therefore say that the earth, by its gleaming light, sent to it from the sun, casts its rays on the opacity or night in the lunar body no less than, in turn (in exactly the same way) the full moon illuminates our nights in earth with its

rays received from the sun, and turns them almost to day in proportion to their brightness. It does this with all the greater clarity in proportion to the earth's circle's being greater than the moon's circle. And the ratio of the one to the other is greater than twelve times. Consequently, just as these two bodies by turns intercept the sun's light for each other, as we have said before, so in turns each lights up to the night of the other. This opinion receives support from that weakening of this light. For, when the moon afterwards moves away from the new, it begins gradually to leave this illuminated central part of the earth and to perceive its remaining part more and more obliquely. At the same time, the strength of the reflected rays is both diminished and dulled. Hence it happens that whatever of this light is reflected to the moon that is halved or swelling beyond that, can be seen on earth either not at all, or with greatest difficulty, because of the excessive attenuation. (OPTICA,[2] pp. 254–255; transl. pp. 266–267; the parts between round brackets are Kepler's interpolations; the original is in Maestlin, 1596, pp. 7–8)

Soon after this long quotation, Kepler mentions one of his own observations which confirmed that capacity of the earth to reflect sunlight and thus supported Maestlin's interpretation.

From Kepler's reference to his teacher's work there is little doubt that, several years before the publication of *Sidereus*, Maestlin had expounded a fairly correct explanation for the dark light of the moon. However, his explanation was not, as in the case of Galileo, inserted into the framework of a thorough discussion of the mechanism of light reflection from unpolished surfaces. Moreover, even though Maestlin was—like Galileo and Kepler—a Copernican (and even if he attempted to use the argument of the moon light as an evidence of the similarity between earth and moon) his reasoning did not have the power of Galileo's arguments in support of a new vision of the world. This was because his work (as well as the works of many contemporary astronomers) remained largely within the limits of specific academic and astronomical texts and did not involve a critical analysis on the way humans acquire knowledge of reality.

Moreover, in his *Disputatio de eclipsibus solis et lunae*, Maestlin does not make a clear distinction between reflection from land and water, and indeed, with his allusion to the light 'which is collected and reflected off all the world's land and water' he seems actually to lump together the diffuse reflection typical of land and the specular one associated to still water.

On his side Kepler, while trying to surmise that many of the themes of *Sidereus* had been anticipated by his own considerations, he was nevertheless obliged to admit that he had wrongly assumed that water reflected sunlight more brightly than land; this was in contrast to Galileo's correct conclusion about the difference between the reflectivity of seas and lands. In his *Dissertatio* Kepler justified his previous conclusions with an observation (fully reported in his *Optical part of astronomy*) made in 1601, during an ascension on Mount Schöckl in the Styria region of Austria. By looking down, from the summit of the mount, he had seen that 'the river Mura, then stagnant and turbid, exceeded by far the cloudy clarity of the nearby lands' (OPTICA, p. 251). He had applied this observation to the interpretation of moon astronomy with these words: 'I conclude then that in the Moon the clear parts are of an aqueous matter, while, on the other hand, the obscure ones are continents or islands' (p. 252).

11.2 **Plutarch and the face which appears in the moon**

Kepler's observation had led him to contradict what Plutarch had said in his *De facie* where the Greek scholar was inclined to attribute the dark spots on the moon to the presence of seas. In his

2 As indicated in the Bibliographic Abbreviations at the beginning of this book, OPTICA is the term by which we will indicate Kepler's 1604 volume on optics in quoting from it.

1604 text, Kepler even mentioned Plutarch's short (and obscure) passage alluding to the poor reflectivity of waters:

> Just as our earth has certain large gulfs, so we judge that the moon too is opened up with great depths and rifts, containing water or foggy. which the sun does not penetrate with its light, but abandons them, making a diffuse reflection [*reflexionem dissipatam*]. (OPTICA, pp. 250–251; transl. p. 262)

In *De facie* this is the statement by which a follower of Plato's philosophy, Lamprias (Plutarch's main spokesman and brother in real life), concludes chapter 21 by developing his argument on the similarity between moon and earth (one of the main themes of the work).

Plutarch's book had a large circulation in the Renaissance, particularly after the edition of the collected works of the Greek philosopher published in the seventeenth century by the German humanist Wilhelm Xylander. It was a fundamental reference for both Kepler and Galileo (and for Maestlin who introduced Kepler to *De facie*). It was similarly so for other contemporary scholars not inclined to accept the prevailing views on the crystal-like perfection of the lunar body. Besides the theme of light reflection from the moon's surface, one of the important elements of Plutarch's work was the idea that, as on earth, there are high mountains and valleys on the moon. A fundamental motif of *De facie* was the similarity of earth and moon, and this accounts for why it would be a reference for the adherents to the Copernican doctrine (including Copernicus himself). The argument of a similar materiality and light reflectivity between earth and moon was connected to the notion (also potentially Copernican *ante litteram*) that, as a consequence of the illumination received from the moon, the earth, seen from the moon, would show monthly phases similar to the lunar phases visible from the earth.

The possible existence on the moon of waters (alluded to by Lamprias in the passage quoted earlier) also suggested the possible presence of some forms of life (one of the themes that had an important echo in Kepler's own work).

To a large extent, the first part of *De facie* tries to undermine the popular belief that the aspect of the moon, with its clear and dark zones, is due to a mirror-like reflection of the earth's surface, with its lands and oceans. The thesis expounded by the two main discussants, Lamprias and Lucius, is that the lunar surface is not regular and polished like a mirror but rough and irregular like earth, with mountains and valleys, seas and islands. Because of that it cannot reflect faithfully the image of external bodies, even though it reflects sun light in a non-mirror-like way.

There are several passages in *De facie* in which the themes of light reflection and irregularity of the lunar surface are considered together. In chapter 17, Lucius attempts to show why, despite its reflecting capacities, the moon does not produce a specular image of the earth. Taking into account the classical, mirror-like reflection regulated by well-defined geometrical laws, he says:

> In the first place, this is likely to occur only in mirrors that have been polished to exact smoothness; but the moon is very uneven and rugged, with the result that the rays from a large body striking against considerable heights which receive reflections and diffusions of light from one another are multifariously reflected and intertwined and the refulgence itself combines with itself, coming to us, as it were, from many mirrors. In the second place, even if we assume that the reflections on the surface of the moon occur at equal angles, it is not impossible that the rays as they travel through such a great interval get fractured and deflected so as to be blurred and to bend their light.[3]

[3] The translation from Plutarch's *De facie*, made by H. Cherniss and W. C. Helmhold, is taken from the online text at the website: <http://www.perseus.tufts.edu/hopper/text?doc=Perseus%3atext%3a2008.01.0357>.

In chapter 23, the theme of reflections returns, this time with Lamprias, who tackles the evident absence, on the face of the moon, of features that could correspond to the reflected image of the sun. After considering the way the image of the sun can be reflected by a water surface, he rebuts the arguments of his adversaries by saying:

> So they must not demand that every kind of mirror or a mirror at every distance produce a similar reflection, since (in doing so) they are at variance with the manifest facts. On the other hand, to us who declare that the moon is not a tenuous or a smooth body as water is but a heavy and earthy one, I do not understand why it is required of us that the sun be manifest to vision in it. For milk does not return such mirrorings either or produce reflections of the visual ray, and the reason is the irregularity and roughness of its particles; how in the world is it possible for the moon to cast the visual ray back from itself in the way that the smoother mirrors do? Yet even these, of course, are occluded if a scratch or speck of dirt or roughness covers the point from which the visual ray is naturally reflected, and while the mirrors themselves are seen they do not return the customary reflection.

In these two passages it seems that in *De facie* the distinction between mirror-like and diffuse reflection is rather clear, although it is not as well-developed as it will be, centuries later, in Galileo's writings. In the two quotations there is an evident awareness of the various directions of the reflected rays after that light hits an irregular surface. There is, however, in no way the conception that an irregular surface can be considered as made up by a multitude of minute, differently oriented mirrors. Moreover, the rest of Lamprias' discourse in chapter 23 (largely based on an extramission-type vision theory, with references to the 'visual ray' emitted from the eye and reverberating through the cosmic spaces) makes the matter rather complex:

> One who demands that the moon either reflect our vision from itself to the sun as well or else not reflect the sun from itself to us either is naive, for he is demanding that the eye be a sun, the vision light, and the human being a heaven. Since the light of the sun because of its intensity and brilliance arrives at the moon with a shock, it is reasonable that its reflection should reach to us; but the visual ray, since it is weak and tenuous and many times slighter, what wonder if it does not have an impact that produces recoil or if in rebounding it does not maintain its continuity but is dispersed and exhausted, not having light enough to keep it from being scattered about the irregularities and corrugations (of the moon)? From water, to be sure, and from mirrors of other kinds it is not impossible for the reflection (of the visual ray) to rebound to the sun, since it is still strong because it is near to its point of origin; but from the moon, even if the visual rays do in some cases glance off, they will be weak and dim and prematurely exhausted because of the magnitude of the distance. What is more too, whereas mirrors that are concave make the ray of light more intense after reflection than it was before so as often even to send off flames, convex and spherical mirrors by not exerting counter-pressure upon it from all points give it off weak and indistinct.

Among the considerations expounded in *De facie* in order to account for the spotted aspect of the moon is that the dark spots can, at least in part, be due to shadows projected by the sunrays hitting prominent reliefs and other irregularities of the moon's surface (the theme of lunar shadows is one of those that would recur in Galileo's work). Of course, unlike the case with Galileo, in *De facie* all reasoning (with shadows and other visual aspects) only concerns appearances to the naked eye. Since the spots visible directly occupy a large extension of the lunar surface, this would require the presence on the moon of extremely high mountains capable of projecting vast shadows. This point is highlighted in chapter 22 by one of the discussants, the mathematician Apollonides, with these words:

> Then by the moon itself, do you people think it possible that any clefts and chasms cast shadows which from the moon reach our sight here; or do you not reckon the consequence, and shall

I tell you what it is? Please listen then, though it is not anything unknown to you. The diameter of the moon measures twelve digits in apparent size at her mean distance; and each of the black and shadowy spots appears greater than half a digit and consequently would be greater than one twenty-fourth of her diameter. Well then, if we should suppose that the circumference of the moon is only thirty thousand stades and her diameter ten thousand each of the shadowy spots on her would in accordance with the assumption measure not less than five hundred stades. Consider now in the first place whether it is possible for the moon to have depths and corrugations so great as to cast such a large shadow; in the second place why, if they are of such great magnitude, we do not see them?

Lamprias replies with an argument based on the idea that the size of a shadow can largely outdo that of the object. Although the argument is in principle justified, however, the way he develops it is rather perplexing. He says that the size of the shadow gets bigger as the distance between the light sources and the object increases, and, in this way, he pretends to account for the large size of the dark spots seen with the full moon (when the sun is at the greatest distance from the moon). Lamprias' argument is largely flawed, both because the size of shadows depends on the relative inclination of the light source with respect to the objects and not particularly on their distance, and also because shadows cannot account for dark spots in the condition of full moon. In the case of a full moon this is because—as Galileo would remark much later—that condition is the most unfavourable for production of shadows on the main part of the lunar surface, due to the perpendicular direction of sunrays. Moreover the shape and extension of the spots visible with the naked eye should change during cycles of the moon, which is not the case (and occurs only for the lunar shadows visible exclusively with the telescope as it will be manifest with Galileo).

It is interesting, however, to consider how Lamprias concludes his reasoning:

Besides, even in the case of mountains the dazzling beams of the sun prevent their crags from being discerned in broad daylight, although their depths and hollows and shadowy parts are visible from afar. So it is not at all strange that in the case of the moon too it is not possible to discern accurately the reflection and illumination, whereas the juxtapositions of the shadowy and brilliant parts by reason of the contrast do not escape our sight.

The last line contains an allusion to the effects of contrast that makes shadows more visible when they are located beside bright zones. This is another of the interesting themes of *De facie*, although it is generally considered as a passing statement. For instance in chapter 20, when Lucius wishes to undermine the opinion of the Stoics that the brightness of the moon is due to an intrinsic fire of star-like nature. To this end, he remarks that if that were the case the moon should be visible during eclipses of the moon. This would be because the shadow of the sun would then make the celestial region surrounding its body darker, and the shining moon should be intensified by effects of visual contrast. This is how he puts it:

We see that from a shadowy place fire glows and shines forth more intensely, whether because the dark air being dense does not admit its effluences and diffusions but confines and concentrates the substance in a single place or because this is an affection of our senses that as hot things appear to be hotter in comparison with cold and pleasures more intense in comparison with pains so bright things appear conspicuous when compared with dark, their appearance being intensified by contrast to the opposite impressions.

For Lucius, the fact that, contrary to these expectations, the moon loses its brightness during eclipses 'implies that it is anything but a fiery and star-like body'.

11.3 Kepler, Averroes, and the complex roots of the diffuse reflection

After this rather long digression into Plutarch's moon, let us come to Kepler and his conversation with Galileo's sidereal messenger. After recognizing his deception in his previous interpretation of the relative darkness or brightness in the reflection from lands or waters, Kepler attenuated his error in the interpretation of his observation of land and river from Mount Schöckl by referring to a marginal note of his *Optical part of astronomy*; this pointed to the presence of 'a diurnal clearness of the air' which 'surrounded the river from any side' (*undique flumen circumstaret*). He thought that this could have been the cause of the river appearing brighter than the lands, partly justifying his incorrect assumption that water might reflect light more effectively than land. Kepler (Figure 11.2) would return to this argument in his *Somnium, seu de astronomia lunari*, written between 1620 and 1630, but published posthumous by his son Ludwig, in 1634. In a long footnote (n. 154, pp. 62–64) he refers again to his Mount Schöckl experiment and to his deception with the atmospheric clarity responsible for the great brightness of the river compared to nearby land. The footnote shows that even many years after the publication of Galileo's *Sidereus* (and his own *Dissertatio*), Kepler did not have a clear concept of diffuse reflection, and he had not grasped fully the interpretation of the phenomenon given by his Italian colleague. The reason was that, in explaining why an irregular surface shines when illuminated by the sun, he writes that the phenomenon cannot be accounted for by the ordinary laws of reflection but must be referred to a different notion, that of 'communicated light', already considered in his *Optical part of astronomy*:

> Celestial bodies illuminated by the sun, and looked at from far, are in no way seen through the solar rays reflected according to the optical law of specular reflection [*repercussis Optica & speculari lege*], but due to a light communicated by the sun, as I called it in the *Optics*, and become properties of the bodies as a consequence of the roughness of their surfaces. And this communicated light is, by the virtue of its definition stronger in lands than in waters [*fortior est in Terris, quam in undis*]. (Kepler, 1634, p. 63)

Kepler's concept of communicated light had an affinity with the interpretation of lunar splendour (and also of the moon dark light) expounded by Averroes in his commentary to *De caelo*. Averroes rejected the idea of a (mirror-like) reflection of sunrays by the moon surface and assumed that the moon shines in the sky because it is somehow imbued or impregnated by the light of the sun. In his commentary he attributed this opinion to 'Abennhata' (i.e. the Hispano-Jewish scholar Abraham ben Ezra), and says that, after receiving the light of the sun, the moon shines 'as shines a body luminous in itself' [*secundum quod luminosum illuminatur per se*] as is the case for the other stars. He adds that:

> If its shining power originated from reflection, it would illuminate on the earth only some specific sites, depending on its position; this is because the reflection is indeed produced only under a particular angle. (From Aristotle, De coelo, Lib. II, Summa III, Caput II, *Motus stellarum motus enuntiat*, 49; see Duhem IX, p. 410)

Averroes insisted that this special kind of light reflection from the lunar surface indicated a kinship between moon and earth, which he attributed (incorrectly) to Aristotle's *On animals*;[4] this was based mainly on the fact that the moon, similar to the earth but unlike most other celestial

[4] Even though Averroes could allude to various of Aristotle's texts (*Historia Animalium*, the *De Partibus Animalium*, and the *De Generatione Animalium*), in none of these did the Greek philosopher seem to consider the affinity between earth and moon invoked by the Arabic scholar.

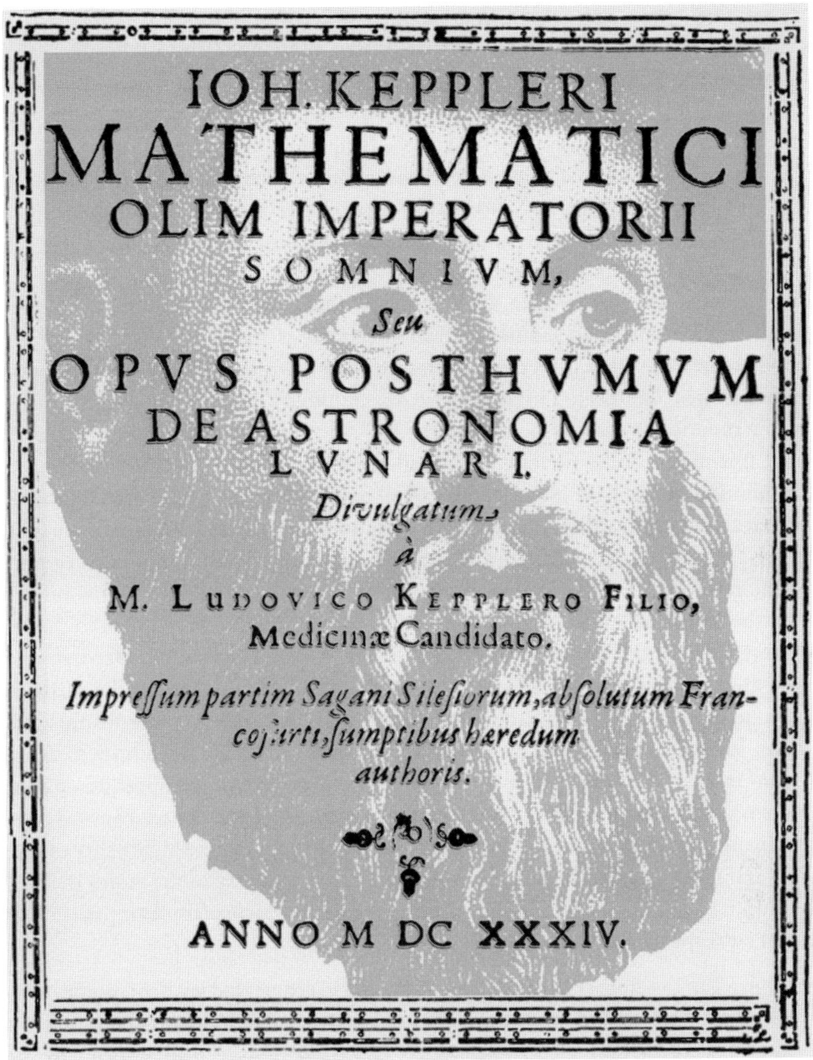

Figure 11.2 *Kepler's Somnium* by Nicholas Wade. Kepler's portrait (derived from an engraving in Knight, 1834) is combined with the title page of his *Somnium*.

bodies, is not endowed with intrinsic light. In the views of the Arabic commentator (and in contrast to the ideas expounded in *De facie*) this did not appear to be a genuine kinship, based on a similarity of composition, but a form of analogy. It was generally considered in this way by subsequent medieval commentators. The analogy would be justified by the fact that the moon, being the lowermost of the celestial bodies, shared properties with earth. As to the spots on the moon, Averroes demonstrated that they could not be due to a reflection of external objects because they did not change with the changes in the relative position of earth and moon.

As highlighted by Pierre Duhem in volume IX of his monumental *Le système du monde*, the opinions of Averroes circulated widely in the Middle Ages through compilations and commentaries by various philosophers (among them the Venerable Bede, Honorius Augustodunensis, the anonymous author of an old-French manuscript entitled *Introductoire d'astronomie*, Albertus Magnus, Thomas Aquinas, Robertus Anglicus, Pietro d'Abano, Giles of Rome (i.e. Ægidius Romanus or Egidio Colonna), Bernard of Verdun, Peter of Auvergne, Jean Buridan, Nicole Oresme, Giovanni Gianduno, and Albert of Saxony) and, afterwards, through the writings of Renaissance scholars. Moreover, as remarked by the Italian scholar Eugenio Garin in an important essay on Leonardo's sources, a large part of medieval knowledge of astronomy became a part of general culture in the Renaissance; a culture that even relatively uneducated people could absorb from conversations, conferences, sermons, technical treatises, various forms of encyclopaedic texts and manuscripts, without the need to go to the original authors (Garin, 1961).

One of the questions considered in the writings of these authors from the Middle Ages concerned the difference between a genuine reflection capable of rendering a well-defined image of external bodies, and the special mechanism responsible for the brightness of the moon under the action of sunlight. Connected to this theme was Plutarch's motif of the nature of the spotted surface of the moon. For the mechanism of the brilliance of moon, Albertus Magnus explicitly negates that this might occur by mirror-like reflection and considers that it involves instead a form of 'imbibition of sun light in her depth' (*imbibitionem luminis solis in profundum eius*).

The spotted aspect of the moon was generally attributed to a variable density of the matter near the lunar surface, with authors differing on which would appear more luminous or darker (the denser or the rarer parts). The opinion expressed by Robertus Anglicus in a manuscript commentary on the *Sphere* of Sacrobosco was that the brighter spots corresponded to the less dense zones whereas the more dense zones appeared darker. In rejecting the popular hypothesis that the spots of the moon surface might be due to the reflection of the image of the earth, Robertus assumed that according to this view 'the parts of the earth covered with water would appear clear on the moon surface, whereas the continents appear dark'. A similar opinion was expressed by Jean Buridan on Averroes. Most of the other commentators were of the opposite opinion, interpreting Averroes' thinking in support of a greater brightness of the denser zones. This was also the opinion expressed in chapter 18 of Plutarch's *De facie* to support the materiality of the moon's substance—and its analogy with the composition of earth, contrary to the Stoics theory that the moon is composed of air and fire. To support this argument Lucius (like Lamprias a follower of the ideas of Plato) specifically says:

> There are no reflections from anything rarefied or tenuous in texture, and it is not easy even to imagine light rebounding from light or fire from fire; but whatever is to cause a repercussion or a reflection must be compact and solid, in order that it may stop a blow and repel it. (Plutarch, 1968, vol. XII, p. 115)

The theme of the nature of light reflection from water with relation to the moon's brightness would recur in the texts of scholars from the Middle Ages and Renaissance. Another theme is the comparison of mirror-like reflection and the reflection from a wall, a comparison that would recur with an especial relevance in the work of Galileo. These themes were discussed by the French scholars Jean Buridan and Nicole d'Oresme, whose works remained, however, in manuscript form (although they circulated widely). Interestingly, Oresme, who thought that the dark spots of the moon corresponded to the less dense parts of the lunar matter, invoked an analogy of the moon with 'the alabaster stone':

> Therefore the parts of the moon by their very nature cannot all be uniformly transparent and clear, but rather in different degrees, as we observe certain differences in other parts of heaven. This is the explanation for the appearance of the spot. But it should be noted that, just as in the case of the alabaster stone, those veins and sections that are most clear and through which one can see almost as clearly as

> through crystal seem darker and less white than the other parts; and the same is true of the parts of the moon. Thus the clearer some parts are, so that the sun's penetration is deeper, the darker those parts appear, and the others proportionally lighter. The shape of the spot on the moon, then, is of this kind just explained. (Duhem IX, p. 423; transl. p. 491)

This is a theme that would have an echo in Sagredo's allusion to mother-of-the-pearl in Galileo's *Dialogue* (Galileo, 1632, p. 79: see our Chapter 3).

One of the texts which had a particular relevance in the transmission of these lines of thought up to Galileo's and Kepler's era was the commentary of Albert of Saxony entitled *Subtilissimae Quaestiones in libros de caelo et mundo*, written in 1368. It addresses both Aristotle's original work and the commentary by Averroes and was circulated widely and underwent several editions in print between the sixteenth and the seventeenth centuries. It is largely based on previous works and particularly on the writings of Buridan (Albert's teacher) and Oresme. In the *Quaestio* XXII of Book II, after excluding that the brightness of the moon could be accounted for by a mirror-like reflection, Albert considers the possibility that in the case of the moon it could correspond to that of a wall illuminated by the sun. He writes:

> But one might object to this reasoning. If the light of the sun strikes a wall, the wall seems lighted on all its surface and not only at a point corresponding to an angle of reflection equal to the angle of incidence. The objection is worthless: The moon is not like a wall. Because of the roughness of its surface, a number of parts of the wall can reflect rays to our eyes; hence a large extent of the wall appears lighted to us. But if the wall were perfectly smooth like a mirror or like the body of the moon, the solar rays would not light up all its surface when striking us, but only at a point where the incident ray from the sun and the reflected ray toward the eye give equal angles of incidence and reflection. That can be seen easily with still water. Only a small part of the surface of the water represents the light of the sun of a star with intensity. But if one troubles the surface of the water a little, it no longer remains perfectly smooth, and the light of the sun is sent to us with intensity throughout a greater region of the surface. (Albertus de Saxonia, 1497, Lib, II, Q. XXII; transl. in Duhem, 1996, pp. 492–493)

On the basis of this reasoning (that seems to anticipate various Galilean motifs), one could perhaps expect that Albert would conclude a similarity between reflection from the moon and from a wall, but he does not. Surprisingly Albert decidedly excludes such a possibility by saying:

> One must therefore utter another opinion. That is why I state that the light of the sun is incorporated in the moon. The moon is translucent and transparent body, at least on its surface, and perhaps in its totality, even though the size of the moon's body does not allow the light of the sun to cross its whole length, so that this light cannot be as intense as on the side of the moon that does not face the sun as on the side of the moon that does. Thus the light of the moon we see is not simply the light of the sun that the moon soaked-up and became incorporated with it [*lumen lune quod videmus non est solum lumen solis reflexum super corpus lune sed lumen solis lune imbibitum et incorporatum*]. (p. 493)

Paradoxically, the theme of 'imbibition' or 'incorporation' seems more apt to account for the moon shining even to a scholar like Albert of Saxony who, with the allusion to the wall and water, seems to have grasped the concept of diffuse illumination. This is to a large extent the consequence of the strength of the received views and of the difficulty of refuting a well-consolidated intellectual scheme like the cosmology of Aristotle. This is confirmed by the next statement where the moon's luminosity is interpreted within the framework of the Aristotelian notions of *in potential* and *in actu*:

> One can express oneself as follows: The moon is not luminescent actually; it cannot itself disturb a transparent medium [*de se possit movere diaphanum*]. However, by its natural disposition, it has a

> proximate potential for luminosity [*est in potentia propinqua per suam naturalem dispositionem ad luciditamem*]. This potential is brought to actual luminosity by the incidence of the solar light on the moon. (Albertus de Saxonia, 1497, Lib, II, Q. XXII; transl. in Duhem 1996, pp. 493)

In the *Quaestio* XXII of his work, Albert also addresses the problem of the luminosity of other celestial bodies, by considering two opposite views, i.e. that they shine because of the illumination received from the sun, or that they are endowed with an intrinsic light like the sun itself (a theme that would be long debated until the time of Kepler and Galileo). After considering the various reasons supporting the two possibilities, he seems to suppose that the first alternative is the most likely. One of the reasons for this preference is the appearance of the moon in the quarter phase. At the outset of the *Quaestio* XXII ('Whether all stars other than the sun, have their luminosity from the sun, or from themselves'), Albert answers:

> This is first demonstrated in the case of the moon. In conditions of clear air, in the phase of first quarter, all the body of the moon is seen, even though the part which looks at the sun appears more luminous than the other part turned away from the sun. (Albertus, 1497; transl. in Grant, 1994, p. 399)

With this assertion it is evident that Albert of Saxony is interpreting the phenomenon of the dark light of the moon as evidence for its intrinsic light. Assuming that the other celestial bodies behave like the moon, Albert needs to explain why they do not exhibit periodical phases similar to those of the moon. To this end he considers that they are more permeable to the sun light which therefore produces a complete imbibition of their entire body.

In order for us to appreciate the persistence, the idea that even the brightness of real stars depends on the illumination from the sun, we must consider that in 1606 it would have an echo in Kepler's *De stella nova*, where the German astronomer explains the scintillation of stars on the basis of a rotatory movement of their globes. This movement would be necessary to allow every single star to enjoy the illumination of the sun (considered as situated at the centre of the cosmos, according to the Copernican perspective) over the totality of its body (see Chapter 14). Kepler's view might have been inspired by some considerations of Oresme, probably through the mediation of following medieval scholars and notably by Nicolas of Kues (Cusanus), a fifteenth-century scholar considered by him as *divinus,* i.e. divine, see later.[5]

11.4 The ambiguous shining of stars and planets, a cosmic dream, and the relativity within the framework of 'Learned ignorance'

Throughout the history of astronomy, a counterpoint to the idea that true stars receive their light from the sun was that planets (including the moon) might possibly shine due to intrinsic light. Prior to (or outside) the system of Aristotle (who attributed the light of celestial bodies to the movement of ethereal spheres or to the reflection of sunlight) the intrinsic luminosity of stars or planets was generally referred to the presence of some fire in them, possibly mixed together with other matter. This second component could be the matter of earth, an idea that goes back at least to Anaxagoras (in the fifth century BC) and was endorsed by Plato as well as by some of

[5] Oresme applies this consideration particularly to the Earth that he supposes to move by a rotatory movement around its axis. In his manuscript *Traité du ciel ed du monde*, he justifies the assumption of this rotatory movement of the Earth around its axis to account for the apparent movement in the sky of the Sun, the main source of heat in the universe: 'This is, to speak in a familiar way, similarly to the thing that is roasted at the fire which receives around it the heat because it is turned, and not because the fire is turned around it' (see Duhem, IX, p. 337).

his followers. A dense component was needed to account for the reflecting capacity of planets, and particularly for the moon: that the moon could reflect sun light is a notion at least as ancient as Parmenides, a contemporary of Anaxagoras. Stoic philosophers were inclined to think that in the body of the moon the element fire was combined with air, an assumption that is criticized in Plutarch's *De facie* (see p. 198 above).

One of the reasons which seemed to justify, on phenomenological grounds, the presence of fire in the moon was the weak light visible on its surface during eclipses of the moon. For this planet, there was indeed a form of transition between different views, going from the assumption of an intrinsic light source (i.e. one independent on sun's illumination), to the idea of light impregnation or imbibition (the luminosity persisting—after absorption—for variable periods) and eventually the idea of genuine, instantaneous form of light reflection.

About one millennium before Albert of Saxony, the idea of a kind of impregnation of the moon by the light of the sun had been expounded by the Roman scholar Macrobius in his *Commentarius in somnium Scipionis* (this being a 'Commentary on the Dream of Scipio', a dream narrated by Cicero in the VI book of his *Republica*). Macrobius's text enjoyed great popularity from the early Middle Ages until the Renaissance (and was among the books read and quoted by Galileo in his works). In the *Somnium*, Macrobius popularized a geocentric theory like that developed in the fourth century BC by Heraclites Ponticus; this assumed that Mercury and Venus revolved around the sun, while the sun revolved around the earth. One of the problems discussed in the *Somnium* concerned the difference of the effect of sunlight on the earth and moon. Macrobius was among those who considered the moon was like the earth because of its low position in the cosmos and its proximity to the earth. For him the stars shine due to an intrinsic luminosity because they are located in the most pure and luminous zone of the celestial ether. The sun is particularly luminous because all this ethereal light is concentrated on it. Being located between sun and earth, the moon is assumed 'not to have intrinsic light' (*lunam non habere lumen proprium*). As Macrobius writes: 'since the Earth is the innermost part of the entire world, and the Moon the innermost part of ether, the moon was called Earth, although an ethereal one'.

One of the problems addressed within this comparison between earth and moon concerns the behaviours of their respective surfaces with respect to the light of the sun. This depends on the difference of their composition, and particularly on the very great density of the matter of earth compared to that of the moon. Because of this extreme density, the light of the sun cannot penetrate the surface of the earth which explains why, in contrast to the moon, 'the earth, upon receiving the light of the sun, only becomes luminous but cannot send back the light (*terra accepto solis lumine clarescit tantum modo, non relucet*)'. On its side, the moon:

> despite being of a denser matter than other celestial bodies, is much less so than the earth, and is then is more permeable to the light received, such as it sends back this light, even though she does not convey the sensation of hotness. (Macrobius, 1848, p. 105)

Within the framework of a very different vision of the cosmos, the motif of a similarity between earth and moon, present in both Plutarch and Macrobius, would return in a particularly intense way at the beginning of the fifteenth century in the book *Docta ignorantia* ('Learned ignorance') by the German philosopher and theologian, Cardinal Nicholas of Kues or Cusanus (Figure 11.3). For Cusanus the world has no definite centre and is potentially infinite. Unlike the case with Macrobius who spoke of the moon as an 'ethereal earth', with Cusanus it is the earth which becomes similar to the moon and stars. Besides being provided with an approximately circular movement, Cusanus's earth is endowed of an internal source of luminosity (also attributed to the moon and—of course—to the sun and stars). In contrast to the moon of Macrobius (and of Aristotle) it could shine towards the other celestial bodies (and also exert on them astronomical and astrological 'influences' similar to those exerted on it by the other celestial bodies).

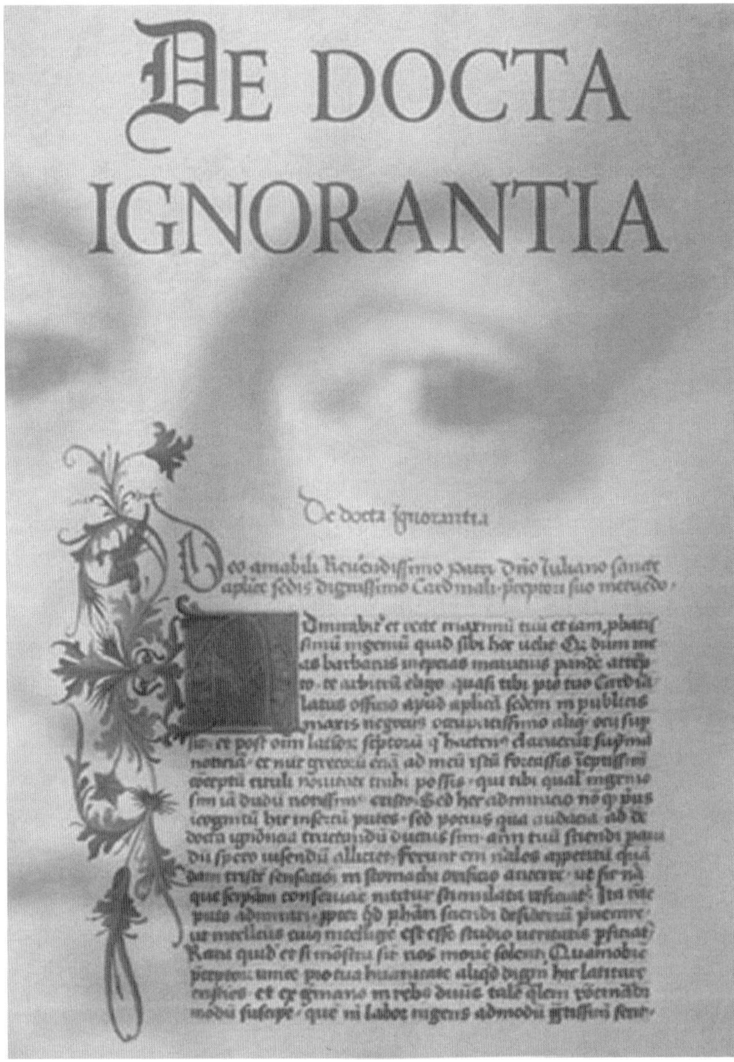

Figure 11.3 *The learned Cusanus* by Nicholas Wade. The portrait of Nicholas of Kues or Cusanus can be seen with the title page of his *De docta ignorantia*.

Within a framework of doctrine strongly permeated by the notion of relativity (which concerns both motion and visual appearance), Cusanus expounds a singular argument to account for the apparent 'black colour' (*color nigredinis*) of the earth's surface. We do not perceive the light of the earth (as we do not see its movement) because we are located on it. 'If one were situated on the sun, he would not see it shining as we do' (*non appareret illa claritas quae nobis*). In Cusanus' views, the reason for this is that, like the earth the sun is made of four spheres, and the origin of its splendour is the most external one, i.e. the sphere of fire. Only looking afar, from the outside we could see the earth shining, as we see the splendour of the sun.[6]

[6] Although, as mentioned in Chapter 1, in his work on the sunspots also Galileo says that we cannot see the splendour of the earth because we cannot observe from afar the earth illuminated by the sun, the physical and perceptual reasons invoked by him are quite dissimilar to those of Cusanus.

11.5 Leonardo da Vinci: the perceptive science of a Renaissance artist

This long excursion through classical and medieval science is now bringing us back to the beginning, that is, to Kepler and his remarks on Galileo's *Sidereus*. It started with Kepler's proposal of Maestlin as the possible first author of the correct theory of the dark light of the Moon (expounded by Maestlin in Tübingen as early as 1597). From an historical point of view, Kepler's caution in assigning the priority of the theory to his teacher can be considered appropriate because about one century before Maestlin, a similar (and even more comprehensive) explanation of the phenomenon had been expounded by Leonardo da Vinci (Figure 11.4).

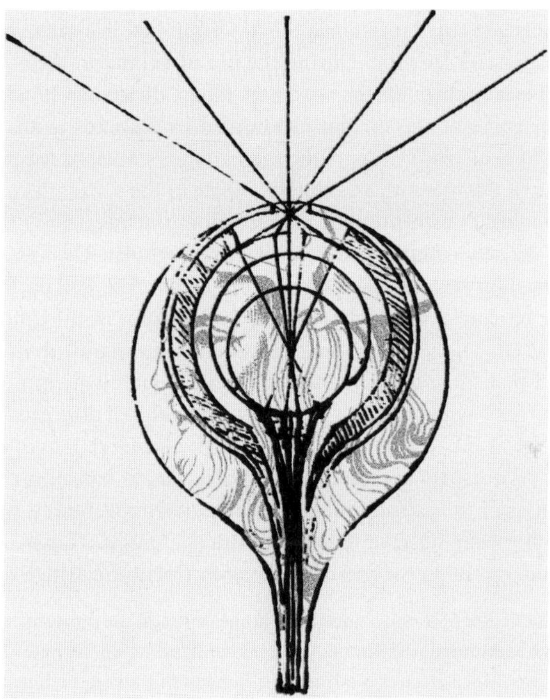

Figure 11.4 *Leonardo's eye* by Nicholas Wade. Leonardo represented the anatomy of the eye in his notebooks and this diagram is derived from one printed in McMurrich (1930). Leonardo's portrait is derived from an engraving in *The historic gallery of portraits and paintings*. Leonardo's eye looked to the past rather than the future. It bears closer similarity to that of Roger Bacon than to Kepler's conception. Leonardo's anatomy did little to inform him of the structure of the eye, let alone its optical properties. He tried to reconcile the passage of light through the eye with the characteristics of his vision: since objects appeared upright so should the image in the eye. In order to achieve this, he had a double inversion in the eye! In terms of the optics of the eye, Leonardo was Ptolemaic rather than Copernican.

Credit: Cutaway view of human eye, from Atlantic Codex (Codex Atlanticus) by Leonardo da Vinci, folio 921 recto, Vinci, Leonardo da (1452–1519) / Biblioteca Ambrosiana, Milan, Italy / De Agostini Picture Library / Metis e Mida Informatica / Veneranda Biblioteca Ambrosiana / The Bridgeman Art Library.

Leonardo, who was interested in the various dimensions of science and technology no less than in art, gave special attention to the problem of visual appearances during both normal (i.e. terrestrial) observation and in connection with cosmology. His considerations on light and shadow, visual contrast, perspective, optics, and particularly on the mechanism of light reflection provided an important background for his interpretation of heavenly appearances. Within this framework, his remarks on the appearance of the moon were of particular importance, and especially those on the dark light visible in the zone of the lunar surface outside the illuminated crescent.

Before considering this aspect of Leonardo's thought, it should be noted that his interest in cosmology involved all the classical themes concerning the constitution of the world, the nature of the celestial bodies (and especially the moon), and it included attention to the possibility of the movement of the earth and of the infinity of universe. These themes had a long tradition which had been particularly vibrant through the Middle Ages with the various scholars and compilers already mentioned. In the Renaissance this tradition had been revived particularly by the wide circulation of Plutarch's *De facie*. During the era of Leonardo these cosmological themes had been diffused especially through the works of Albert of Saxony (that Leonardo undoubtedly knew). Moreover some of the themes expounded by Cusanus in his *De docta ignorantia* were directly relevant to Leonardo's ideas. Although Cusanus's work had appeared in print several times between the end of the fifteenth and the beginning of the sixteenth century, the recurrence of these motifs in Leonardo's astronomical interests does not necessarily mean that the Italian artist was acquainted directly with the text of the German scholar. This is because he might have absorbed them from various texts in the idiom current in Florence, and particularly those dealing with astrology and esoteric matters which were inspired by some of the conceptions of Cusanus.

Whatever the transition might have been, undoubtedly Leonardo shares some themes with Cusanus, like the idea that there is no definite centre in a potentially infinite universe, that the earth is simply the centre of aggregation of its elements and that it does move like the other celestial bodies do. Moreover, as in the work of Cusanus, in his considerations of the earth, moon, and sun, Leonardo makes recourse to a relativistic approach. This is based on the idea that, in order to understand the causes of the astronomical and terrestrial appearances, we should change our viewpoint and metaphorically observe the earth from the moon. This is what he writes at the beginning of his consideration on the moon in a manuscript at the British Museum:

> The Earth is not in the centre of the Sun's orbit nor at the centre of the universe, but in the centre of its companion elements, and united with them. And any one standing on the moon, when it and the sun are both beneath us, would see this our earth and the element of water upon it just as we see the moon, and the earth would light it as it lights us. (LNB II, p. 136, para. 858)

According to Leonardo, like the earth, the moon is made up of the four elements (earth, water, air, and fire), and it shines exclusively because it reflects external light, but not only that from the sun. This intrinsic opacity of the moon is asserted in various passages of his manuscripts and particularly in the Leicester Codex where there is a drawing (Figure 11.5) which clearly portrays the phenomenon of the secondary light of the moon, that Leonardo correctly attributes to a reflection from the earth.

Leonardo's interpretation of the mechanism by which moon and earth illuminate each other is based on the idea that water is particularly effective in reflecting sunrays, and (similarly to Plutarch) on the assumptions that vast areas of the moon's surface are covered with water. In his view the spotted aspect of the moon is due to the different reflectivity of oceans and lands. As we know, the notion of a more effective reflectivity of water compared to land would not be endorsed by Galileo, who correctly considered the mirror-like reflection of a surface of still water

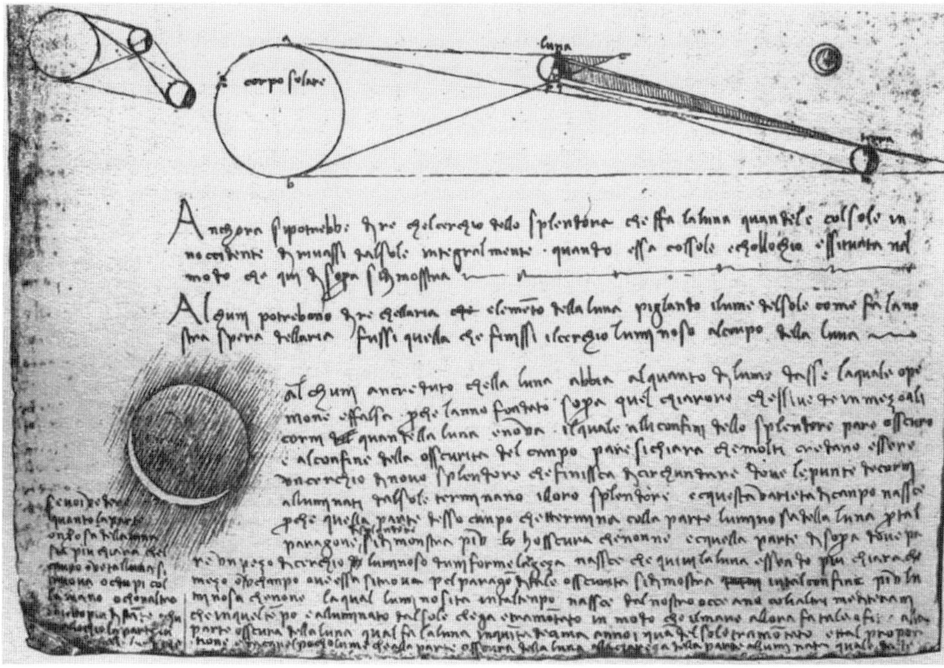

Figure 11.5 A detail of the Leicester Codex with the drawings illustrating the secondary light of the moon and Leonardo's explanation of it based on the reflection by the earth onto the moon of the light of sun. The image has been reflected horizontally in order to facilitate the comprehension of the scheme above the writing. In both the small and big scheme above the handwriting, are represented, respectively from left to right, the sun (*corpo solare*—i.e. sun body), the moon (*luna*), and the earth (*terra*). Notice how in drawing the image of the moon, Leonardo makes its surface darker near the illuminated crescent. This is an appearance that—as he, and also Galileo after him—noticed, resulted exclusively from a perceptual phenomenon.

Credit: Astronomical diagrams, fol. 2r from the Codex Leicester, 1508–1512 (pen & ink on paper) (b/w photo), Vinci, Leonardo da (1452–1519) / Private Collection / The Bridgeman Art Library.

as inappropriate to account for the shining moon and invoked instead the notion of diffuse reflection from lands (see Chapter 5).

Developing the tradition of Middle Age perspectivists, like Alhazen, Witelo, and especially Peckham, of which he seems to have had direct knowledge (possibly due to the presence of Peckham's optical manuscript in the library of San Marco in Florence), Leonardo investigated the phenomena of reflection experimentally. He was aware, moreover, of the various hypotheses put forward over the centuries by various scholars to account for the brightness of the moon and the spotted aspects of its surface. From his knowledge of the mechanisms of reflection Leonardo was well aware that the aspect of the moon's face could not be explained on the basis of a mirror-like reflection, either in the version of a flat or spherical mirror. Among the hypotheses that he refuted are those accounting for the moon spots as a result of the interposition of vapours or clouds between it and the earth as well as on the variable density of its matter. This is how he argues on the topic in two passages from a notebook held at the Institut de France: as to the first hypothesis he writes:

> Some have said that vapours rise from the moon, after the manner of clouds and are interposed between the moon and our eyes. But, if this were the case, these spots would never be permanent, either

> as to position or form; and, seeing the moon from various aspects, even if these spots did not move they would change in form, as objects do which are seen from different sides. (LNB II, F84a, p. 165)

As to the second possibility he writes:

> Others say that the moon is composed of more or less transparent parts; as though one part were something like alabaster and others like crystal or glass. It would follow from this that the sun casting its rays on the less transparent portions, the light would remain on the surface, and so the denser part would be illuminated, and the transparent portions would display the shadow of their darker depths; and this is their account of the structure and nature of the moon. And this opinion has found favour with many philosophers, and particularly with Aristotle, and yet it is a false view for, in the various phases and frequent changes of the moon and sun to our eyes, we should see these spots vary, at one time looking dark and at another light: they would be dark when the sun is in the west and the moon in the middle of the sky; for then the transparent hollows would be in shadow as far as the tops of the edges of those transparent hollows, because the sun could not then fling his rays into the mouth of the hollow which however, at full moon, would be seen in bright light, at which time the moon is in the East and faces the sun in the West; then the sun would illuminate even the lowest depths of these transparent places and thus, as there would be no shadows cast, the moon at these times would not show us the spots in question; and so it would be, now more and now less, according to the changes in the position of the sun to the moon, and of the moon to our eyes, as I have said above. (pp. 65–66)[7]

In proposing a particularly effective reflection of sunlight from the watery regions of the moon surface as an argument to account for its spotted appearance, Leonardo realized that, in the case of the reflection of sunlight from the surface of still water, the zones of the water outside the image of the sun would appear dark, and thus his explanation could not correspond to visual appearances. Because of this he attributed the shining of the water zones on the moon to the waves which usually ruffle the surfaces of vast water extensions. This is how he puts the matter in an important passage of a notebook at the British Museum:

> The moon has no light in itself; but so much of it as faces the sun is illuminated, and of that illumined portion we see so much as faces the earth. And the moon's night receives just as much light as is lent it by our waters as they reflect the image of the sun [*simulacro del sole*], which is mirrored in all those waters which are on the side towards the sun. The outside or surface of the waters forming the seas of the moon and of the seas of our globe is always ruffled little or much, or more or less and this roughness causes an extension of the numberless images of the sun which are repeated in the ridges and hollows, the sides and fronts of the innumerable waves; that is to say in as many different spots on each wave as our eyes find different positions to view them from. This could not happen, if the aqueous sphere which covers a great part of the moon were uniformly spherical, for then the images of the sun would be one to each spectator, and its reflections would be separate and independent and its radiance would always appear circular; as is plainly to be seen in the gilt balls placed on the tops of high buildings. But if those gilt balls were rugged or composed of several little balls, like mulberries, which are a black fruit composed of minute round globules, then each portion of these little balls, when seen in the sun, would display to the eye the lustre resulting from the reflection of the sun, and thus, in one and the same body many tiny suns would be seen; and these often combine at a long distance and appear as one. The lustre of the new moon is brighter and stronger, than when the moon is full; and the reason of this is that the angle of incidence is more obtuse in the new than in the full moon, in which the angles

[7] As already seen in Chapter 8, a similar reasoning would be used by Galileo against the argument of the variable density of moon surface adduced by Locher and Scheiner in their *Disputatio*. In a passage of the *Dialogue* where this theme is addressed, Salviati correctly says that the authors of the *Disputatio* could not even be excused for their error as being the first to propose a similar explanation.

[of incidence and reflection] are highly acute. The waves of the moon therefore mirror the sun in the hollows of the waves as well as on the ridges, and the sides remain in shadow. But at the sides of the moon the hollows of the waves do not catch the sunlight, but only their crests; and thus the images are fewer and more mixed up with the shadows in the hollows; and this intermingling of the shaded and illuminated spots comes to the eye with a mitigated splendour, so that the edges will be darker, because the curves of the sides of the waves are insufficient to reflect to the eye the rays that fall upon them. Now the new moon naturally reflects the solar rays more directly towards the eye from the crests of the waves than from any other part, as is shown by the form of the moon, whose rays a strike the waves b and are reflected in the line b d, the eye being situated at d. This cannot happen at the full moon, when the solar rays, being in the west, fall on the extreme waters of the moon to the East from n to m, and are not reflected to the eye in the West, but are thrown back eastwards, with but slight deflection from the straight course of the solar ray; and thus the angle of incidence is very wide indeed. The moon is an opaque and solid body and if, on the contrary, it were transparent, it would not receive the light of the sun. (LNB 2, pp. 157–158, n. 896)

In this passage it is clear that, despite the incorrect assumption that water would appear more brilliant than land upon receiving sun light, Leonardo understands that a mirror-like reflection similar to that occurring from still water (and also from 'gilt balls'—*palle dorate*) could not account for the shining of the moon. This is even more explicit in another passage of a notebook held at the Institut de France:

The image of the sun [again *simulacro del sole*] in the moon is powerfully luminous, and is only on a small portion of its surface. And the proof may be seen by taking a ball of burnished gold and placing it in the dark with a light at some distance from it; and then, although it will illuminate about half of the ball, the eye will perceive its reflection only in a small part of its surface, and all the rest of the surface reflects the darkness which surrounds it; so that it is only in that spot that the image of the light is seen, and all the rest remains invisible, the eye being at a distance from the ball. The same thing would happen on the surface of the moon if it were polished, lustrous and opaque, like all bodies with a reflecting surface. Show how, if you were standing on the moon or on a star, our earth would seem to reflect the sun as the moon does. And show that the image of the sun in the sea cannot appear one and undivided, as it appears in a perfectly plane mirror. (LNB 2, pp. 155–156)

In the notebook at the British Museum, where he proposes the reflection from the ruffled water as a mechanism useful in accounting for the moon shining, Leonardo adds further annotations to explain how the presence of waves on the sea widens the reflected image of the sun and thus corresponding to the diffuse shining of the moon:

The innumerable images [*inumerabili simulacri*] of the solar rays reflected from the innumerable waves of the sea, as they fall upon those waves, are what cause us to see the very broad and continuous radiance on the surface of the sea.

That the sun could not be mirrored in the body of the moon, which is a convex mirror, in such a way as that so much of its surface as is illuminated by the sun, should reflect the sun unless the moon had a surface adapted to reflect it—in waves and ridges, like the surface of the sea when its surface is moved by the wind.

The waves in water multiply the image of the object reflected in it. These waves reflect light, each by its own line, as the surface of the fir cone does.

The moon, with its reflected light, does not shine like the sun, because the light of the moon is not a continuous reflection of that of the sun on its whole surface, but only on the crests and hollows of the waves of its waters; and thus the sun being confusedly reflected, from the admixture of the shadows that lie between the lustrous waves, its light is not pure and clear as the sun is. (LNB II, pp. 159–160)

Before leaving Leonardo we must recall that the notion of a more apparent reflection from a rough sea compared to still water is present in medieval scholars like Albert of Saxony and his teacher Buridan.

11.6 Galileo and Leonardo

There are many themes in the passages quoted earlier that would resurface in the works of Galileo, like the reflections from the surface of a wavy sea. Among Leonardo's motifs that we have already seen in Galileo is the impossibility of accounting for the splendour of the moon on the basis of mirror-like reflection from a perfectly polished surface. There are also some linguistic correspondences like the repeated use of the term *simulacro* (of Lucretian origin) to indicate the reflected image of the sun instead of *specie* (species) more common in the tradition of the medieval perspectivists; *simulacro* is present in *Saggiatore*, in the context of the reflection of the sun from the surface of the sea at various degrees of regularity (see Chapter 1).

There are other aspects of visual relevance in which the themes developed by Leonardo in his notebooks would recur in the texts of Galileo; these include dark–light contrast and the variable play of shadows. To deal with the Leonardo–Galileo correspondences in some detail would require more than a chapter, and possibly an entire book. Even though in Galileo's time no printed edition of Leonardo's manuscripts was available, the scientific and artistic culture derived from these manuscripts was widespread in Italy, and particularly in Florence where several textbooks used for teaching art were largely inspired by Leonardo and particularly by his *Trattato della pittura*. In the sixteenth century at least 20 manuscript copies of this text were in circulation in Florence; they were based on a lost text written by him, and compiled—in the extant form—by Leonardo's pupil Francesco Melzi around 1530. The *Trattato* is a collection of Leonardo's considerations on painting in its various dimensions, vision, perspective, light, and shadows. His elaborations on these various themes were the basis of several practical or theoretical treatises on perspective and painting that circulated widely in Galileo's era in manuscript and printed form, like those of Giacomo Barozzi da Vignola and Egnatio Danti (Vignola & Danti, 1611), Giovanni Paolo Lomazzo (Lomazzo, 1585), Daniele Barbaro (Barbaro, 1569), and many others. Galileo absorbed this culture during his youth when he attended the course of Ostilio Ricci at the Florentine Accademia del disegno (see Chapter 13). Among his fellow students was his friend Ludovico Cigoli who would write a treatise of practical perspective that circulated in manuscript form. In addition, a practical treatise prepared by Pietro Accolti for the students of the Accademia (and published in 1625) was largely based on Leonardo, with ample passages faithfully copied from the *Trattato della pittura*.

Galileo might have continued absorbing Leonardo's science during his residence in Padua, because he had ready access to the library of Gian Vincenzio Pinelli, a gentleman of Neapolitan origin, who was in contact with many exponents of the European intelligentsia and held one of the most important private libraries of his age, which included one of the early manuscript copies of the *Trattato della pittura* (the so-called Codex Pinelliano). In this same period he might have also benefitted from the wide circulation of Leonardo's texts in Venice, the chief city of the *Serenissima* Republic, where he used to spend some of the vacation periods from his university duties in Padua.

There is little doubt, on the basis of both historical circumstances and comparison of texts by Galileo and Leonardo, that Galileo was deeply inspired by the work of his predecessor; this is evident in his lunar thoughts, and especially those on light reflection from the moon's surface and on the cause of the weak luminosity on the dark zone of the moon. However, as we shall see in Chapter 12, Galileo was strongly innovative with respect to his precursors, including Leonardo, particularly because he abandoned the idea that water surfaces were the main source responsible for moon (and earth) shine. In elaborating a comprehensive and coherent theory of diffuse reflection from solid surfaces, Galileo was able to make the fundamental step that freed him from assuming the presence of seas on the moon's surface. He probably benefitted from Leonardo's observations and experiments on reflections from water under different conditions. On his side Leonardo was probably unable to rid himself of the idea that dense and opaque bodies without a polished surface could not produce a shining splendour. This happened despite the fact that he was well aware that the reflection from a wall struck by sunlight was capable of illuminating an opposite wall. In the *Trattato della pittura*, in noting that an illuminated body can communicate its illumination and its colour to nearby bodies, he remarked that the effect might include the communication of 'black shadows'. He concluded the argument with this a significant statement 'Darknesses do likewise, for they envelop with their obscurity whatever is included in them' (Leonardo, *Treatise*, McMahon, I, p. 268). Possibly Leonardo's reluctance to attribute the capability of light reflecting from land was due to a persisting idea of the intrinsic opacity of earth, whereby the darkness of an unilluminated part of its surface might quench the reflectivity of the nearby illuminated regions. This was probably the reason of his tenacious adherence to the idea that the exchange of light between earth and moon relied on the presence of water, an idea that Galileo was ready to abandon, perhaps after personally discussing the matter with a singular theologian strongly interested in science, as we shall see in Chapter 12.

Chapter 12

A moon circle: celestial reflections and illusions with Sarpi, Galileo, and Castelli

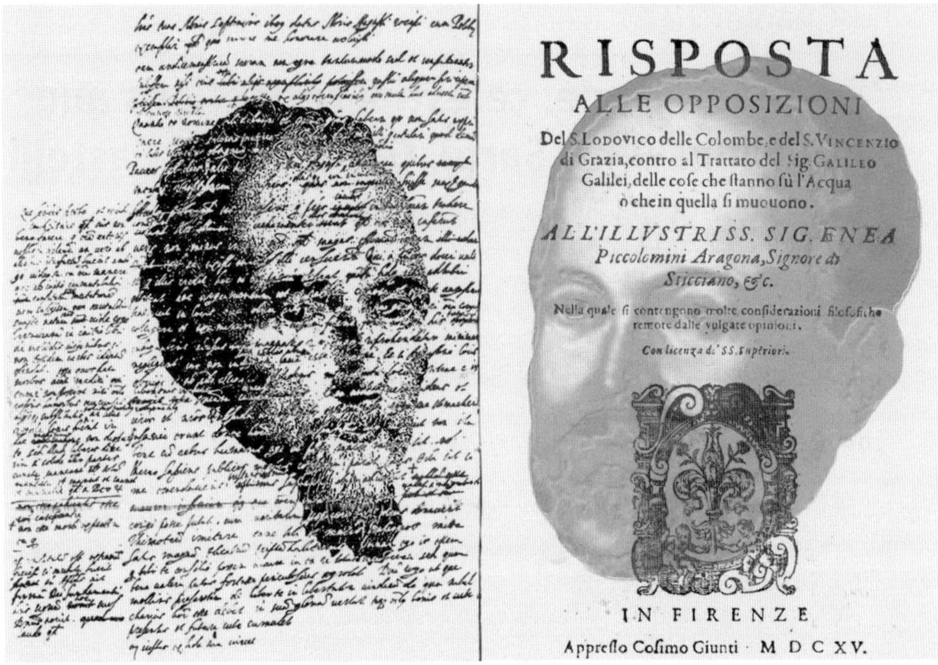

Figure XII *Sarpi's thoughts and Castelli's Risposta* by Nicholas Wade. Paolo Sarpi's features are visible within a copy of a handwritten series of his thoughts. Benedetto Castelli's features are presented with the title page of his *Riposta* to the objections voiced against Galileo's work.

This chapter continues our analysis of the sources Galileo used in his interpretation of the appearances of the moon. It is mainly centred on Paolo Sarpi, a theologian belonging to the order of Servites (*Servi di Maria*) who had strong interests in science, and to lesser extent on Benedetto Castelli, a Benedictine who was perhaps Galileo's most devoted pupil. Sarpi was a contemporary of Galileo and had scientific discussions with him. He collaborated with Galileo on some experiments, including the complex and poorly known pathways leading to the invention of the astronomical telescope. There is indeed little doubt that Sarpi and Galileo influenced each other over wide fields of their common scientific interests. It is also very likely that the friar, who was competent in optics and vision, influenced Galileo's interpretation of telescopic observations. Despite the importance of his achievements, Sarpi is little known among historians of science. Thus, we will widen the scope of this chapter to reconstruct some part of Sarpi's scientific work within the context of the Venetian culture when Galileo was in Padua.

12.1 **Intellectual societies in Padua and Venice**

Gian Vincenzio Pinelli (Figure 12.1) and his well-endowed private library in Padua were mentioned in Chapter 11, in the context of Galileo's possible acquaintance with Leonardo's texts. Pinelli was erudite and interested in science and especially botany; he corresponded with some of the important naturalists of his age (like Luca Ghini, Andrea Mattioli, and Ulisse Aldrovandi). He was also interested in optics as is documented by the notes in his hand on the papers of Giuseppe Moletti, Galileo's predecessor in the chair of mathematics in Padua. Pinelli also annotated the copy of the manuscript *Trattato della pittura* of Leonardo that was in his library.[1] Through Moletti other texts arrived at Pinelli's library, and among them the papers of Ettore Ausonio, a Venetian physician and instrument maker, who was particularly interested in optics and astrology of whom much will be said in Chapter 13 with relation to the optical background of Galileo.

Pinelli's palace in Padua, which also held an important collection of mathematical and astronomical instruments (in addition to naturalia, numismatic, and archaeological items), was a centre of attraction for a literary circle which included members of the local aristocracy and intellectuals and also foreign visitors to Padua or Venice. Pinelli was in correspondence with many exponents of the European intelligentsia and with various scholars connected in a directed or indirect way to Galileo (like Justus Lipsius, Nicolas Fabri de Peiresc, Mark Welser, Roberto Bellarmino, Joseph Justus Scaliger, Guidobaldo dal Monte, Girolamo Mercuriale, Fabricius ab Aquapendente, Paolo Sarpi, and many others).

Among the Padua residents who were connected to Pinelli (and through him to Galileo) there were Antonio Querengo (dedicatee of the *Cecco de Ronchitti*), Paolo Gualdo (author of Pinelli's biography: Gualdo, 1607), Lorenzo Pignoria (an archaeologist who collected paintings, antiques, naturalia, and exotic material), and Martino Sandelli and Vincenzo Contarini (both learned scholars acquainted with classical texts). With these and other members of the Paduan intelligentsia Galileo became an active member of the Accademia dei Ricovrati, founded in 1599 by the Venetian nobleman (and future Patriarch of Venice) Federico Cornaro. Some of the members of this academy produced literary compositions in the language of Padua (the *pavano*), and it is thus likely that they warmed to the *Cecco de Ronchitti* (written in *pavano*); this was the first printed work on astronomical themes associated with Galileo (see Chapters 2 and 9).

[1] Pinelli's manuscript copy of Leonardo's *Trattato* was one of the sources for the first printed edition of the work published in Paris in 1651.

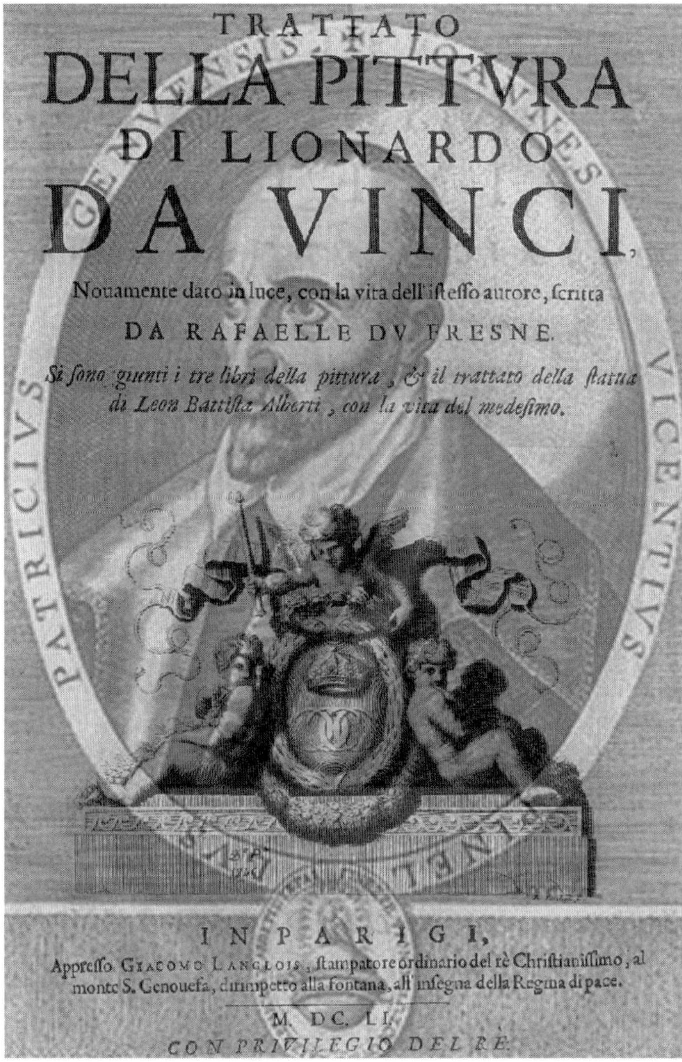

Figure 12.1 *Gian Vincenzo Pinelli and Leonardo's Trattato* by Nicholas Wade. It was largely because of Gian Vincenzio Pinelli's dissemination of Leonardo da Vinci's treatise on painting and its publication in Paris that it became more widely recognized. Pinelli is shown together with the Paris publication of Leonardo's treatise.

On a more scientific note, Galileo associated with some of the intelligentsia and aristocracy of Venice, where the circle established by Andrea and Niccolò Morosini (the so-called *Ridotto Morosini*) was of significance in framing his familiarity with eminent people. Among those who attended the *Ridotto* was Giovan Francesco Sagredo (inspiration for the homonymous discussant of the *Dialogue*); he was important for Galileo's intellectual history because he was interested in various aspects of science and notably in optics and magnetism.

12.2 A perceptive friar and his scientific circle

Paolo Sarpi was especially significant in the context of Galileo's interest in vision and its relevance to astronomical observations. Besides being connected to the various circles of the most progressive cultural milieu of Venice, Sarpi was the leading member of a small group of associates interested in science and pursuing theoretical and experimental studies in various fields. Among the members of this circle, in addition to those already mentioned, were Sebastiano Vernier and Agostino Da Mula, both important exponents of the dominant class of the *Serenissima*, with significant civil or military roles in the administration of its territories.

In Chapter 8 we noted that Sarpi collaborated with Fabricius ab Aquapendente, especially in the field of comparative physiology of vision. Also connected to Sarpi's circle was another physician, Santorio Santorio, the author of *De statica medicina*; this was perhaps the first text based on a quantitative approach to the study of physiology and medicine.

Sarpi's main interests and public activities were largely concerned with religion, politics, and history rather than science. He was the official theologian of the Venetian Republic and is famous mainly for his religious and political attempts to reform the Catholic Church at the turn of the sixteenth and seventeenth centuries. He played an important part in conflicts between Venice and the Vatican (leading to the excommunication of the town, the so-called 'Venetian Interdict' of 1606). Sarpi is generally known for his *Historia del Concilio Tridentino* ('History of the Council of Trent'), which focuses on the strong political motives underlying the action of Papal Curia regarding the Counterreformation. Interestingly this book (soon included in the *Index Librorum Prohibitorum*) was first published in London in 1619 (in Italian and pseudonymously).

Less is known about Sarpi's wide interests in science. This is so despite recent accounts of his connections with Galileo in Padua, and on the possible role of Sarpi (and other members of his scientific circle, especially Da Mula) in the development of the telescope and in the first astronomical observations of the moon made with the new instrument.

Problems in establishing the range of Sarpi's interests and achievements in science, and of his relations with Galileo, arise from Sarpi's reluctance to publish the results of his investigations. Moreover and sadly, many of his manuscripts were lost as a consequence of the destruction by fire in 1769 of the Servite library in Venice. Among the '*Cinque tometti*' (five small tomes) in which most of his papers were bound together, only one is extant, in the form of a copy derived from the lost original. This includes short annotations (*Pensieri*, i.e. 'Thoughts') written for private use, many of which are of a scientific nature, reflecting Sarpi's multifaceted commitment to science. Part of the lost material was available to the early biographers. We largely rely on their (possibly unreliable) witness to broaden our knowledge of the investigations of Sarpi and his circle. Some reference to Sarpi's scientific work can also be found in his vast correspondence with some members of the European intelligentsia.

Even more than in the case of Leonardo, Sarpi's scientific writings were for private use and not intended for publication. They are therefore often difficult to interpret and generally very succinct. In several circumstances it is difficult to understand if Sarpi is reporting a personal observation or reflection or simply transcribing what he has read in his voracious appetite for science. To add to the difficulty, we must consider that the extant parts of Sarpi's scientific papers remained in manuscript form until the end of the twentieth century, accounting for the limited knowledge among science historians of his personality and achievements.

Among the lost material mentioned by one of his biographers, Francesco Griselini, were three drawings of the moon to be used—according to Griselini—to prepare what could be the first detailed selenography. Moreover, one of the lost manuscripts was a text dealing with blood circulation, a subject that attracted Sarpi's interest since he collaborated with Fabricius and made studies of comparative anatomy. According to the Griselini, the main result of these dissections was the discovery of the valves in the veins, an achievement generally ascribed to Fabricius, but which was due—also according to some authoritative contemporaries—to Sarpi's genius. In the description of the pupillary light reflex, Fabricius did overtly recognize the importance of Sarpi's merit in his discovery. He wrote: 'This was observed and communicated to me by the Reverend Father Master Paulus Venetian, Theologian belonging to the Order of Servites, a distinguished philosopher, particularly expert of mathematics, and especially of optics, that I mention here with the purpose of honouring him' (Fabricius, 1600, p. 93).

The priority of this discovery is usually accorded to Leonardo da Vinci rather than Sarpi or Fabricius. As happened with Sarpi, Leonardo wrote about the pupillary reflex only in his notes and it is thus possible (but not certain) that the friar was unaware of the achievement of his predecessor. Leonardo himself had been anticipated by the observations made at the beginning of the tenth century by Persian scholar, al-Razi, who described it in a treatise (written in Arabic) entitled 'On the reason why the pupil contracts in light and dilates in darkness' (see Lindberg, 1976)

It is interesting to note here that in the Third Day of his *Dialogue*, Salviati would attribute to Sagredo the observation on the change of pupil diameter with light and darkness. It has been suggested that, by doing so, Galileo wished to pay homage to the friar, who he could hardly mention by name in a book undergoing the censorship of Vatican authorities.

In the course of his experiments on vision (leading to the description of pupillary reflex) Sarpi made another important discovery. It concerned a long-debated discussion on whether animals (particularly cats) are capable of seeing in complete darkness. Connected to this question was the belief that the phosphorescent aspect of the cat's eye in near darkness might be due to the emission of an intrinsic light. Sarpi correctly noticed that cats (and other nocturnal animals) are able to see in dim light but not in complete darkness. He discounted the supposed emission of an intrinsic light which could account for their ability to see in complete darkness. He remarked that, if this were the case, in the presence of a cat then we should also be able to see in the total absence of light. Sarpi obtained similar results with other animals (like dogs and horses) which can also see in dim light. He accounted for the nocturnal luminosity of the cat's eye on the basis of reflecting ambient light. He confirmed this by an experiment in which the apparent brightness of animal eyes disappeared upon masking the light of candle used to illuminate them (*Pensiero* 10). In his research on the vision of nocturnal animals, Sarpi went beyond the achievements of Leonardo who stated that the vision of cats and other nocturnal animals worsened drastically when the ambient illumination became very dim (LNB II, para. 834, pp. 124–125).

Sarpi's competence and interest in mathematics (which included geometrical optics, astronomy, mechanics, and other provinces of physics) was probably of a very high standard. Galileo was an authoritative witness and referred to him as *Mio Maestro* (My Teacher). When speaking of 'gentlemen…extremely expert of mathematical sciences' he made this statement about the friar: 'With no hyperbole I can assert that in Europe nobody beats him in these sciences' (OG II, p. 549). This high praise was probably reciprocal, particularly if we believe Sarpi's former student and biographer, Fulgenzio Micanzio. In a letter addressed to Galileo on 4 November 1634 (11 years after Sarpi's death) he expressed the considerations of his former teacher for Galileo:

> It remains always impressed in my mind what the said good Father was used to saying, that in certain ages nature produces intelligences suitable for certain speculations, and if these speculations are not tackled by them, there would not be any more hope that they could be attained. And he brought the

example of Your Lordship in [the study of] motion, and said to anybody that you had not had any equal in that, nor he believed that you could have any. (OG XVI, p. 150)

Micanzio would reiterate Sarpi's special appreciation for Galileo in subsequent letters, and similar statements on the extraordinary capacity of the Tuscan scientist to penetrate the laws of motion are present in the extant correspondence directed to him until May 1637.

12.3 Similarities and differences between Sarpi and Galileo

It is possible that the first contact between Galileo and Sarpi occurred in 1592, soon after Galileo's arrival in search of an appointment as professor of mathematics in the University of Padua. The first documented evidence of their acquaintance is, however, from a later period; it is based on Galileo's signed note dated 30 July 1600 stating that 'an instrument without quadrant had been donated to F[ather]. M[aster] Paulus' (OG XIX, p. 149).

Concerning their common scientific interests, a significant point is that, despite the difference of their cultural backgrounds and professional responsibilities, Sarpi and Galileo shared a general mistrust of Aristotelian philosophy, particularly in the way it had been developed along the medieval tradition. Both sought an intellectual change in science and culture at large. As with Galileo, Sarpi's main reference in the mechanical and hydrostatic sciences was Archimedes rather than Aristotle. Moreover, for Sarpi too the atomistic philosophy of Democritus, Epicurus, and Lucretius represented the general background for the elaboration of a new conception of the world, at philosophical, physical and biological levels. Sarpi was also influenced by Stoicism.

An obvious difference between Sarpi and Galileo concerns the role attributed to science in their respective personal and social endeavours. By reading Sarpi's *Pensieri* one gets the impression that for the friar the scientific interest was mainly the expression of an intense and pervasive intellectual curiosity. Unlike Galileo, it was certainly not the main reference for an intellectual (and also moral) reformation of humankind. Perhaps more aware than Galileo of the complexities and intricacies of politics and history, Sarpi did not share the deep conviction of the Tuscan scholar for the intrinsic force of scientific truth.

The important point is that, especially after the telescopic discoveries, Galileo's life programme turned to be one based on scientific investigations associated with an intense publication agenda. Sarpi, however, left in manuscript form all his scientific writings and only in some cases did he write with the possible (though unrealized) plan of publishing what he was investigating.[2]

12.4 Sarpi's reflections on the moon, waters, light reflection, and vision

From the comparison of Sarpi's and Galileo's manuscripts, and published and unpublished texts it appears that the influence (possibly reciprocal) between Sarpi and Galileo concerned many scientific dimensions and particularly the laws of motion, astronomy, tides, and visual perception. We will

[2] In addition to Grisellini, Micanzio, who wrote a biography of the friar, also mentions some of Sarpi's texts that were suitable for publication (Micanzio, 1646; Grisellini, 1761, 1785). Among the extant manuscripts there are a few more elaborate writings putatively conceived for publication, as, for instance, a treatise on the 'Art of good thinking' (*Arte di ben pensare*). But these are only a modest fraction of Sarpi's writings, and they do not have the scope or the literary qualities of the texts that Galileo produced after his first telescopic observations.

concentrate now on the theme of interpreting astronomical images. The main point of interest will be the aspect of the moon and its dark light and, more generally, the mechanisms of light reflection from surfaces of different regularity. This is a recurrent and important theme in Sarpi's *Pensieri*, and would become the subject of some letters that the friar would write after the publication of *Sidereus nuncius*.

Sarpi was acquainted with the texts of perspectivists from the Middle Ages, particularly from the reading of *Opticae thesaurus* published in 1572 in Basel by Frederic Risner with the assistance of Peter Ramus, which contained the Latinized form of the *Kitab al-Manazir* (i.e. optical treatise written in Arabic at the beginning of the eleventh century by the scholar Ibn al-Haytham—Alhazen: see Figure 12.2). It was printed together with a short treatise, *Liber de crepusculis*, also attributed to Alhazen,[3] and with Witelo's *Perspectiva*; this last one was an optical text written in the thirteenth century by the Polish-German scholar Erazmus Ciolek (known as Witelo, and already published in two editions in 1535 and 1531, respectively). Sarpi was also familiar with medieval works on motion, astronomy, and cosmology written by various scholars and commentators on Aristotle (especially through the texts of Albert of Saxony). He was also aware of more recent exponents of Western culture, like Cusanus, Leonardo, Giordano Bruno, not to mention Thomas Digges who adhered to the Copernican conception and supported the notion of the infinity of the world (see Chapter 8).

Sarpi's literary acquaintance with Leonardo emerges from one of the opening citations to his unpublished treatise on the *Arte di ben pensare*, which was derived from one of Leonardo's notebooks, now at the Institut de France.[4] Of obvious importance for Sarpi was the work of Copernicus. The *Pensieri* reveals a progressive attraction to the cosmological theories of the Polish astronomer, which developed on the basis of initial considerations on the celestial bodies observed from a viewpoint different from that of a terrestrial observer. Francesco Maurolico (1494–1575) could also be included among the authors who could have influenced Sarpi's work on optics and vision. Maurolico (Figure 12.3) was a Sicilian of Greek origin, who wrote a treatise *Photismi de lumine et umbra* ('Visual phenomena concerning light and shadow') in 1521. This text circulated in manuscript form before being published, in 1611, by Clavius. Another important text by Maurolico that Sarpi might have known in a manuscript form was the *Diaphanorum libri tres* ('Three books on lenses') inserted in the 1613 edition of Maurolico's optical works. This treatise contained an explanation of the corrective action of lenses in the common optical defects of the eye. Very likely Sarpi was also acquainted with the optical studies of the Venetian mathematician Ettore Ausonio, possibly through the mediation of the Sicilian astronomer Giuseppe Moletti, who was an estimator of Galileo and, as mentioned, his predecessor for the chair of mathematics at the University of Padua.[5]

---

[3] As shown by Abdelhamid I. Sabra this text which deals with the astronomic effects of atmospheric vapours is a Latin translation made by Gerard of Cremona from an Arabic text written by the Andalusian mathematician Abū 'Abd Allāh Muhammad ibn Mu'ādh (Sabra, 1967).

[4] This is, in translation, the text of the quotation: 'Man has got a big discourse, most of which is vain and false; animals have got a small one, but useful and true; it is better the small certitude than the great lie. As a kingdom gets destroyed when divided, so it happens when the intelligence divides itself in different studies' (Codex F, Institut de France. F. 96*v*).

[5] As we shall see in Chapter 13 both Sarpi and Galileo had made a copy of a diagram of Ausonio on spherical burning mirrors *Theorica speculi concavi sphaerici* which had a certain circulation in manuscript form before being published, with editorial modifications, in 1602 and in 1611 by the Bolognese astronomer, Giovanni Antonio Magini. In the last years of the sixteenth century the original of Ausonio's work, now lost, belonged to Pinelli's library.

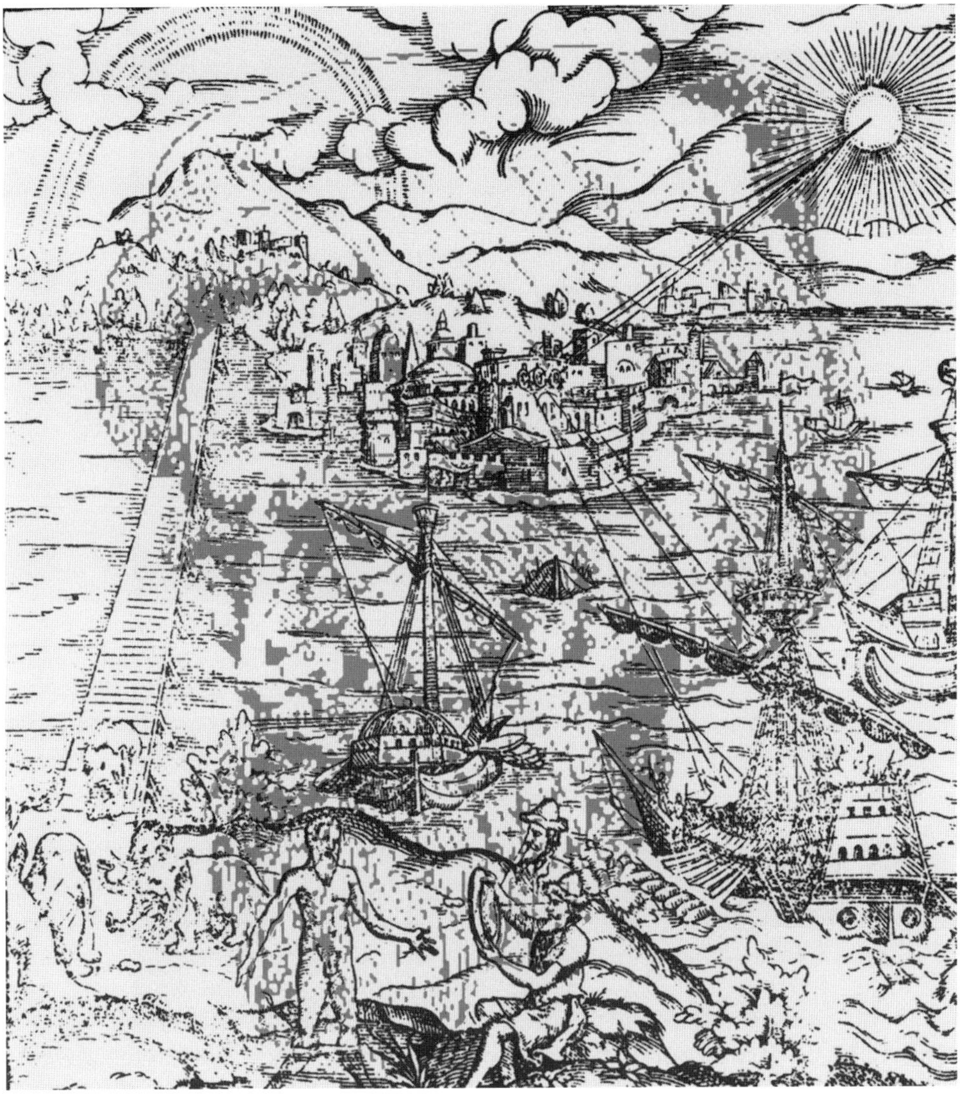

Figure 12.2 *Alhazen's Opticae thesaurus* by Nicholas Wade. It is likely that all portraits of Alhazen are somewhat fanciful, as is the case with the one dimly discerned in the illustration. Alhazen is shown in the frontispiece image of the book published in Basel in 1572. Among the symbolic elements underlining the importance of the optics in its triple dimensions of vision, reflection, and refraction, in this image there are also elephants crossing a bridge. These allude to an episode of the Carthaginian wars in which Hannibal deceived his enemies by simulating a great army by setting fire in the night to faggots and torches tied to the horns of a herd of two thousand oxen. The terrific impression was amplified by the dark of the night which enlarged the perceived image of the flames.

In Sarpi's *Pensieri* the theme of light reflecting from the moon appears among annotations which can be ascribed to the year 1578. It is developed within the framework of various considerations on light, senses, and the mechanism of knowledge, in an anti-Aristotelian manner. The first annotation concerned explicitly with the mechanism of reflection (*Pensiero* 9, p. 17) deals with the problem, long debated in the Middle Ages and Renaissance, of the differences in light

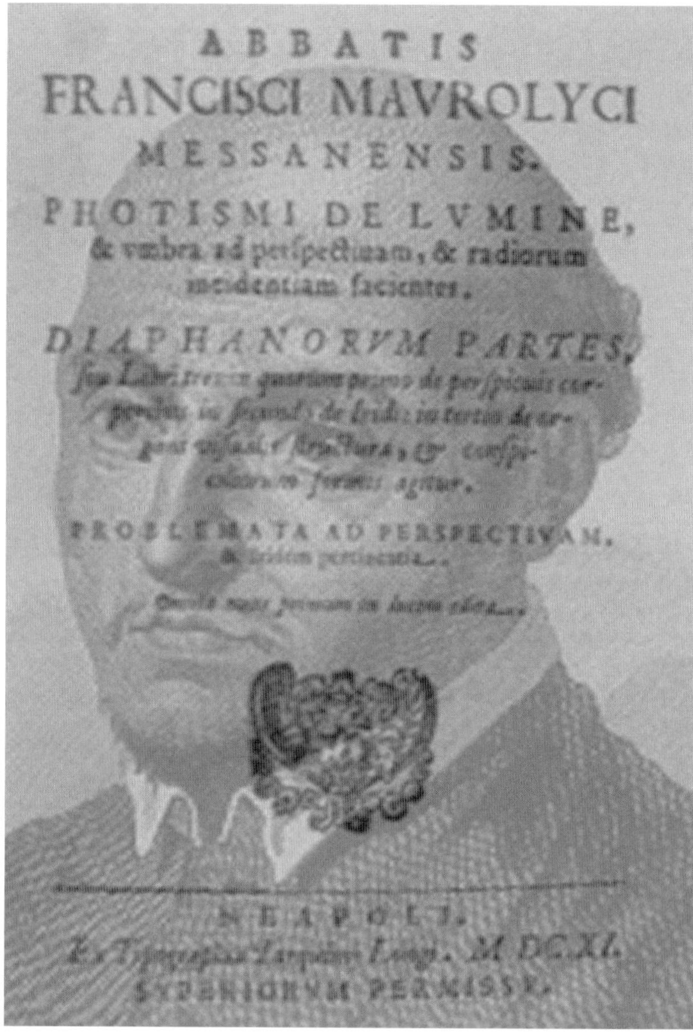

Figure 12.3 *Maurolico's Photismi* by Nicholas Wade. The portrait of Franciscus Maurolico is derived from an illustration in Schmitz (1981) and combined with the title page of his *Photismi et Lumine*.

reflection from bodies of various optical density. Sarpi writes in Italian and uses the word *trasparente* (transparent) to translate the Latin term *perspicuous*, and *opaco* (i.e. opaque but with a somewhat different connotation) for the Latin *opacus*. After saying that 'the [light] rays penetrate inside the transparent bodies, while in the opaque ones they are reflected', he makes the distinction less clear by saying:

> Since we see that in any transparent body some rays are reflected, and, similarly, some rays penetrate into any opaque one, we conclude that no transparent body is devoid of opacity, and no opaque of transparent; but any of them has always some mixture of the other. It is well true that such mixture is generally minimal and by itself insensible to us, but light proves it because the rays which hit transparent bodies pass across whereas those which hit the opaque ones are reflected. (p. 17)

Sarpi's intention is to undermine the classical distinction between transparent (or tenuous) and opaque (or dense) bodies; it should be noted that a similar position was taken by Galileo from the time of his first astronomical writings. This is evident from many of the annotations used by Galileo in the preparation of the three public lectures on the new star of 1604. For example:

> Show that in order to reflect the light of the sun it is sufficient to have a very slight condensation over the tenuity of the ether, as it is exemplified by the dry clouds; these appear as very vast mountains hanging in the air, being illuminated by the sun above the luminosity of the Moon and all stars, etc.; in a similar way much weaker condensation could win the luminosity of the stars. (OG II, p. 282)

In Sarpi's extant scientific writings, the first explicit consideration of light reflection from the moon is in *Pensiero* 26 and involves the difference in the reflection from ordinary opaque bodies, and from opaque bodies whose surface is polished (*tersa*). It makes reference to an example already debated by medieval scholars (and particularly well developed by Leonardo), that of the reflection from a spherical mirror. Sarpi writes:

> That the Moon receives the light from the sun is manifested by the lunar eclipses; that she is not like a convex mirror (*specchio colmo*) is manifested from the fact that the Sun is not seen in her, as [on the contrary] is seen in other convex mirrors. Thus she makes the reflection similar to our secondary lumen, that is similarly to the reflection made by things not polished [*cose non terse*]; because of the great distance her luminosity is very faint, being less than our secondary lumen, and even of the lumen of crepuscules. Were the Moon a polished mirror she would shine even during the day, and not only in the shadows; on the contrary she would make a duplicate lumen, similar to the solar lumen itself,[6] because the mirrors and the waters do make so, and thus make the solar lumen duplicated. (pp. 33–34)

It is not clear to what extent Sarpi's ideas are his own or derived from previous texts, possibly passages in which Leonardo shows why the moon's reflective properties cannot be likened to a spherical mirror. Compared to what Galileo would write, particularly in the *Dialogue*, Sarpi's text differs in his stating that 'were the moon a polished mirror she would shine even during the day'. Salviati and Sagredo describe the 'mirror experiment' on the First Day of Galileo's masterpiece. If the moon was a spherical mirror its brilliancy would be undetectable by terrestrial observers because of the relatively small size of the light cone from the great distance of the moon (see Chapter 5). On another issue, Sarpi repeatedly uses the expression 'secondary lumen' (*lume secondo*) as a possible explanation for reflection from the moon and this term appears in the treatises of Italian artists and humanists (including Leonardo). It was probably derived from the phrase *lux secunda* which appeared in the Latin version of Alhazen's optical treatise and in Witelo's *Perspectiva* (both published in the *Opticae Thesaurus*).

Interestingly the next consideration (*Pensiero* 27) shows that, while speculating on the mechanism of light reflection from the moon, Sarpi was ruminating on the variable appearances of cosmic bodies depending on the relative position of the observer:

> If one were on the Moon and looked at the Earth, because of the monthly motion he would see [in the Earth] all the appearances of the Moon, all the figures and both eclipses. (p. 36)[7]

---

6 This passage is difficult to interpret. The Italian original reads: '*Se ella fosse specchio terso, lucerebbe ancor di giorno, e non solo nelle ombre, anzi lume doppio, se ben nell'istesso lume solare*'.

7 A similar argument would return, at least partially, in a marginal annotation inserted by Sarpi near *Pensiero* 99: 'Perhaps the Earth itself also moves, and the monthly motion can similarly be of the Moon as of the Earth'.

Sarpi's considerations about the brightness of celestial bodies were influenced by medieval and Renaissance scholars. This is particularly evident from *Pensiero* 29 where the friar rejects the opinion of Albert of Saxony that ordinary stars shine because they receive the light from the sun. In Sarpi's statements neither a mirror-like nor a diffuse-type of reflection could account for the appearance of the stars:

> If stars were to receive the light from the sun, being polished and opaque, not only would they be seen during the day in a lively way, but it would also occur that the Sun would be seen in them. Nor can we ascribe to their smallness the fact that we cannot see them. This is because every mirror whose distance is proportioned to its size can be seen, and in it can be seen the sun; on the other hand, the size of stars is proportional to the distance, since they can be seen in the night; so the matter is. Not even can it be said that the stars are opaque but not polished, because then they would be seen like the Moon, despite their smallness, for the said reason.[8] They are therefore self-luminous bodies [*lumi propri*], and—being so small—they can be occulted by the great lumen of the Sun. This is because, operating both onto the eye, the action of the smaller lumen becomes insensible. (pp. 38–39)

This passage deserves some comment. Sarpi applies to the stars the partially faulty argument that, were they reflecting the light of the sun like spherical mirrors, they should shine very intensely so that they would be seen during the daytime. Moreover, he does not show a clear understanding of the problem of vision of luminous bodies at distance. This emerges particularly where he writes that 'every mirror whose distance is proportional to its size can be seen, and in it can be seen the sun', and when he says that 'the size of stars is proportioned to the distance, since they can be seen in the night'. At this stage the friar seems to be unaware of the fact that distant luminous objects might appear much larger than can be accounted for by the geometrical laws of vision. With regard to the expression 'occulted' (*occultati*) used to describe the phenomenon leading to the invisibility of stars in the presence of the sun, it is to be noticed that Sarpi was alluding to the effects of light adaptation produced by sunlight which make the stars invisible in daytime; he was not referring to real occultation like that occurring at eclipses.

The argument of the possible reflection between Earth and Moon as an explanation of the spotted aspect of the moon (and of her dark light) is addressed by Sarpi directly for the first time in the intervening consideration (*Pensiero* 28), which also addresses the theme of the reflection from the surface of the sea. The difficulty is that in this circumstance Sarpi's wording is particularly obscure and ambiguous, and it is not even clear whether he attributes a greater reflecting power to the surface of waters or lands:

> The Moon being an opaque but not polished body, she would be more rough where she has the spots; or else, where are the spots, she would be transparent [*perspicua*] to some depth, the sea making to her the spot in this way. Because of the sea, whose surface is even [*che è terso*], the Earth shines more onto the Moon than the Moon to the Earth; and perhaps from the Earth comes the lumen that is seen in the dark part of the Moon when she has the horns. This cannot originate from the Moon, because it would then be even during the eclipses; nor from the sun [directly] because it would be there just before the total eclipsing [*perfetta eclissazione*], when the Moon shows uniquely the horns. (pp. 37–38)

If, in our translation, we have correctly interpreted Sarpi's rather obscure and elliptic wording, in writing down this consideration the friar was convinced that seas were more reflective than

[8] With these words (*si vedrebbon come la Luna, non ostante la loro piccolezza, per la detta ragione*), perhaps Sarpi was alluding to the possibility that if the stars were not self-luminous they should exhibit the periodic phases like the moon. The argument is similar to that previously developed by Albert of Saxony, but the conclusion is different (see Chapter 11).

lands, and that the earth shone more towards the moon than reciprocally, because of the greater proportion of oceans on its (i.e. earth's) surface.

The theme of light reflection (and also of other forms of physical reflections) would return with other arguments connected to the theory of vision in many of the subsequent *pensieri*. In *Pensiero* 75 Sarpi elaborates on the way we evaluate the size and distance of objects with particular reference to the stars:

> The distance is known by means of the interposed bodies. This is why it seems that the stars appear to be all on one surface, that chimneys and mountains touch the sky, and that a very distant light, amid the fog or in the night, seems a star. The same happens also looking across a blowgun. (p. 84)

Sarpi's argument (partly derived from Alhazen, Peckham, and Witelo) would return in the theory of an intriguing visual phenomenon (the 'moon illusion'), whereby the moon—or sun—appears of greater size when near the horizon than when at the zenith. These arguments are important in the context of the scientific exchanges between Sarpi and Galileo, because Sarpi's interpretation appears to be the more effective.

Despite the continuous reference to visual and optical themes in the *Pensieri* of the first period, the argument of the dark light of the moon would be returned to in Sarpi's later writings (in item 490, probably written about 10 years after the first mention of the dark light of the moon). This short *pensiero* concerns the astronomical aspects underlying the reciprocal illumination between the moon and the earth:

> The Moon is illuminated by such a great part of the Earth, so much as in her is of obscurity; therefore, as she is near the full Moon phase, she is illuminated by a smaller part [of the Earth]; and by greater one so much as she is near the new Moon phase. Consequently, the part of the Moon that is illuminated by the Sun is as brilliant as the Moon is more new. (p. 363)

In the *Sidereus nuncius*, Galileo would use a somewhat similar wording to account for the astronomical relationships responsible for the variable brightness of the dark part of the moon:

> The Moon receives more or less light by reflection from the Earth as she faces a larger or smaller part of the illuminated terrestrial hemisphere. For the relative positions of those two globes are always such that at those times when the Earth is most illuminated by the Moon the Moon is least illuminated by the Earth, and vice versa. (SIDEREUS, pp. 15–16; transl. pp. 56–57)

12.5 Reflections and contrasts after the *Nuncius*

It is without doubt that the publication of *Sidereus nuncius* represented a new dawn in the history of cosmology. On a more personal note, it acted as a dramatic break in Galileo's scientific and intellectual relations with Sarpi and his circle. Scholars have suggested various reasons for this. On one side, there was in Galileo's text no explicit mention of the role played by Sarpi and his associates (especially Da Mula) in the improvement of the telescope and in the first observations of the sky. It is also probable that, given his personal interest in visual processes, Sarpi might also have contributed to the interpretation of the images of the moon and of the other celestial bodies. In this context it is to be remarked that Galileo probably made some of his telescopic observations in Venice, from the Convent of the Servites, possibly in the company of Sarpi and his associates.

Another important reason for the break in the relationship is connected to Galileo's scientific and career plans following the publication of *Sidereus*. By dedicating the revolutionary book to Cosimo II, the Grand Duke of Florence, Galileo was hoping to leave Venice and become Cosimo's official mathematician. With this in mind, Galileo had been developing contacts with important officials in the Florentine court. Very likely Sarpi, and other members of the Venetian intelligentsia (among them Sagredo), saw Galileo's decision as a form of ingratitude towards the *Serenissima*, which had enabled Galileo to develop his investigation in an atmosphere of intellectual freedom. Together with this ingratitude, Galileo's decision appeared politically insensitive because it seemed to be opposed to Venice, and especially to the anti-Vatican party headed by Sarpi himself; it was an option judged as favourable to the Catholic Church to which Florence was tightly connected politically.

These aspects arising from publication of *Sidereus* are mentioned in order to appreciate Sarpi's and Galileo's interpretations of the mechanisms of light reflection from the moon and the earth, and especially the causes of the dark light of the moon. In *Sidereus*, Galileo uses a rather indirect wording concerning the reasons why some parts of the moon's surface appear dark and other clear:

> So if someone wanted to revive the ancient Pythagorean theory namely that the Moon is like another Earth, its land surface would be more fittingly represented by the brighter region, and the expanse of water by the darker one. I have never doubted that if the terrestrial globe were observed from afar, bathed in sunlight, the land surface would appear brighter and the expanse of water darker. (SIDEREUS, p. 9; transl. p. 60)

Galileo's circumspection, and particularly his reference to an ancient conception, probably derives from his reluctance to enter into a direct discussion on whether there are seas on the moon (in his future texts he would be decidedly inclined to negate such a possibility[9]). On the other hand, he is rather explicit and straightforward in saying that, being illuminated by the sun, the surfaces of seas would appear darker than those of lands, even though he does not provide any explanation for his strong (and apparently long-maintained) conviction.

We find much more developed arguments on the issue of the moon's reflection, and particularly on the different appearance of waters and land, in some letters that Sarpi wrote after the publication of *Sidereus* to his correspondents, and particularly to the French lawyer, Jacques Leschassier (Sarpi, 1961). Leschassier had received a copy of *Sidereus* from Sarpi and had the opportunity to confirm some of Galileo's observations with a telescope built in Paris. In the letter in which he communicated to Sarpi his own observations of the moon, he asked the friar to provide explanations of the appearance of the moon and particularly on the difference of light reflection between lands and waters which were not clear to him.

In his response (the third of Sarpi's letters written to his correspondent after the publication of *Sidereus*), the friar begins the part concerning the moon's appearance in a surprising way, which clearly betrays the difficulties created by the publication of Galileo's book in Sarpi's circle. He says that, concerning the moon, he had not read 'what the mathematician [i.e. Galileo] wrote about it'. This statement seems really difficult to believe in view of his close collaboration with Galileo and of the excitement produced in Venice (and elsewhere) by the publication of *Sidereus*. Sarpi wrote to Leschassier that in his letter he would deal only with things that he could verify personally. What follows is a long and detailed explanation of the astronomical conditions which lead to a more or less effective illumination of the moon by the earth (and vice versa). Afterwards, Sarpi enters in the problem, aroused by Leschassier, of the different reflectivity of water and land, with these words:

> If you will look at a very great mass of water, such as a lake exposed to the sun, you will see the particle of water on which the sun is reflected, luminous as the sun itself, and rather returning its image and

[9] See, for instance, the letter written by Galileo to Giacomo Muti on 28 February 1616 (OG XII, pp. 240–241).

> if the interposed place (as you say) would shine almost as the sun itself, while the other parts where the sun does not fall would appear to you dark. If instead you observe a part of earth of the same size illuminated by the Sun, it will appear all luminous; less, however, than the water particle from which the ray was reflected, but more than the remaining water. I will make use of these things, but in a way more appropriate to the example. If you place a stone ball and a spherical mirror of the same size in the Sun and at some distance from you, you will see that the hemisphere of the stone ball is bright, while the mirror, by contrast, will be completely dark, apart from the minute area in which you will observe the tiny image of the reflected Sun. If you were to move further away, such that the visual angle (i.e. of the small sun) was extremely small, you would barely be able to see the mirror, but the stone would appear very brilliant indeed. [The Earth's] oceans and land masses form a sphere, and the Moon has a bright part and a spotted part; apply these principles to the problem, and you will see the point. (PENSIERI, p. 80; partial transl. Reeves, 1997, p. 107, revised)[10]

In this passage Sarpi describes light reflection from the surface of still water, probably on the basis of both personal observations and critical understanding of the previous literature on the subject. There is an appreciation of the reasons why the reflection of a small source from a spherical mirror could result in the mirror appearing completely dark. In this respect, Sarpi's understanding has progressed relative to *Pensiero* 26 (and also 29), where he was assuming that the reflection from a spherical mirror would result in a shining splendour, clearly visible from afar even during the day. Sarpi's argument seems to anticipate that developed by Salviati and Sagredo in the First Day of Galileo's *Dialogue* by showing why the reflection of the sun from a spherical mirror (and from the moon, if its surface was perfectly polished) would be practically undetectable from afar.

In the letter to Leschassier, Sarpi also elaborates on the reasons why the observation of the moon, and particularly the variable appearance of small luminous or dark spots near the terminator, can be interpreted as evidence of the play of light and shadow due to the variable inclination of the sun's rays illuminating reliefs or depressions on the lunar surface. Of interest in this context is a consideration that clearly derived from his personal interest in vision and possibly from his knowledge of optics and painting techniques; it anticipates some of the themes developed by Galileo in the *paragone* between painting and sculpture developed in his letter to Cigoli (and also in his letter to Grienberger, see Chapters 6 and 7). Responding to Leschassier who had expounded the traditional argument of the rare and dense parts of the moon to account for the spotted aspect of its surface, Sarpi writes:

> If you were to say that those things that look like cavities to me are really rarer parts of the Moon, and the apparent peaks its denser parts, I will prove to you that this is not so. A body's solidity, as you know well from optics, can only be perceived because of light and shadows, and thus paintings imitate solidity through lights and shadows. I can make anything appear solid, as if it were three- dimensional, through lights and shadows rendered through variations of colours [*luminibus, & umbris per colores*

---

[10] In the translation of this passage provided by Eileen Reeves in her *Painting the heavens* there is a mistake that leads the author to misinterpret Sarpi's argument and to attribute to the friar the supposed 'shortcomings of his explanation'. Reeves writes 'If you were to move further away, such that the visual angle was extremely small, you would barely be able to see the mirror, but the reflected Sun would appear very brilliant'. This translation clearly does not correspond to the Latin original inasmuch as it exchanges the reflected sun (which actually becomes invisible when looked at from great distance) with the illuminated stone ball which appears brilliant seen from afar: '*Quod si tantum elongaveris, ut insensibilis sit angulus, i.e. ille parvus sol, speculum vix videbis, lapidem autem maxime illustrem*'.

> *variatis*]. I say now that the light and shadow of those parts prove that there are peaks and valleys. (PENSIERI, p. 80; transl. Reeves, 1997, p. 110, modified)

To conclude with Sarpi's considerations on the theme of light reflections applied to the appearance of the moon, we must say that, although this theme had been central to his *Pensieri*, it is in the letter to Leschassier that it reaches its most clear and developed elaboration. It is true that this letter was sent about three weeks after the publication of *Sidereus* (on 5 April 1610). However, Sarpi deals with the matter in a much more diffuse manner than did Galileo in his text. This is the case concerning the reason why a water surface and a spherical mirror might appear dark when viewed from a distance. There is little doubt therefore that Sarpi had a very clear understanding of the problem and it could be an important source of information for Galileo in his interpretation of the moon's appearances.

It must be recognized on the other hand that in none of the extant Sarpi's texts is there an explanation of the mechanisms of diffuse reflection comparable to that expounded by Galileo in his more mature works. Galileo assumed eventually that a rough surface is able to produce a reflection in a different way to that of a mirror because it can be conceived as composed of 'very many little surfaces' oriented in various directions. No such notion is present in Sarpi, nor in Leonardo, and we have not been able to find it in other authors prior to Galileo. As we have seen in Chapter 11, in his search for a model capable of accounting for the splendour of the moon, Leonardo struggled intensively with the idea that it could be due to the various surfaces in which the lunar sea was divided by the presence of waves. In some of his *Pensieri*, Sarpi develops the theme of the so-called 'discontinued reflection', i.e. that occurring in the bodies that are neither perfectly transparent nor perfectly opaque. In doing so he arrives close to the idea that the phenomenon might be due to a multitude of reflections (this occurs, for instance, in *Pensiero* 11 and 54). However, what he writes is rather oblique and surely not so developed that it could be considered a genuine explanation of the phenomenon. This appears, for instance, from *Pensiero* 54:

> Tenebrous and invisible bodies are of two kinds, the transparent [*perspicuo*] and the opaque body. This last one comes from the discontinuity, while the first originates from the continuity; this is because the lumen passes everywhere if it is not reflected or refracted. However, in the continued body it does not do either of the two things, and it makes both in the discontinued body; therefore, if it encounters a continued thing it passes across, and if it encounters a discontinued one it makes so many reflections and refractions that it cannot pass across, and the small portion that passes cannot be perceived. (pp. 66–67)

A similar type of elaboration is present in other *Pensieri* in which Sarpi invoked the concept of discontinuity to account for the origin of the sensation of white (50 and 487). This is how *Pensiero* 50 reads:

> The white is the discontinued transparent; this appears in the water, either when it breaks off and makes the foam, or when it is mutated into fogs or snow: the same thing appears from the glass, either simply grinding it to a white powder, or by depriving it of his continuation humour and making a lime of it. On the other hand the sugar and salt become transparent when they are candied; also the wood knots have some transparency as they are more dense, and therefore more continued. (p. 62)

Galileo's descriptions of light reflection are surely along the lines of discussions by medieval and Renaissance scholars with a particular influence from Leonardo and Sarpi. As already mentioned, particularly in Chapter 1, Galileo repeatedly considered a sea in different degrees of motion as a model of a reflection which goes from a perfectly polished mirror to a rough surface like that of a wall, or of the moon; this resonates with Leonardo's motifs. As to Sarpi, it is difficult to believe that in the course of their scientific collaboration, and particularly at the time of the first telescopic observations, Galileo did not benefit from the continuous ruminations on visual themes that the friar had been developing since the time of his first *Pensieri*. However, it is worth reading again a passage from the *Dialogue* that we have already quoted in Chapter 5 in order to perceive the importance of the transition from Leonardo and Sarpi to Galileo on light reflection. This passage is inscribed in the framework of the experiment of the 'dark mirror' performed during the conversation between the three discussants. To Simplicio who has difficulty in imagining how a rough surface like a wall 'is able to reflect light more powerfully and vividly than a smooth and well-polished mirror', Salviati replies:

> Not more vividly, but more diffusely. As to vividness, you see that the reflection of that little flat mirror, where it is thrown there under the balcony, shines strongly; and the rest of the wall, which receives a reflection from the wall to which the mirror is attached, is not lighted up to any great extent (as is the small part struck by the reflection from the mirror). If you wish to understand the whole matter, consider how the surface of this rough wall is composed of countless very small surfaces placed in an innumerable diversity of slopes, among which of necessity many happen to be arranged so as to send the rays they reflect to one place, and many others to another. In short, there is no place whatever which does not receive a multitude of rays reflected from very many little surfaces [*moltissime superficiette*] dispersed over the whole surface of the rough body upon which the luminous rays fall. From all this it necessarily follows that reflected rays fall upon every part of any surface opposite that which receives the primary incident rays, and it is accordingly illuminated. It also follows that the same body on which the illuminating rays fall shows itself lighted and bright all over when looked at from any place.
>
> Therefore the Moon, by being a rough surface rather than smooth, sends the sun's light in all directions, and looks equally light to all observers. If the surface, being spherical, were as smooth as a mirror, it would be entirely invisible, seeing that that very small part of it which can reflect the image of the sun to the eyes of any individual would remain invisible because of the great distance, as we have already remarked. (DIALOGO, p. 69: transl. p. 77)

From the considerations made in this and the previous chapters we can undoubtedly conclude that Salviati's words are in no way a solitary creation of Galileo. From that point of view we can endorse the opinion of von Bekesy reported at the beginning of Chapter 11 on the difficulty for humankind in inventing and creating new things, or even simply imagining them. On the other hand, there is little doubt that, in Galileo's hands, diffuse light reflection becomes a mature and clear scientific notion. Moreover, it also becomes a powerful tool contributing to rejecting the crystalline immutability of the moon and to fostering a new vision of the world.

12.6 **Looking at the moon and sun on the horizon, illusion, and deception**

Despite the clarity and exhaustive interpretation of the mechanism of diffuse reflection and its application to the appearances of the moon, it must be remarked that Galileo's views on visual problems do not prevail over those of Sarpi in all circumstances. Sarpi's *Pensieri* that consider the moon or sun illusion (more accurately the 'celestial illusions', because they also involve constellations) are certainly more perceptive (and substantially more correct) than those expressed by Galileo.

We will use the term moon illusion because it is in common currency in visual science; it refers to the apparently larger size of the moon when observed near the horizon compared to the zenith. It is a visual illusion because the geometrical size of the moon at the horizon is very similar to that at the zenith (Ross & Plug, 2002). This can easily be verified by taking a photograph of the moon in the two positions. In Sarpi and Galileo's day it could be assessed by means of astronomical measurement. As a matter of fact the projected image of the moon at the horizon is slightly smaller that that high in the sky (see Figure 12.4) but this difference is imperceptible.

There is evidence that the moon illusion came to human attention in prehistoric times and various interpretations have been advanced since the classical Greek epoch. Two main types of explanation were provided by Greek scholars. The first ascribed it to some type of optical phenomenon due to terrestrial vapours interposed between the eye and the celestial body. The second pointed to the importance of a purely perceptual process. Sometimes, as in the case of Ptolemy (and of Alhazen, Peckham, Roger Bacon, Witelo, and others several centuries later) the two contrasting explanations are found in different texts by the same author (Ptolemy) or in different places of the same text (Alhazen, Peckham, and Witelo).

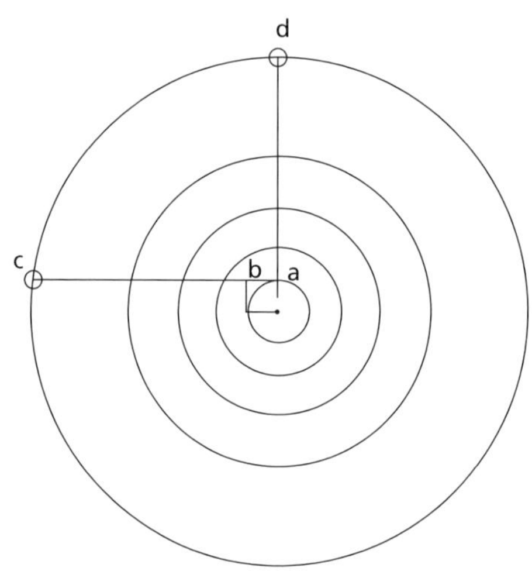

Figure 12.4 One of the diagrams drawn by Leonardo to show that the geometrical image of a celestial body would be smaller for a terrestrial observer when above or towards the horizon. This is because the viewpoint is situated on the surface of the earth (and not in the centre of a supposedly circular orbit of the Sun, moon, and other planets). In the diagram a is the position of the observer, while c and d indicate the celestial body at, respectively, the horizon and the zenith; a–b, a length corresponding to the Earth's radius, is the excess of the horizon distance compared to the distance at the zenith. The three circles surrounding the earth are the sphere of water, air, and fire that Leonardo supposed encircled all cosmic celestial bodies. Based on the modern values of the diameter of the earth and its distance from the moon or the sun, this geometrical effect is, however, very small (about half a minute of arc for the moon and about 400 times smaller for the sun) and thus it has no relevance to the appearance of the celestial bodies in the two conditions of observation, apart from being in the opposite direction to the illusion. Reproduced from the notebook now at the Institut de France: Leonardo da Vinci, *The notebooks of Leonardo da Vinci (vol II)/compiled and edited from the original manuscripts*, Jean Paul Richter, Dover Publications, para. 913. A similar diagram is also present in the same notebook; see Leonardo da Vinci, *The notebooks of Leonardo da Vinci (vol II)/compiled and edited from the original manuscripts*, Jean Paul Richter, Dover Publications II para. 867.

The optical explanation, which assumed various forms from Aristotle until relatively recent times, is based on the greater optical magnification supposedly resulting from the greater thickness of the layer of vapours surrounding the earth along the line of sight towards the horizon than towards the zenith. Alternatively it was related to the fact that the vapours at the horizon were more dense or humid. The magnification could be attributed simply to the effects of vapours by themselves, on the idea that dense vapours—or other optically dense materials (like water)—could magnify objects when interposed between them and the observer because of dioptric effects. After Aristotle, this idea is found in one of the works of Ptolemy (second century AD), Cleomedes (third century), Macrobius (fifth century), and in Alhazen (eleventh century). A variation of this hypothesis was that the optical effect might depend on the shape of the surface of the vaporous layer. Leonardo, who was interested in the phenomenon and speculated about it in various places of his notebooks, alluded to a more defined optical effect in two of his reflections.

The first, illustrated by the image shown in Figure 12.5, was as following:

> Why the sun appears larger when setting than at noon, when it is near to us?
>
> Every object seen through a curved medium seems to be of larger size than it is. (LNB II, p. 153)

In another annotation (in a manuscript now at Royal Library of Windsor), Leonardo elaborates a little more his optical hypothesis, by writing:

> If you want to prove why the moon appears larger than it is, when it reaches the horizon; take a lens which is highly convex on one surface and concave on the opposite, and place the concave side next the eye, and look at the object beyond the convex surface; by this means you will have produced an exact imitation of the atmosphere included beneath the sphere of fire and outside that of water; for this atmosphere is concave on the side next the earth, and convex towards the fire. (LNB II, p. 168, para. 909)

Leonardo was attempting to attribute the magnification at the horizon to the optical effect produced by the two spherical surfaces of different curvatures delimiting the sphere of fire

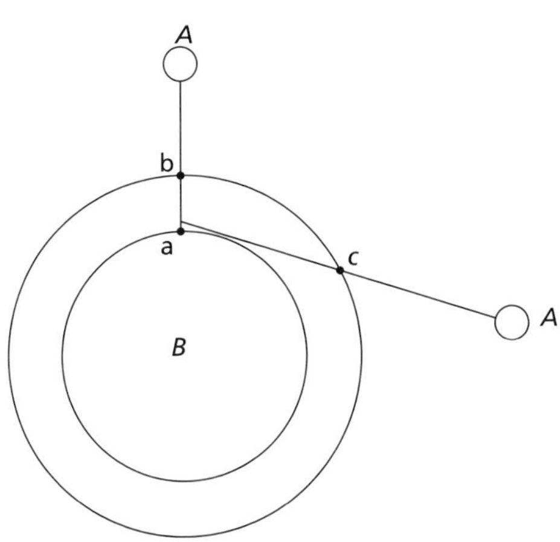

Figure 12.5 The image by which Leonardo wished to account for the increased apparent size of celestial bodies at the horizon, in one of his reflections annotated place of a notebook now at the Institut de France. See the text for explanation. Reproduced from Leonardo da Vinci, *The notebooks of Leonardo da Vinci*, vol. II, edited by Jean Paul Richter, Dover Publications [etc.]

(with the internal surface having an angle of curvature smaller than the external surface). In terms of modern optics, he is conceiving the sphere of fire as a negative lens and attributing a magnifying power to it. Not having a clear idea about the laws of refraction, Leonardo does not develop his hypothesis in geometrical terms. It is possible that such an idea might have been reinforced by manipulating various sorts of lenses. An annotation contained in the Codex Atlanticus (now at the Biblioteca Ambrosiana of Milan) suggests that Leonardo might have been assembling lenses for enlarging astronomical images: 'Construct glasses to see the moon magnified' (LNB II, p. 168, para. 910).

It is an idea based on an optical effect due to the terrestrial vapours, somewhat similar to that of Leonardo, which would resurface more than a century later in the work of Galileo. The Pisan scientist expounded this view first in a pseudonymous pamphlet published in 1606, the *Considerazioni di Alimberto Mauri* (mentioned in Chapter 2), and he repeated it in *Saggiatore*.

It should be noted at the outset that any kind of hypothesis for the moon illusion based on geometrical optics is faulty. This is because, as remarked earlier, there is virtually no physical difference between the images at the horizon and the zenith. In this context we must consider that even though the phenomenon varies between observers and circumstances, it is a large and robust visual illusion. The moon (and the sun) at the horizon appears to be almost twice as large as at the zenith. If such image magnification had an explanation based on the laws of geometrical optics, certainly it would not have escaped the detection of astronomers who had been measuring small differences in the geometrical images of celestial bodies during their movements. This statement is especially true for astronomy after the second half of the sixteenth century, initiated particularly by Tycho Brahe with his very precise instruments.

One of the first demonstrations that the phenomenon could not be attributed to optical refraction but was of a perceptual nature is found in a work published in 1545 by the Dutch astronomer, physician, and instrument maker Reinerus (Reiner) Gemma Frisius in his *De radio astronomico & geometrico*. The 'astronomic and geometric radius' described in this book was an instrument, similar to other devices of the epoch, developed by Gemma Frisius for astronomical, navigation, and surveying purposes. Among the applications suggested by the author in the astronomical field there was one that allowed demonstration of the deceptive nature of the celestial illusions. Gemma Frisius first considers the case of the moon:

> Whoever wished to destroy this impression [*phantasia*] can do so easily with the Radius: let him measure the diameter of the Moon emerging from the horizon when it is full, in northern signs [of the zodiac] or at any other time, and then measure its diameter on the same night when it reaches culmination. When he finds that the diameter does not differ by even a minute from that found at first, he can surely and without doubt believe that the density of the air in no way changes the size of the stars. For although the luminaries seem larger near the horizon, when they are measured with the instrument no difference is perceived. Though it is true that images of things which appear in air that is denser seem larger, in fact they do not become larger as one can see from ordinary experience. (Gemma Frisius, f. 30r.; transl. Goldstein, 1987, p. 173)

For what concerns the stars he writes:

> For, though the distances between stars near the horizon appear to be greater than when they are high in the sky, nevertheless, when they are measured with the Radius, they do not differ at all. (Gemma Frisius, f. 30r.; transl. Goldstein, 1987, p. 173)

Kepler, in *Astronomiae Pars optica* published in 1604, considers various visual deceptions and deals with the moon illusion in a 'Proposition' entitled 'Considerations of those things that Witelo advised to be necessary for astronomy' (Chapter 4, Proposition 7). He attributes the phenomenon to perception and says that the illusion does not interfere with objective measurements taken by astronomers. He writes:

> This cause does not affect astronomers much, because the observation that is carried out with instruments does not introduce any error from this source. The only important thing is this: when we read that the ancients carried out their observations, not with instruments but by estimation of the distances, we know that they might have been in error in this matter, since the faculty of estimation itself is egregiously in error through this cause. This was taught by Tycho Brahe, and by Ptolemy himself in Book 9 Ch. 2. (OPTICA, p. 134; transl. p. 146)

And in the Proposition 5 in chapter 5 of the same book ('Those things that recoil upon Astronomy from the means of vision; or, on flawed vision') he applies similar considerations to the distances between stars:

> And so, when the distances of stars are to be taken using astronomical instruments, the more careful astronomers, as has been said, do not trust the eye. (p. 212; transl. p. 226)

After the invention of the telescope, a variation in the optical size of the sun with its position on the sky would not be missed by the accurate method of projection of the solar image on a paper based on the use of telescope. This was first devised by Galileo's student Benedetto Castelli and largely used in the study of sun spots. In his *Discorso sulla visione* ('Discourse on Vision') written in 1639 (but published posthumously in 1669), Castelli verified the matter and showed with an astronomical instrument that the change in the visual size of the celestial bodies is not the consequence of effects attributable to geometric optics. He did that for the constellation of *Ursa major* (Big Dipper) after having noticed that it appeared much larger when seen near the horizon than in the middle of the sky:

> I repeated this observation many and many times for the two positions, and [the constellation] always seemed to me much larger when I observed it toward near horizon, than when I observed it overhead. Moved by such an oddity, I wished to make sure by measuring with an instrument how much the said constellation subtends in the one and in the other posture. I always found that it subtended the same space and thus I felt sure that such a phenomenon (being not a deception of the eye) of necessity had to be a fallacy of judgment and of apprehension. (Castelli, 1669, pp. 28–29)

The observation of Castelli, on which we will come later in this chapter (section 12.10), was such as to dismiss any theory of the moon illusion based on purely optical effects.

12.7 **A vaporous lens in the sky, and the deception of a perspicacious observer**

As mentioned earlier, Galileo expounded the idea of a refraction effect as an explanation of the celestial illusion for the first time in 1606. The hypothesis emerges in the context of a discussion concerning a theory advanced by his antagonist Ludovico delle Colombe in order to account for the appearance of the new star of 1604. According to delle Colombe it could be explained on the basis of magnifying the image of a pre-existing, but almost invisible, star due to the optical effect produced by a particularly dense part of the 'Crystalline sky'. Galileo dismisses this hypothesis with various arguments and accuses his adversary of a logical fallacy. In particular, he criticizes the idea than an optically dense medium is per se capable of producing magnification. It is in order to produce an example of his views on the optical action of a dense medium that he elaborates a

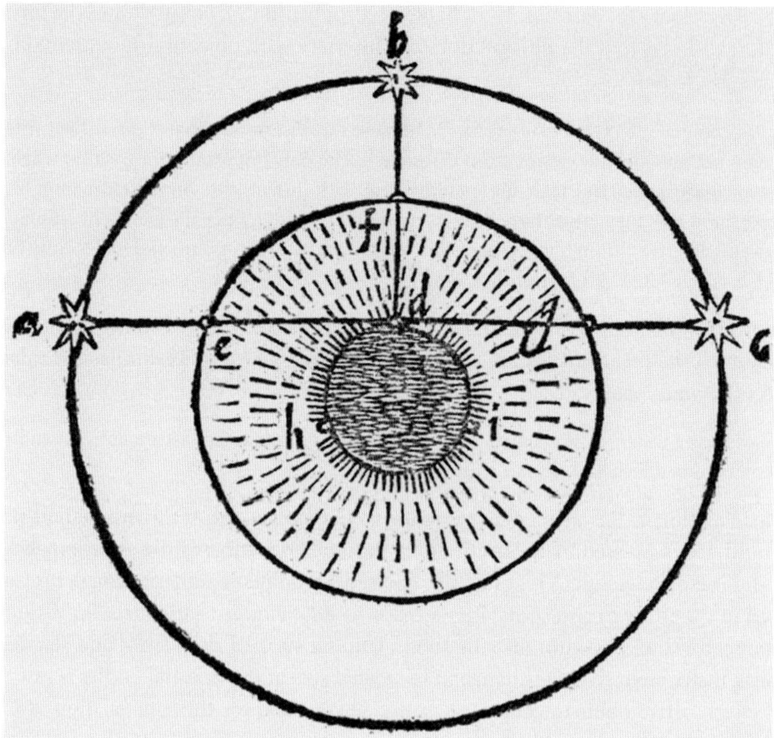

Figure 12.6 The image from the *Considerazioni di Alimberto Mauri* illustrating the optical hypothesis supposedly responsible for the Sun illusion; a, b, and c are the position of the sun at, respectively, dawn, midday, and sunset; hdi represent the surface of the earth; and efd the surface of the dense zone of atmosphere around the earth to which are attributed the optical effects responsible for the illusion. Reproduced from Galilei, G. *Considerazioni d' Alimberto Mauri sopra alcuni luoghi del discorso di Lodovico delle Colombe intorno alla stella apparita 1604*. Firenze, appresso Gio. Antonio Caneo.

hypothesis for the sun illusion. This hypothesis is illustrated by a diagram somewhat similar to Leonardo's (see Figure 12.6).

The main difference is that in the scheme of Figure 12.6 the earth is said to be surrounded only by a layer of vapours and not by the three external spheres of the elements of Leonardo's diagram (Figure 12.4). Galileo attributes the cause of the larger magnification with the horizontal view to the larger distance of the observer from the external surface of the vapours sphere at the horizon, compared to the distance in the vertical view (a–e exceeding a–b by the radius of the earth). This is how he puts forward his explanation of the phenomenon after having rejected the idea that vapours per se might have a magnifying action:

> Before I tell my opinion on this, it should first be known that moistures and vapors drawn on high by celestial power from any place on the surface of the earth are lifted not infinitely high, but only out to a certain definite boundary, which many people say is a height of 52000 paces.
>
> Since the earth is spherical, so also the concave surface formed by the boundary of all those vapors. Second, when we look at an object through a crystal of a concave shape, experience teaches us that the farther we remove the said crystal from ourselves, the larger the object will appear to us, provided that there shall be in between us and the crystal some quantity of water or vapor.

I come now to the purpose. In order for us to see the sun when it is situated anywhere in the sky, it is necessary that our vision shall pass through the said concavity originating from the earthly vapors, and that the concave surface is everywhere equidistant from the globe of the earth. Hence the concave surface through which our visual rays pass is farther away from us when we look at the sun situated in the east or west, than when we look at it at noon. Therefore I say it is no wonder that the sun looks larger at rising and setting, since to see it at any other place our sight, our vision need pass through a surface closer to us, as plainly seen in the next diagram [our Figure 12.6]. (MAURI, f. 24 r & v; transl. p 121)

Rather surprisingly (and incorrectly) in the *Cosiderazioni di Alimberto Mauri* it is positively asserted that the horizontal magnification concerns only the sun and not the moon.

In *Sidereus* Galileo would make a brief mention of the same hypothesis by putting together two completely different phenomena, the magnification at the horizon of the moon and the sun (now supposed to underlie a comparable magnification), and the reduction of the apparent size of stars, by alluding for this last effect to the action of crepuscular light considered as particularly effective near the horizon.

It is, however, in the *Saggiatore* that Galileo would elaborate more diffusely on the hypothesis of vapours in order to account for the magnification of both sun and moon. This occurred again within the context of a debate on the subject of comets. He used his hypothesis against his new adversary (Horatio Grassi) and accused him of the same type of logical fallacy imputed to delle Colombe in 1606 (i.e. having derived an erroneous conclusion by connecting in an uncorrected way two apparently sound premises). The argument is in this case slightly more developed than in the 1606 text, even though it is not accompanied by a figure. After discussing the proposition of his adversary, Galileo concludes his reasoning by saying:

Place between your eye and any object a convex crystalline lens, at various distances. You will see that when this lens is close to the eye it increases but little the size of the object viewed, but moving it farther you will see the enlargement progressively grow. And since the vaporous region terminates in a spherical surface not much elevated above the convexity of the earth, all the straight lines drawn from our eyes to that surface are unequal, the one toward the zenith being the shortest of all and the others being gradually longer the more they point away from the zenith and toward the horizon. (SAGGIATORE, pp. 208–209; transl. p. 316)

In continuing his arguments, Galileo attributes a phenomenon long remarked on by astronomers to the optical effect of the terrestrial vapours, that of the oval shape of the sun and moon at the horizon:

Let it be remarked in passing that here one may easily deduce the cause for the apparently oval shape of the sun and moon when they are near the horizon by considering the great distance of our eyes from the center of the earth, which is the center of the vaporous sphere. Whole books have been written about this appearance, as I believe you know, though the entire mystery requires no doctrine more profound than to understand why a circle seen straight on looks round to us, while looked at in foreshortening it appears oval. (SAGGIATORE, p. 209; transl. p. 316)

Galileo was correct in attributing the oval shape of the sun to the optical effects of terrestrial vapours. These effects had been a great concern for astronomers of the period, starting from the astronomical measurements of Tycho Brahe (see also Chapter 14). It must be said that in the *Saggiatore* Galileo did not produce any real optical theory of the effect leading to the appearance of the oval sun. This can be justified by his apparent desire of treating the matter just 'in passing'.

On the main theme, in both *Considerazioni di Alimberto Mauri* and *Saggiatore*, Galileo was definitely wrong in attributing the magnification of the moon and sun in the horizontal view to an effect of geometric optics. His attitude in this circumstance is perplexing. First, it seems that he never measured the physical dimensions of the images of the two celestial bodies (or of the constellations) with any type of astronomical instrument. This is a puzzling shortcoming, especially because he was well aware of the possible deceptive nature of visual appearances. It must be remarked, moreover, that in his texts Galileo often reproached other scholars or laymen for their superficiality in assuming something as true on the basis of common beliefs without verifying it personally. This is the case with Tycho Brahe and other anti-Copernicans. One of their suppositions was that the body would not fall perpendicularly when dropped from a moving boat (see OG VI, pp. 545–546). Experience—as Galileo could repeatedly certify with his experiments, sometime rather spectacularly—showed the contrary, provided that the boat was moving with a rectilinear and uniform motion (see Conti, 1990).

Another puzzling aspect of the problem is that Galileo seemed to ignore what Kepler had said on the same subject (both in *Optical part of astronomy* and in *Dioptrice*). Although it is likely that he had not read the work of Kepler when he wrote *Considerazioni*, it is much less so at the time of *Saggiatore* (as we shall discuss in Chapter 13). It is also puzzling that his optical theory of the moon and sun illusion is similar to one of the explanations provided by medieval perspectivists, notably by John Peckham in his *Perspectiva communis*. Galileo might have read this text (possibly in Pinelli's library) because at least 10 printed editions had been published by the end of the seventeenth century (two in Venice). If this was the case, the problem is that Galileo seems to have read only the passage in which Peckham expounded his optical version of the moon and sun illusion (Proposition 12 of Part III) and not the other parts of *Perspectiva communis* in which he accounted for the phenomenon on a purely perceptual basis (Propositions 63–65 and 82 of Part I). In his Propositions, Peckham was following arguments largely derived from Alhazen (*Opticae Thesaurus* Book II, section 25, pp. 39–41). Peckham's explanation was based on the idea of a better appreciation of distance in the horizontal view made possible by the presence of intervening bodies. After having said (in Proposition 63) that 'the comprehension of the magnitude of distance is derived from the magnitude of the intervening bodies' (from Lindberg, 1970, p. 141), he applies the argument to the vision of celestial bodies in Proposition 82 entitled 'Stars appear larger in the horizon than in any other part of the sky'. He writes:

> This is proved because, as is evident from Proposition 65, they [i.e. the stars, meaning in fact especially Moon and Sun] appear more distant when they are on the horizon and because an object is judged larger by the correlation of and equal angle with a greater distance, as Proposition 74 shows. Since an object on the horizon is perceived by the eye under the same angle as [that under which it would be perceived] elsewhere in the sky and since it appears to be at a greater distance, the object is judged larger when on the horizon. However, if the distance were really greater, the angle would be smaller, and the object would appear smaller; but that is not the case. On the contrary, an equal angle correlated with an apparently greater space makes the object to be judged larger. (Lindberg, 1970, p. 153)

Surprisingly this proposition concludes with a statement which refers to a later passage (Proposition 12 of Part III) in which the phenomenon is interpreted on the basis of an optical phenomenon (similar to the Galileo's): 'The interposition of vapors which will be touched on below, concerns the same'.

By comparing Peckham on celestial illusions with what Galileo wrote more than four centuries later, one gets the impression that he had read only a part of the treatise by the medieval perspectivist and completely neglected the others. A negligence that could be perhaps explained by the rhetorical requirements of his theory in *Considerazioni* and in *Saggiatore* but it can in no way be justified in a scientist of Galileo's calibre. It is also possible, however, that he had not read any of the explanation of the celestial illusion provided by the medieval perspectivist and was relying on his old (and somewhat inaccurate) memories as a student, at the time in which he was attending the course of 'perspective' given by Ostilio Ricci in Florence (see Chapter 13). Among the didactic material of Ricci's course there was a manuscript treatise *Della prospettiva* ('On perspective') which dealt with this subject in the form of a dialogue between a teacher and a student (Polixeo).

Dealing with the atmospheric vapours of different density which interfere with the appreciation of the 'quantity, distance and true place of stars and planets', the teacher says:

> In a similar way the reason why the sun appears greater in the morning and evening, as also moon and stars on the east and west appear greater and nearer than in the middle of the sky, this is the refraction of the rays [*fractione de' razi*], in which they first pass through coming from the sky toward us, and then, passing through the dense medium come together toward the perpendicular and show [the moon and stars] greater than they are. And this dense medium is nothing else than the vaporous air, which is near the water and always receives haziness [*fumi*] one time more than the other. And always we see through that vaporous air when we look at east or west; whereas, when we look upward, there are not so many vapours in the clear weather.; this is why we judge the thing with a better reason, except in the case there are many fogs, which do the same because they are vapours. (Parronchi, 1964, p. 638)

Although the magnification is attributed to the vapours, in the words of the teacher there is no allusion to the optical explanation of the *Considerazioni* or *Saggiatore* based on the distance of the observer from the inner boundary of vapours. Galileo could have derived this from the common experience with convex lenses which (within certain limits) magnify the object seen in proportion with the distance from the eye. As we shall discuss in Chapter 13, this was a well-established notion in the practical optics of the Renaissance and Galileo was very likely familiar with it.

Before concluding with the complex relation between Galileo and the celestial illusion we need to return to Sarpi, and, after him, to Castelli. These two scholars have two significant qualities to claim a significant role in our story of Galileo vis-à-vis the moon illusion. Both were closely related to Galileo (Sarpi being his senior and Castelli his junior), and both seemed to have a better understanding of the celestial illusion than their celebrated fellow.

12.8 **Sarpi, moon, sun, blowguns, and afterimages**

The phenomenon whereby the moon and the sun appear larger at the horizon recurs in Sarpi's *Pensieri* to such an extent that it is taken as a common example of possible sensory fallacies and their origins. It is evident that Sarpi's interest in vision and its deceptions are important aspects of his general approach to the acquisition of knowledge. Although Sarpi was mainly inspired by atomism and stoicism, he shared with Aristotle the idea that sensory errors were not generally due to deceptions of the primary sensory processes. Rather, they involved an act of judgement. Following Alhazen and the perspectivists, Sarpi recognized that with experience acts of judgment tended to become automatic.

In *Pensiero* 75 (see section 12.3) Sarpi alluded to the theory of interposed bodies as an explanation of the way we can know the distance of objects at the horizon. What Sarpi says is basically a very rapid résumé of reflections that he could have read in Alhazen, Witelo, or Peckham. However, the final statement shows that he has probably verified the importance of the intervening objects with an observation based on the use of a blowgun (*ciarabottana*, i.e. *cerbottana*) to exclude the vision of peripheral objects. In doing so Sarpi was probably inspired by Alhazen who examined vision through an aperture as a way of restricting the vision of intervening objects (see Sabra, 1989, I, pp. 154–155).

In the period in which Sarpi annotated this consideration (about 1578), he was particularly interested in the complex problem of the perception of distance and the size of objects, which had been at the centre of attention for scholars since the classical era. He might have been reading Witelo (in the 1572 edition of the *Opticae thesaurus*). This is because in the following *Pensiero* (n. 76) he reflects on the various cues to resolving the ambiguity of objects having different sizes but subtending the same angle due to their different distances. He quotes a statement from Witelo which essentially summarizes the title of Proposition 19 of Book 4 of his *Perspectiva*:

> In two ways is judged the magnitude of a thing: the first [was is] by the simple eye, which judges from the quantity of the angle, and knows this one by the quantity of crystalline humour that is painted [*tinto*] by the colour of the object; the other way is by involving [in the task] the reason, or by making recourse to the universal species, or comparing then basis of the [visual] triangle with its sides, which correspond to the length of the [light] rays; these are known exclusively through the intermediate bodies when the reason has not a role. All the things seen under the same angle appear equal; this is why Witelo says 'Visa sub eodem angulo, quando distantia non videntur, videntur equalia'[11]; but it must be added 'Neque figura animadvertitur alias visa'[12]; this is because with the said discourses of reason, or with one of them, even though we see under the same angle a finger or a bell-tower [*campanile*], we judge this larger than the other. That the eye judges by the angle alone is manifest in the case of stars, which are judged so small because it is not possible for them to apply one of the two discourses; it appears for the things represented in perspective (and this is a demonstrative argument), because these things appear as they appear only by the angle; therefore on the basis the angle alone also the solid things would appear.[13] It appears from the spectacles and other transparent optical devices [*altri perspicui*], which magnify or reduce the thing, simply by making the angle large or small. Finally it appears manifest from seeing a uniform thing without intermediate [bodies] (I say that in order to avoid two ways in which reason might be involved), because it is judged as the hole; and in seeing the rule very far from the mirror, because it was uniform, and no intermediate bodies were seen, nor on the surface [of the mirror], and at the mirror was judged equal. Therefore, the true magnitude is known by comparing the angle to the distance and obliquity, or to the universal species residing in the soul: if the distance is not immeasurable, the reason can know it [i.e. the magnitude] in either of the two ways: if it is immeasurable [the reason] can know it on in the second way, that is by comparison and making recourse to the universal species; certainly not in the first way; this is because the line of the [visual] pyramid in unknown. (PENSIERI, pp. 85–86)

In this unusually long *Pensiero* Sarpi develops Witelo's arguments (in turn derived from Alhazen who repeatedly remarked on the importance in perception of judgement—the *virtus distinctiva* in the Latin terminology of the *Opticae thesaurus*). Most probably, Sarpi verifies these arguments with personal experiments. As to the vision of a uniform thing (that is, a thing whose size and distance are not immediately apprehended by simply identifying its figure) made through a hole [*buco*], Sarpi is probably alluding to some of the experiments by Alhazen. The Arab scholar pointed to the visual deceptions caused by looking through a hole in order to exclude the vision

11 'Things seen under the same angle, when the distance is not seen, are seen equal.' The title of Witelo's proposition derived from Euclid's *Optics* is a little different: '*Omnia visa sub eodem angulo, quorum distantia ab invicem non perpenditur, videntur equalia. Euclides 7 opticorum*'.

12 'And the figure seen is not recognized by other ways.' Sarpi wishes to add another condition to Witelo's statement, meaning that the things seen under the same angle are perceived as equal if the two conditions are given, namely the distance is not perceived directly, nor the figure recognized in some other way.

13 Here Sarpi wishes to say that the argument considered for the things represented in perspective also applies to the real things when there are no other cues to tridimensionality.

of the intervening ground or objects in the space in between. However, not all of the experiments of the original manuscript *Kitab al-Manazir* were translated in the *Opticae thesaurus* (compare Sabra, 1989, I, pp. 154–155 with the corresponding sections Alhazen's Book II in Risner, 1572 and Smith, 2001).[14] The same experiments might have inspired Sarpi's use of the blowgun in the observation reported in the previous *Pensiero*. In the case of the mirror experiment, he was probably considering the possible deceptions caused by the vision of a 'uniform' thing in a mirror depending on whether it was perceptually localized on the mirror surface or in the illusive depth created by the reflection.

It is in pursuing these personal experiments, made in order to verify what he was reading in the texts of medieval perspectivists, that Sarpi arrives at an important observation that he reports in the next *Pensiero* (n. 77):

> Having looked at the sun, or other very brilliant thing, in such a way that the image remains in the eye, if you look at a distant thing, she [the image in the eye] is big, if [you look at] a near one, [the image of the sun] is small, and [if you look] at your eyelids it is very small; there her size appears according if the [visual] angle is compared to a long or short distance.

In order to clarify the complex problem of the size–distance perception Sarpi is here exploiting the after-image of the sun, i.e. the brilliant image of the solar disc that remains visible for a relatively long time after having fixed the sun for a brief instant. Afterimages have a venerable history, being described by scholars since antiquity and by medieval perspectivists.[15] Sarpi is demonstrating how the perception of distance potentially resolves the ambiguity of the visual size. Or, to use his own words (relating to the old theory of vision which considered the crystalline lens as the visual organ) Sarpi was declaring how the ambiguity of objects of different size, located at different distances was perceptually resolved, even though they were to 'paint' the same 'quantity of crystalline humour'.

Finally, in the next *Pensiero* (n. 78), and particularly in a marginal annotation added to it, he draws conclusions from the after-image experiment for the vision of objects at the horizon and at the zenith (celestial bodies included):

> Things with right angles, elevated above the horizon, appear smaller at the top [*paiono in alto più piccole*]. This is not because they are seen with a smaller angle; in fact they do not appear so small to the people that looks at them on the horizon with the same angle. This is made by making them far away. Similarly it happens if they are elevated by a quarter of a circle [*quarta di cerchio*] and the eye is in the centre. They would appear then smaller, as also it is seen in the stars. Nor can it be said that vapours make the stars to be seen in different size, because vapours are not interposed among the elevated magnitudes [*grandezze elevate*]. Therefore not even the effect on the appearance can be ascribed to vapours [*perciò né men de' vapori alla figura può attribuirsi*].
>
> [*Marginal note*] The things [are] seen larger on the horizon, because it appears distant the part of the terrestrial horizon which is seen in the sky, and what is there of the height of houses, not because it makes a larger angle. This appears by the solar image that remains in the eye [*Consta per la solare imagine che nell'occhio resta*].

The rather oblique wording of this *Pensiero* makes its interpretation rather difficult. Nevertheless, it can be grasped that Sarpi wished to dismiss any role of vapours in the phenomenon whereby

---

[14] In some way those experiments seem to anticipate Ames' room, i.e. the popular visual illusion in which the design of a room is manipulated in an artificial manner such as to distort the perception of sizes and distances inside it when looked from outside through a hole.

[15] After-images were known, for instance, to Aristotle who discussed their changing colours and invoked them as an evidence against the extramission theory of vision.

things at the horizon appear larger than overhead. The marginal annotation is, however, particularly significant, especially in the final statement. With the phrase 'the solar image that remains in the eye', Sarpi is invoking the result of the after-image experiment in order to account for the different size of the same object observed at the horizon or at the zenith. In that regard it must be remarked that the initial word of the last sentence, *consta*, can also be translated as 'it comes out' or 'it is proved'. It is fortunate that Sarpi's extreme conciseness and obscurity in this sentence could be clarified by the comparison with the considerations expounded in the other *Pensieri* of the same period.

12.9 **A group of prelates in a dark room reciting the Miserere in front of a luminous window**

Many years later, the after-image experiment and its possible relevance to the celestial illusion would recur in the writings of another important member of Galileo's entourage, Benedetto Castelli, the author of the aforementioned *Discorso della visione*.

At the beginning of the *Discorso* Castelli describes some optical experiments he is doing for the entertainment of some of his acquaintances (several *Monsignori*) based on a simple version of the pinhole camera (the *camera obscura*, i.e. literally the 'dark room'). Afterwards, he uses the results of these experiments to relate the functioning of the eye, considered as a 'live' dark room opposed to the 'dead' dark room of the experiments. In contrast to Sarpi, Castelli knows (most probably from the diffusion of the optical works of Kepler and Scheiner) that the organ of vision is the retina and not the crystalline lens. He says that images of external objects are painted on the 'retinal tunic' of our eye. To prove that assumption he makes a further experiment that he describes in this way:

> I got all those present to fix their eyes on a glassed window illuminated by the sun with the following precaution: that they would not let the eye wander over the window but would hold their sight on a determinate spot of one of the panes and keep the eye steady for as much time as it takes to say, for instance, the Miserere psalm. Once this was done, I did so that all those who had done the operation closed their eyes and on questioning them as to what they were seeing with the eyes thus closed all answered that they were seeing the very same window with its glass panes differentiated one from the other by their lead [frames] and by small details [*particolari minuzie*]. [But] what was amazing to all was that the window appeared as painted in very diverse hues, now with yellow colours, then green, now red, then peacock blue [*pavonazzi*]. Then it would vanish, reappear, and fade away again. The wonder of everyone increased even more when the same operation was repeated with open eyes and these eyes were turned now toward one part, now toward another part of a white wall, all saw the image of the same window but with the following additional wonder: when they looked at a wall further away from their eyes than the window, they saw an image larger than the real window; when they looked at a wall nearer and nearer, the image of that same window appeared smaller, and smaller in such a way that when looking at a sheet of paper placed three spans away from the eyes the same image appeared very small on the paper. (Castelli, 1669, pp. 9–10; Ariotti, 1973, p. 7)

On the basis of these results Castelli concludes that the image of the sun has been 'printed [*stampata*]' on the retina in the same way as images previously produced in the dark room experiment. He adds that these observations would be useful to account for several visual phenomena, one of which is the celestial illusion. As a matter of fact the afterimage experiment provides the most important clues to understanding the celestial illusions.

Before examining Castelli's reflections on this theme, let us return to Sarpi and his scientific manuscript. As already mentioned, the celestial illusion is considered to be a deception based on judgement. In his unpublished short treatise on the *Arte di ben pensare*, he elaborates on the fact that an error in a specific sense, due to the intervention of *discorso* (that is 'reasoning' 'judgement'), would recur if it is not corrected by the same sense, but by opinions (*ipolipsi*) derived from another sense or emerged in a different context.

The sun illusion is among the examples that he produces to illustrate his conviction:

> ...the correction is not effective [*la correzzione non apparisce*]; even though we have made the demonstration of the sun magnitude, nevertheless it appears to us exactly as before; and despite we have made clear that it subtends the same angle in the horizon than in the middle of the sky, nevertheless the same appearance comes again. And even though, before seeing for the first time the sun, one had the demonstration of this equality, even so he would see it larger at the horizon. In a similar way the things seen by reflection would appear in front of him, and those refracted would appear broken, and the trees along the rivers to move, even though before seeing them he had a demonstration of truth. (PENSIERI, p. 590)

In a similar vein, the theme of the celestial illusion returns in *Pensiero* 203 within the context of a reflection on the relation between sensation and 'discourse':

> If the distance is perceived only by the intermediate bodies, why does it not seem to us that stars touch our eyes? This is because of the prejudgement [*prevenzione*] that we have learned with the discourse (and that stays in the mind) that the stars stay above the houses, towers and mountains; because of this we always judge them higher than other things seen by us. (PENSIERI, p. 184)

This and other passages in Sarpi's manuscript show that for the inquisitive Venetian friar the celestial illusion was one of the most relevant and recurrent themes with respect to the problem of the complex relationships between sensation and reasoning. If we consider that the phenomenon is still one of the most studied and interesting in all sensory psychology, we could not but see in this interest another instance of Sarpi's scientific and philosophical acumen. We are, moreover, led to regret that Sarpi has not written more clearly about this illusion and published his considerations on the theme, so that the results of his experiments and his reflections were available for posterity.

On another issue, the fact that Sarpi had such an insightful view of the celestial illusion, and treated it as a perceptual phenomenon, makes Galileo's contrary interpretation all the more perplexing. It seems that, although the two scholars had possibly worked together on several occasions, the collaboration was probably episodic, and did not have the character of strong continuity and close association.

12.10 **Castelli, the moon, and the nocturnal science in the carriage**

As repeatedly mentioned, some of Sarpi reflection's on the celestial illusion occurred in the 1570s and were likely to precede Galileo's interest in the phenomenon. The other important character in the celestial illusion saga, Castelli, wrote about the phenomenon in 1639, towards the end of Galileo's life. As already mentioned, Castelli was a close associate of Galileo (who considered him his most beloved and devoted student: see Figure 12.7). The paradox in this story is that Galileo seems to have adhered to an incorrect and obsolete view of the celestial illusion despite having been associated throughout his scientific life with the two scholars who had expounded a much more perceptive view of the phenomenon.

The situation is, however, even more intriguing. To know why, we have to return to Castelli's *Discorso della visione* and particularly to Section XXIV of this text in which he deals expressly with

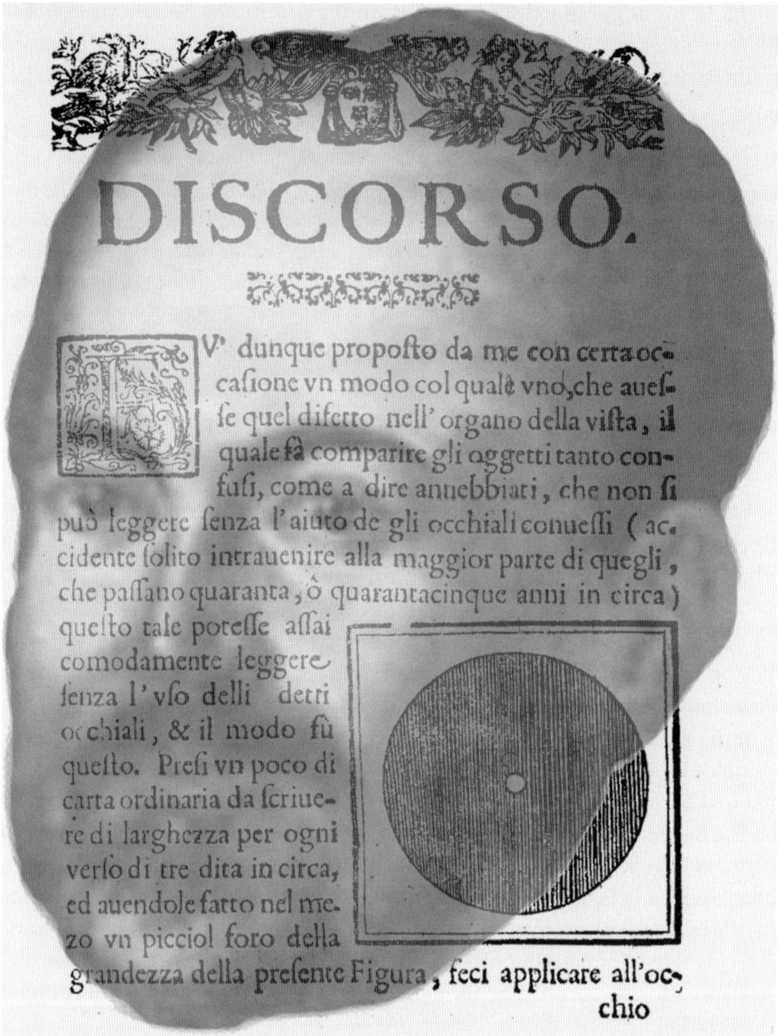
DISCORSO.
V' dunque propoſto da me con certa oc-
caſione vn modo col qualè vno, che aueſ-
ſe quel difetto nell' organo della viſta, il
quale fà comparire gli oggetti tanto con-
fuſi, come a dire annebbiati, che non ſi
può leggere ſenza l'aiuto de gli occhiali conueſſi (ac-
cidente ſolito interuenire alla maggior parte di quegli,
che paſſano quaranta, ò quarantacinque anni in circa)
queſto tale poteſſe aſſai
comodamente leggere
ſenza l'vſo delli detti
occhiali, & il modo fù
queſto. Preſi vn poco di
carta ordinaria da ſcriue-
re di larghezza per ogni
verſo di tre dita in circa,
ed auendole fatto nel me-
zo vn picciol foro della
grandezza della preſente Figura, feci applicare all'oc-
chio

Figure 12.7 *Castelli's Discorso* by Nicholas Wade. The portrait of Castelli is derived from a painting and combined with the first page from his discourse on vision. He describes a wide range of phenomena including afterimages, dark adaptation, distinct vision, moon illusion, size perception, and visual persistence.

the celestial illusion. We have already quoted the passage in which he wrote that the image constellation of the Big Dipper had the same physical dimension when measured in the two positions with an astronomical instrument. In the *Discorso*, as a possible explanation on the phenomenon, Castelli writes:

> After having reflected much and carefully it came to my mind that this business of the large and small is by our mind managed always in relation to some other magnitude better known to us than that which is the magnitude of the object about which we must form an idea of whether it is larger or small. In our case, as we look at the regions of the Heaven that are located near the zenith, we are led to compare

> them and to relate them to the summit of the roofs of our buildings, for we have nothing else near the zenith with which we can compare them. For this reason the constellation of the Dipper, when it is looked at in similar circumstances, will seem to us as occupying a portion of space equivalent to that of the top of a house or of a temple, which space is well known to us and does not attain more than a few tens of cubits [*braccia*]. In that manner we can form a rough idea of the size of the Dipper which we judge and estimate as [rather] small. But when we see it near the horizon we compare it with the long chains [*tirate*] of mountains and with the wide countryside, which we know very well are sometimes tens of miles. In such a case we judge the Dipper to be much larger than what we had thought in the other disposition. In this way the object whose magnitude must be judged is appraised by us sometimes larger and sometimes smaller as we compare with different magnitudes. (Castelli, 1669, pp. 29–30; Ariotti, pp. 15–16)

The explanation of the celestial illusion that Castelli is proposing here belongs to the type of hypothesis based on 'perceived size' in modern psychological theories of the phenomenon. After expounding his explanation, Castelli reports, as a verification of it, a curious episode that we could qualify as entertainment science involving a group of Vatican prelates one evening in Rome:

> An interesting case comes to me as a further confirmation of the same doctrine. While in an evening as customary I was in a carriage with Monsignor Cesarini and other of his noble party and we were going along the Tiber, the full Moon was rising and appeared to peep out over the Aventine hill on the other side of the river. Almost everyone in a single voice said at the Moon—how large it is, how beautiful. I, taking advantage of the opportunity, asked how large it appeared. I was answered that it seemed as of four or five cubits in diameter. At this point, by interposing the brim of my hat between the hat of Monsignor and the Moon, I completely covered the view of the Aventine hill but in such a way that the moon could be seen over the edge of the hat brim and again asked how much the diameter of the Moon appeared to be. The Monsignor, then, almost in amazement, answered that it did not seem to be two fingers breath. The same observation was made by everyone of the party and thus there was an opportunity to consider the illusion again. All conceded that as we compare the Moon and the Aventine and as the Moon seems to us to cover a segment of it which is judged by us to be of four or five cubits, so is the Moon judged of this size. But when the view of the hill is covered up, and the same Moon is compared and referred to the brim of the hat, it results that the Moon is judged to be much smaller even though in both cases the Moon which affects our eye over the retina by impressing it with its image, always has to make exactly equal images on the retina. (Castelli p. 39; Ariotti p. 16)

The description of this amusing scene of *Notturno romano*, ends in a rather surprising way because unexpectedly Galileo re-enters. This is how it happens, in Castelli's words that follow immediately the just quoted passage:

> I felt much satisfied by the thought above, until on communicating it to my teacher [*Maestro* i.e. Galileo] he unveiled to me a much more subtle and artful deception in which our judgement is tangled up and deluded. Although I do not have the ability [*animo*] to explain it with the felicity of expression by means of which it was clarified to me by the great man, as he ever used to do in all his discourses about obscure and recondite matters of Nature, however difficult, I shall attempt to represent it on the best way possible to me while begging whoever reads to excuse me if I shall not be able to reproduce as clearly what I was then taught. Thus, I first consider that of two unequal objects placed at various distances are judged to be equal, it must be that the judgement about their size is fallacious. For example, the Sun according to the most exact astronomical observations is 17,060 times larger in diameter than the Moon; nevertheless the diameter of the Moon seems to us and is commonly judged [by us] to be equal to that of the Sun. Similarly, if two objects are truly equal and truly placed at equal distances from our eye but one of them is judged farther away, it will be appraised larger. On this account, were a painter to draw a picture, and because of the same distance from the eye, two equal figures of men,

> but were such figures represented against the background [*sopra quel grado*] in such a way that one appeared in a place far away from our eye and the other nearer, we would then judge that the one that is represented as much further away as, so to speak, a giant even though the two figures are of equal height. In sum, in these operations of our judgement, to be deceived with respect to distances results in being deceived in our judgment of magnitudes, and also because of the latter we come to a form of false judgement about the distance. But to go back to our purpose, when we lift our sight to the contemplation of the heavens and of those objects that are commonly seen in them we form a very false conception of their disposition. For we reckon those parts that are near the vertex as very near to the eye and those that are placed along the horizon as very far away. Thus the same constellation of the Big Dipper—to stay with the same example—which really and truly is as far away from our eye when it is near the vertex as when it is located and spread out over the horizon, is judged by us larger in the latter than in the former posture. Yet the truth is that the image [*simulacro*] over the retina in the eye is always equal so that the area of the corporal eye is affected by the object in the one and on the other posture is always the same and the illusion consists of and depends on our judgement. (Castelli, 1669, pp. 31–33; Ariotti, pp. 16–17)

The dedicatory letter of Castelli's *Opusculi filosofici* in which *Discorso della visione* is published is dated 29 August 1639. From this letter directed to Monsignor Giovanni Ciampoli, (one of the members of Galileo's and Castelli's entourage), we learn that the scene of the moon on the Aventino was then recent. This is because Castelli indicates that he promenades almost daily in the carriage of Monsignor Cesarini (the dedicatee of *Saggiatore*) and Cittadini (a theologian). The party 'spent the great part of the time in noble and virtuous discourses' between science and theology. Galileo was then in his house-prison of Arcetri near Florence, following the condemnation by the Roman Inquisition. In October 1638 Castelli was given permission to visit Galileo in order to discuss scientific matters with him and his presence is indeed attested in Florence in that period. It is thus likely that the conversation in which Galileo provided his former student with a 'much more subtle and artful deception' took place before October 1638.

The rather ironic conclusion to the story is that near the end of his life Galileo, contrary to his earlier views, gives an accurate explanation of the visual processes involved in the perception of form and distance and thus of the celestial illusions. This was despite the fact that he was then becoming almost completely blind (as Castelli remarked in *Discorso della vision*; see Chapter 4). As Galileo had explained to his pupil, the celestial illusion reveals the complex and bidirectional relation that exists between the perception of form and distance. With reference to the recent studies on the moon illusion, we could conclude that, despite his previous fallacies on the theme of celestial illusion, Galileo was astute in saying (in Castelli's words) that: 'In sum, in these operations of our judgement, to be deceived with respect to distances results in being deceived in our judgment of magnitudes, and also because of the latter we come to a form of false judgement about the distance'.

The fact that he made reference to the technique of painting in his 'discourse' to Castelli is—we believe—of no surprise for any reader who has arrived at this advanced phase of our book.

Chapter 13

Alternative visions

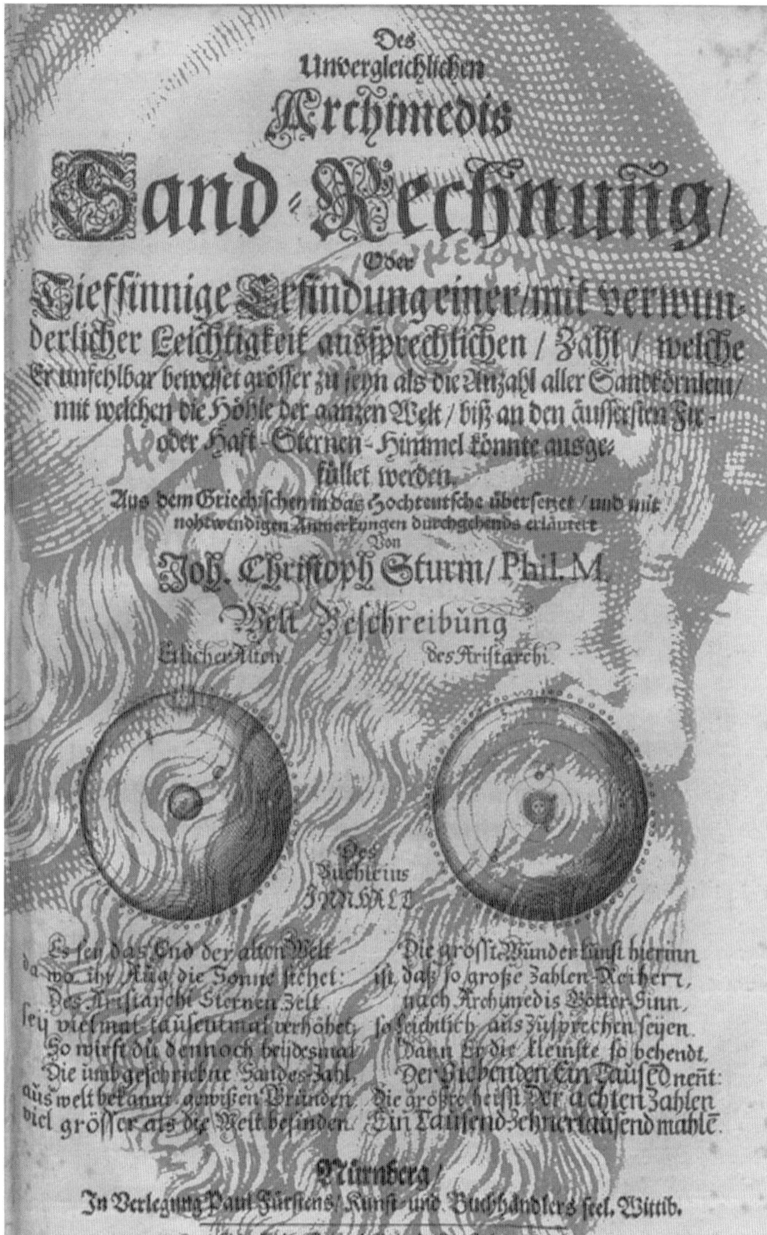

Figure XIII *Archimedes' reckoner* by Nicholas Wade. Archimedes' downcast gaze can be seen in the title page of a German version of the *Sand-reckoner*.

When considering Galileo's predecessors dealing with vision in Chapter 11, we followed Kepler's rapid reactions to *Sidereus nuncius*. However, up to now the German astronomer has played a relatively minor role in our analysis of the origin and context of Galileo's deliberations on celestial appearances. He will come now to the front stage of the present chapter in which we will consider the problem of the apparent size of the stars relative to the geometrical size of their images from the point of view of the observer. In this and other respects, it is important to compare Kepler's ideas with those of Galileo because these two champions of the scientific revolution placed different emphases on the powers of optics and observation. This will lead us to broaden the scope of our consideration to the optics of the Renaissance in which Galileo's enterprise appears to be deeply rooted.

13.1 A new century, an optical century

In Chapter 12, in dealing with Galileo's interpretation of the moon illusion we have remarked about his apparent neglect or ignorance of the geometrical laws of optics, at least of the physiological optics that emerged from the beginning of the seventeenth century largely due to Kepler. Starting from his *Astronomiae, Pars optica* (1604), Kepler had developed a very insightful knowledge of the processes whereby an image of the external world is formed on the retina through the agency of the optical components of the eye. In the history of physiological optics, the publication of this book represents a milestone, not unlike what would occur for astronomy and cosmology with the publication of Galileo's *Sidereus*. After the appearance of the booklet of his colleague (and competitor), Kepler would continue his optical research and would publish in 1611 a more mature optical work, *Dioptrice* ('Dioptrics') containing a theory of the construction of the telescope and a complete theory of lenses (Figure 13.1).

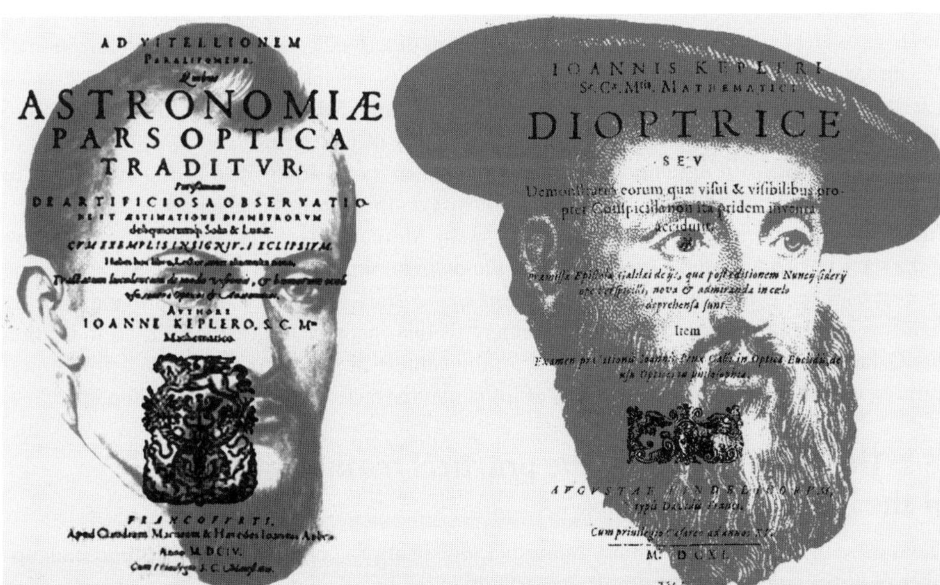

Figure 13.1 *Kepler's optics and dioptrics* by Nicholas Wade. Two portraits of Kepler combined with the title pages of his two major works on optics.

Credit: (Left hand side) Kepler, Johannes (1571–1630) German mathematician and astronomer. / Photo © Tarker / The Bridgeman Art Library. (Right hand side) Johannes Kepler (1571–1630) from 'Gallery of Portraits', published in 1833 (engraving), English School, (19th century) / Private Collection / Ken Welsh / The Bridgeman Art Library.

These two works would be an important source of inspiration for Scheiner in his composition of *Oculus, hoc est, fundamentum opticum* ('The eye, that is, the optical fundament') published in 1619 which provides an accurate anatomical and functional representation of the eye which goes much further than the anatomy of the Renaissance, still largely dominated by the conceptions of Galen and his medieval followers. In the old conceptions the crystalline lens was located in the centre of the eye and the optic nerve was situated on the optic axis.

Scheiner (Figure 13.2) gave the first accurate drawing of the eye (see Chapter 8, Figure 8.1): the lens and its curvatures are appropriately represented and the optic nerve leaves the eye nasally. Scheiner appreciated that an equation of artificial and natural image formation could be made and he described how an artificial eye could be constructed in his monumental *Rosa ursina* (1630). In order to make one, he determined the curvature of the cornea by comparing the size of images reflected from it with those of glass spheres of varying sizes, and he estimated the refractive indices of the humours of the eye. Scheiner presented a pictorial analysis of optical image formation in the camera and the eye—with both inverted and upright images due to the addition of convex and concave lenses. He noted that an upright retinal image resulted in inverted vision. Furthermore, Scheiner described how an image could be seen on the exposed surface of an excised animal's eye—an experiment he 'had often performed'.

The demonstration of an inverted and reversed image cast on the retina of an animal's eye, together with those from artificial eyes hastened optical analyses of vision. Scheiner's analysis was rapidly absorbed by both anatomists and philosophers, as is evident from Descartes's *La dioptrique* ('Optics') published in 1637 in the celebrated *Discours de la méthode pour bien conduire sa raison* ('Discourse on the method of rightly conducting the reason'). His diagram of the cosmic observer inspecting the inverted and reversed retinal image is shown in Figure 13.3. In *Dioptrique* the theory of refraction is expounded on the mathematical basis of the sine refraction law, later referred to as Snell's law because it had been described earlier by the Dutch astronomer Willebrord Snellius (or Snel) in 1621.

In this phase of progress and excitement for optical studies, also attested by the publication of other treatises in the field (as, for instance, in 1613 that of *Opticorum Libri Sex*—'Six Books of Optics'—by François d'Aguilon or Aguilonius), Galileo seems insensitive to the attractions of geometrical and physical optics. Nevertheless, he invents the astronomical telescope and uses it in a masterly way to decipher the appearances of the sky. Moreover, as in the case of the apparent size of the stars, he prevails on the experts of optics and astronomers of his (and previous) ages, being the first to reveal the deceptively large apparent size of stars and planets, by improving by more than two orders of magnitude the measurement of their geometrical size. This is an indication that Galileo's interest in vision, particularly in the context of the interpretation of astronomical features, was different from that of many of his contemporaries and notably from Kepler's.

13.2 **The useful optics of the practical mathematicians of the Renaissance**

The success of Galileo in his optical and visual investigations contrasts with his supposed ignorance of optics and of the advances in this science in the pre-Kepler era. Nowadays, this is indeed a matter of debate, with opinions that differ among historians about the importance of the progresses in optical science in the period between the medieval perspectivists and the beginning of the seventeenth century, when Kepler published his milestone work. A dominant opinion until the last decade, particularly after the studies of the American historian David Lindberg, was that optical studies have undergone a phase of significant stagnation after the time of Alhazen, Roger

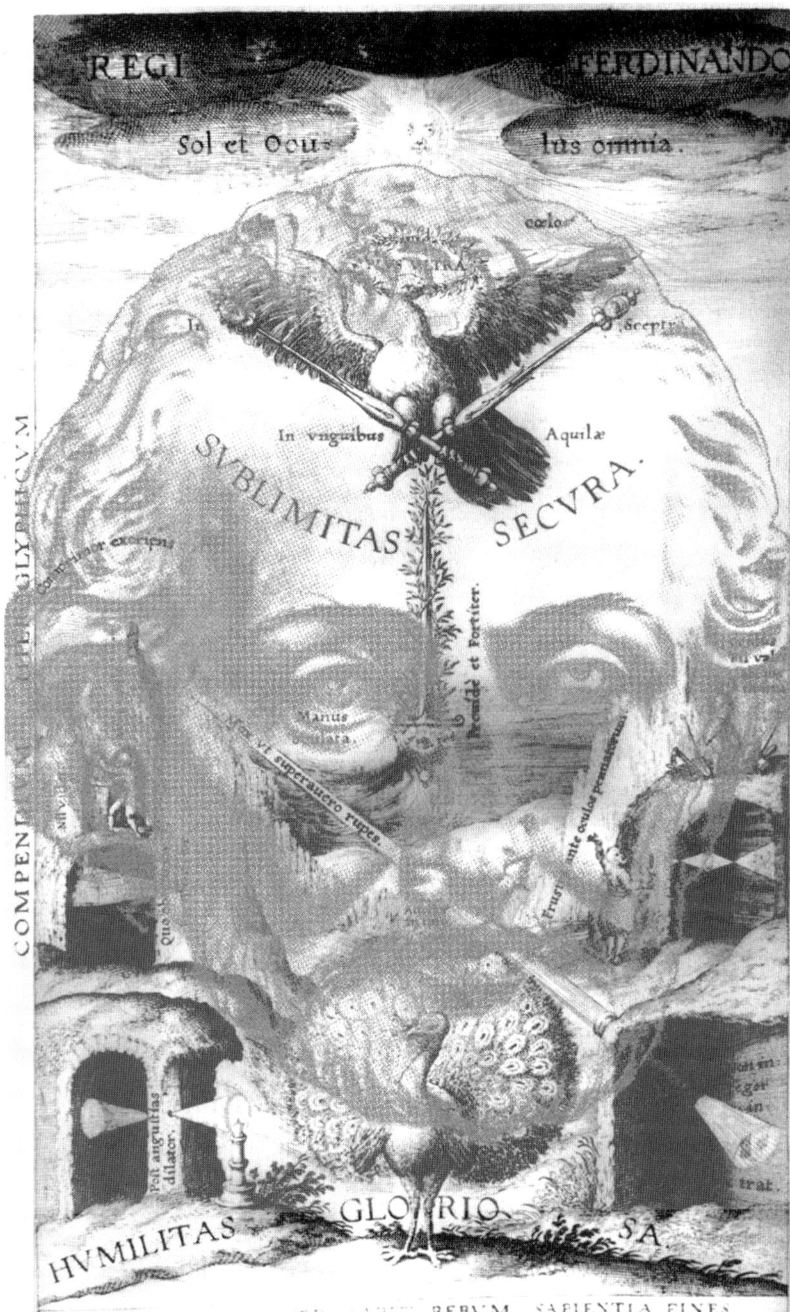

Figure 13.2 *Scheiner's Oculus* by Nicholas Wade. A portrait of Scheiner (from a nineteenth-century bust illustrated in Daxecker, 2004) combined with the frontispiece of *Oculus*. Several optical phenomena are shown in the frontispiece including pinhole imaging in a dark chamber and focusing light with lenses.

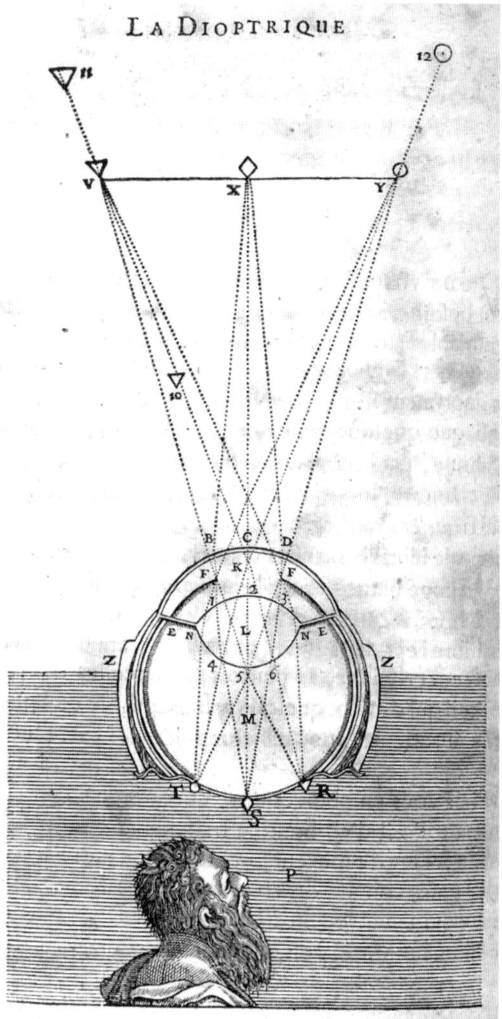

Figure 13.3 Kepler's inverted and reversed retinal image as depicted in René Descartes' *La Dioptrique* illustrating Christopher Scheiner's experiment of observing the retinal image on the translucent retina of a freshly enucleated animal or human eye from which the back of the sclera had been removed.
Credit: Illustration from 'La Dioptrique' by Rene Descartes (1596–1650), following the 'Discours de la Methode' first published in Leiden in 1637 (engraving) (b/w photo), French School, (17th century) / Bibliotheque de l'Academie de Medecine, Paris, France / Archives Charmet / The Bridgeman Art Library.

Bacon, Witelo, Peckham, and other medieval perspectivists of both the Near Eastern and Western tradition. Kepler himself gives this impression in his treatise presenting it as a kind of supplement to the *Perspectiva* of Witelo, intended to correct the errors of his distant predecessor (with the implicit view that nothing important had meanwhile happened in the field). This comes at the outset of the book, its full title being:

> *Ad Vitellionem paralipomena, quibus astronomiae pars optica traditur; potissimum de artificiosa observatione et aestimatione diametrorum deliquiorumque solis & lunae. Cum exemplis insignium eclipsium*

habes hoc libro, Lector inter alia multa nova, Tractatum luculentum de modo visionis, & humorum oculi usu, contra opticos & Anatomicos, Authore Ioanne Keplero, S[acrae] C[esareae] M[aiesta]tis Mathematico.

In this title the initial phrase—*Ad Vitellionem paralipomena*, by which the book is often referred, can be translated as 'Supplements to Witelo', or perhaps better 'Matters left over by Witelo'. With this phrase Kepler wished to relate his volume to the medieval perspectivist tradition, while at the same time mark the limits of this tradition in providing a theory of optics and vision useful for astronomers.

In recent years, thanks particularly to the researches of Sven Dupré (2002, 2005), a somewhat different view of the development of optics before Kepler is emerging; this places Kepler's achievement and the progress of optics in the Renaissance within a wider historical and sociological context. According to this new view, significance should be given to the development of an optical tradition with strong practical dimensions; it blossomed within the framework of technical and intellectual developments in the sixteenth century. Various aspects of Renaissance culture concurred to the progress of this particular optical tradition, in a complex and intertwined way from which the different components are often difficult to disentangle. On one side there was a strong practical interest for the new machines and instruments necessary for a world that was enlarging its physical and intellectual dimensions, and thus required a more sophisticated technology. It suffices to consider just the needs of navigation, cartography, astronomy, and military technology to understand how powerful this interest could be. The practical concern went together with a great revival of the studies of theoretical and practical mathematics which grew within the framework of the great expansion of the printing industry and the related interest in classical and medieval authors. The dimensions of the Renaissance culture went indeed much beyond an exclusive concern for literature, poetry, or philosophy. Among the works of relevance in a mathematical context which were published, read, and studied more keenly were those of Archimedes, Euclid, Ptolemy, Apollonius of Perga, and also of Vitruvius, from the classical era, and those of Alhazen, Witelo, and Peckham from the medieval tradition.

With the demanding intellectual needs imposed by the more sophisticated machines and instruments, the separation between expert craftsmen and theoretical mathematicians or natural philosophers became somewhat less distinct. Indeed many of the protagonists of the optical progress in the Renaissance were mathematicians or were interested in mathematics (in the modern sense) and, at the same time, instrument makers or designers. The need of combining practical and intellectual competence was particular strong in the construction of complex instruments like astrolabes, diopters, and other astronomical devices, scaphe dials, clocks, and other time measuring devices, various surveying and prospecting instruments (known by the general term of 'radius' or 'compass', but also with a wide variety of local names) having diverse applications (architectural, military, artistic, computational: see Figure 13.4).

Within the context of Renaissance optics, the birth of the artistic perspective was of relevance because of the related interest in practical and theoretical mathematics and vision. The astrological dimension was also significant; it went beyond the need of precise astronomical observations supposedly necessary for the precision of prognostications. At least in the conceptions of John Dee, an Englishman who was at the same time an important mathematician and a celebrated astrologer and magician, it also implied the idea that the influx of stars and planets could be transmitted to human beings according to the same laws governing the propagation of light (and could accordingly be modified with the same methodology and instruments, like the use of suitable mirrors).

On the theoretical side, the optics of the sixteenth century was particularly concerned with the geometry of visual projection and it was strongly related to artistic perspective. In addition to its importance for instrument makers, astronomers, cartographers, artists, and a great variety of other practical mathematicians of the age, geometrical optics was important for young people

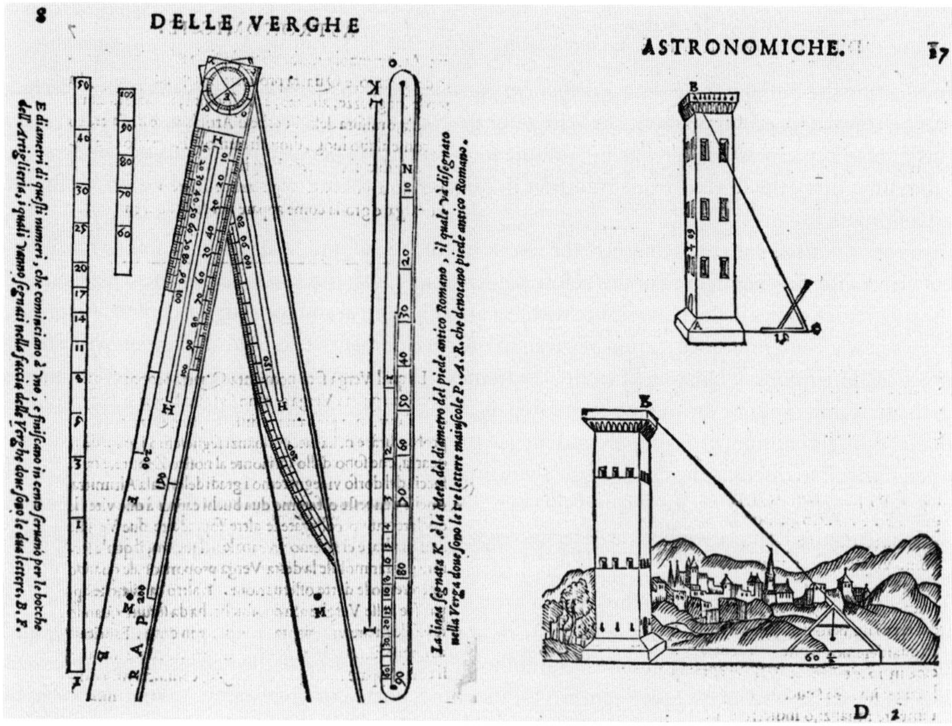

Figure 13.4 A multipurpose prospecting and astronomical instrument (dubbed *verga astronomica*) and its use for the measurement of the height of a tower from a practical manual published in 1582 by Antonio Lupicini, a civil and military engineer at the service of the Grand Duke of Florence.

interested in pursuing careers as military or civil officials at the service of sovereigns. No surprise then that a great number of treatises concerning 'perspective' in its broad senses, in printed or in manuscript form, circulated widely in this period, with ample differences in their quality and scope, from the more scientific and theoretical volumes (largely derived from classic and medieval texts) to more practical manuals useful for instrument makers or artisans, painters, architects, and engineers.

Since his youth Galileo was deeply rooted within this cultural tradition. As already mentioned, in the 1580s together with his friend Cigoli, and important members of the Florentine society, he attended the course of perspective and *disegno* (i.e. 'drawing' but having a broader meaning than the modern word) given by Ostilio Ricci in the house of Bernardo Buontalenti, an artist, stage designer, and military engineer. Besides developing Galileo's taste for art and especially for painting, Ricci's teaching was fundamental in directing him away from the medical studies in Pisa, towards mathematics in its theoretical and practical dimensions.

On the mathematical side Ricci's teaching was based mainly on Euclid and Archimedes, and on Leon Battista Alberti for artistic perspective (Alberti's *Ludi matematici*—i.e. 'Mathematical divertissements'—being one of the course textbooks). Like many mathematicians of his age, Ricci had invented a tool for prospecting and topographical purposes, known as *archimetro fiorentino*. Galileo, who would later teach perspective, prospecting, military architecture, and various other aspects of the practical mathematics, also invented, produced (and sold) various mathematical instruments, and particularly a 'compass' (see section 13.8).

13.3 **Mirrors and lenses in the sixteenth century**

In the period from Witelo to Kepler, the fabrication of mirrors and lenses progressed as did the theories concerning their functioning. As to the lenses, the main stimulus was the need for correction of the common defects of vision (presbyopia, myopia, and hypermetropia). In the Middle Ages, practical optics was mainly the prerogative of corporations or guilds but their secretiveness hampered its development. In the Renaissance, practical optics attracted the interest of more scholarly mathematicians, like Maurolico and Della Porta, who outlined the basic principles of concave and convex lenses and their application to correcting optical defects of the eye.

The interest was mainly in concave mirrors because of their burning capabilities. These had a potential use in military applications according to an idea nourished by the legend, largely flourishing in the Renaissance, of Archimedes burning the Roman fleet on the sea of Syracuse with a powerful concave mirror (see Figure 13.5). On the mathematical side, the study of mirrors was stimulated in 1577 by the translation, carried out by the French mathematician Jean Pena, of the optical works of Euclid (Pena, 1577). Pena's edition also included the pseudo-Euclid *Catoptrics* which dealt with plane and spherical mirrors. And also by the translation, in 1566, of some books on *Conics* by Apollononius of Perga published by Federico Commandino (the teacher of Galileo's sponsor, Guidobaldo Dal Monte). The study of conical sections (among which is the parabola) enabled the design of parabolic concave mirrors. These were much more effective in their burning properties than spherical mirrors because they could concentrate the rays of sun in a single point—the 'burning point' or focus. There was a growing awareness that concave mirrors could be used not only as burning devices but also for their image-forming properties (and even for vision at distance, as was the case for Ettore Ausonio, Thomas Digges, and William Bourne). This turned out to be of great importance in the progress of optics in the period between Witelo and Kepler, according to a tradition that likely represented Galileo's main optical background. A great contributor to this tradition was the already mentioned Venetian practical mathematician, cartographer, and instrument maker, Ettore (or Hectore) Ausonio (*fl.* 1520–1570), a physician with strong interest in alchemy and astrology.

Ausonio is of importance here especially because his 'Theory of the concave spherical mirror' (*Theorica speculi concavi sphaerici*) was copied by Galileo (and also by at least one member of his entourage-Paolo Sarpi). Ausonio was closely related to Giuseppe Moletti, who was Galileo's predecessor in the chair of mathematics at Padua. Moletti inherited Ausonio's papers and eventually bequeathed them to Pinelli's library in Padua, where Galileo probably had the opportunity to copy the *Theorica*, possibly from the now lost original (Figure 13.6).

Teaching was also one of Ausonio's activities (probably at a private level or perhaps within the framework of the Venetian Accademia della Fama to which both he and Pinelli belonged). His teaching, largely based on Witelo, stressed the practical utility of mathematics and perspective for a variety of applications and notably astrology (and astronomy). Ausonio's optics was in the tradition of Euclidean geometry from the theoretical point of view but relied heavily on an experimental and practical approach. From his manuscripts it appears that, with relation to his design of sun dials, he studied refraction, and it is possible that his achievements were transmitted to Commandino (a correspondent of Ausonio), and through Commandino, to Guidobaldo Dal Monte (Commandino's student and Galileo's sponsor), who was also interested in the theory of sundials.

In his practical approach to the design of concave mirrors, Ausonio was able to correct the error of Witelo who assumed (on the basis of the pseudo-Euclid *Catroptics*) that the burning point of a spherical mirror was the centre of curvature of the sphere and he located it instead at a distance of

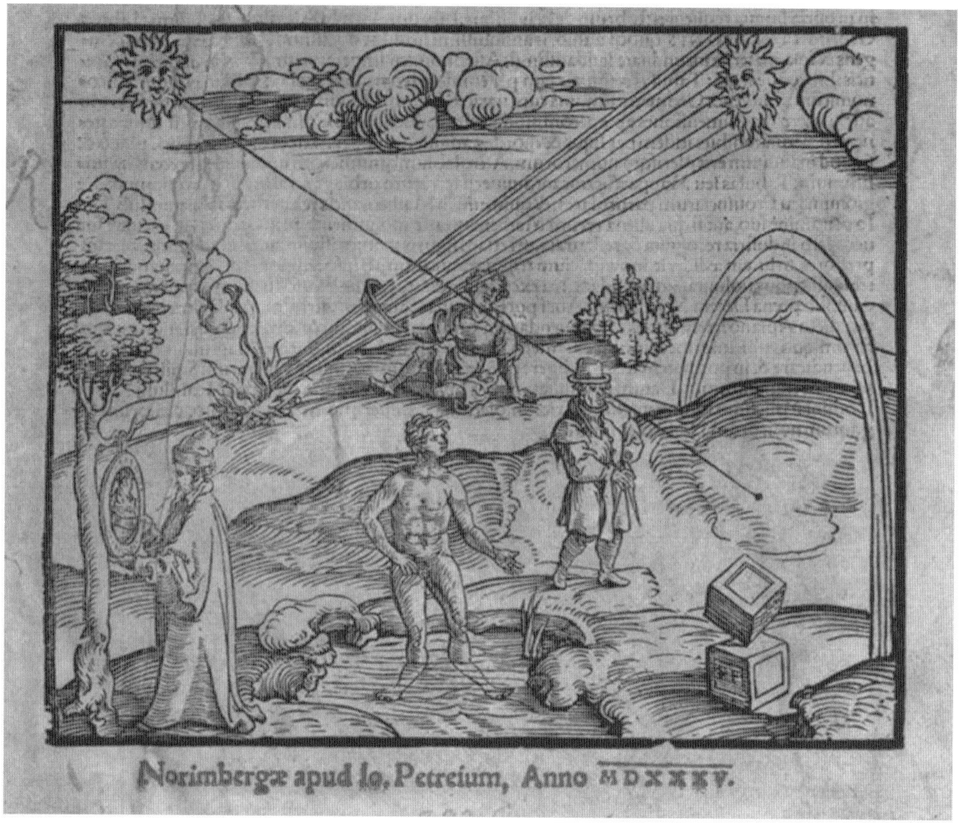

Figure 13.5 Archimedes and the burning properties of his concave mirror in the frontispiece image of the first edition of Witelo's *Perspectiva*. Beside the concave mirror the other aspects of optical science of the age portrayed in this image are refraction (the man in the water with optically broken legs), drawing a regular solid in perspective with the use of a compass, and the formation of the rainbow. As illustrated in Chapter 12 (Figure 12.1) the reference to Archimedes and to the episode of the burning mirror is even more explicit in the edition of Witelo and Alhazen works published in Basel in of 1572. Reproduced from Witelo, *Vitellionis... Peri optikēs, id est de natura, ratione, & proiectione radiorum uisus, luminum, colorum atq[ue] formarum, quam uulgo perspectiuam vocant, libri X*. 1535, Norimbergæ, Apud Io. Petreium.

half of the radius.[1] He showed, moreover, that the burning (or concurrence) point corresponded to the point beyond which images of the external objects could be produced by reflection and become visible by using 'some little scented smoke' (they were in our modern terminology 'real images'). As Ausonio writes in his *Theorica*, when the visual object is placed between the mirror and concurrence point, a virtual image is formed which is upright and visually situated behind the surface of the mirror; its distance from the mirror in the virtual space behind the mirror decreases when the distance of the object from the internal surface is decreased and vice versa. In the case

[1] Prior to Ausonio other authors (like the third-century Greek mathematician Diocles, and—after him—Alhazen, Roger Bacon, and Leonardo) had arrived at the same conclusion (see Dupré, 2002).

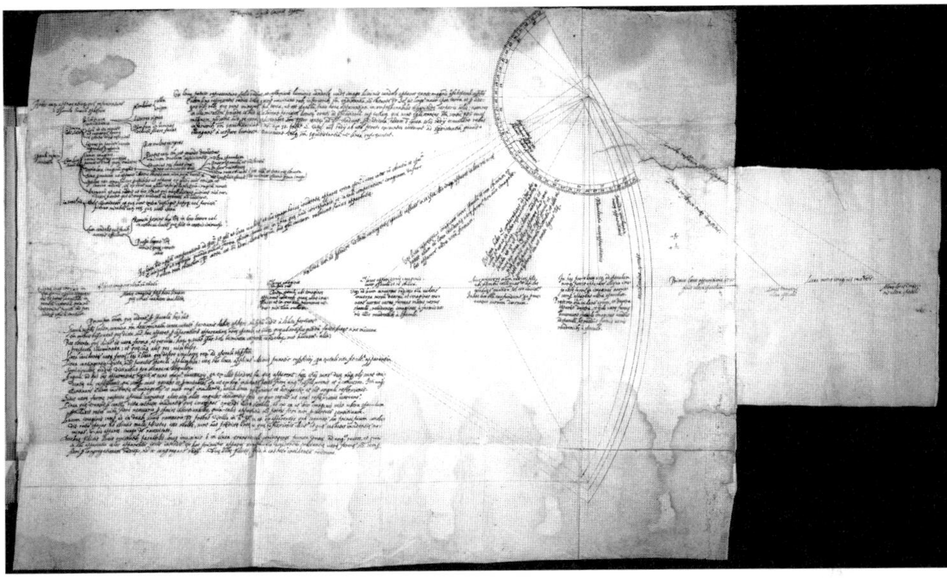

Figure 13.6 The copy in Galileo's hand of the *Theorica speculi concavi sphaerici* by Ausonio. The diagram represents (on the right) a section of a spherical mirror with a goniometer at its top for the measure of angles, and the various loci important in the image forming (and burning) property of the mirror, duly explained with legends (BNF Gal. 83, f. 4r.; © Biblioteca Nazionale of Florence, Italy).

where the object is situated between the concurrence point and the centre of curvature, the image is real, larger that the object and inverted (upside down). It remains inverted and real, but of the same size as the object and co-localized with the object when the object is in the centre of curvature of the mirror. When the object is more distant the image is still real and inverted, but smaller than the object and becomes progressively smaller as the object is moved farther from the mirror.

Principles basically similar to those defined by Ausonio in the image formation in mirrors were developed for lenses by Maurolico in his *Diaphanorum libri tres* which discussed the concept of inversion point in the case of refraction processes, and again without a geometrical treatment of optics (in Kepler's sense). As had occurred with Ausonio in the case of mirror reflections, Maurolico was aware of the existence of spherical aberrations in the lenses (the rays far from the optical axis concur nearer to the lens surface).

On a practical point of view, Ausonio's rules of image formation in a spherical mirror (and those of Maurolico for lenses) correspond basically to those given by modern optics, although they were derived from a sensible and open-minded combination of the principles elaborated by the medieval perspectivists on the basis of the Euclidian geometry and the issues of practical experiments (using smoke to visualize the real images corresponding to Kepler's *picturae*). Like the practical mathematicians of his age, Ausonio (and Maurolico) did not develop a theory for the functioning of mirrors or lenses based on the principles of optics within a framework similar to that that will be afterwards developed by Kepler, Scheiner, and Descartes (and after them Huygens, Hooke, Newton, Young, and Helmholtz). The practical mathematicians of the age were capable of building rather sophisticated optical devices and developed a practical or functional approach to the correction of the common dioptric deficits of eyes, with no reference to any correct theory of image formation in the eye (in a modern sense). This was not only the approach of lens makers but also of natural philosophers and practical mathematicians of the calibre of Maurolico and Della Porta. In this context it is interesting to consider a practical rule elaborated by the lens makers in order to define the 'grade' of the lenses used for the correction of visual defects, in the absence of a modern geometrical theory of their behaviour. This rule was particularly needed for the concave lenses because of the absence of a conception of focal distance in the virtual space necessary to understand the functioning of these particular lenses; for the convex ones the matter was made easy by determining the burning point on the surface of a paper or on smoke.

This practical rule for measuring the power of the lenses was based on the magnification or reduction of the image of an object caused by a convex or concave lens, which depends on the distance of the lens from the observer's eye. From a given distance, the observer should look at a target with the right eye through the lens whose power needs to be measured, while with the left eye the other target was viewed. In the case of concave lenses the target on the right was made smaller than that on the left (and the opposite happened for the concave mirror). The power or grade was found by ascertaining the position of the lens along a graduated scale at which the size of the two targets appeared the same. The operation was similar for the convex lenses, with the difference that in this second case, the measurement of the grade was based on the magnifying power of these lenses (Figure 13.7).

The important point in this method is that it had practical utility even though it did not require any assumption about the functioning of the eye, nor even of the optical properties of the lenses (except for a measure of their degree of concavity or convexity). It was nevertheless a method, not simply a trial-and-error procedure. As remarked by Dupré, in *Sidereus* Galileo

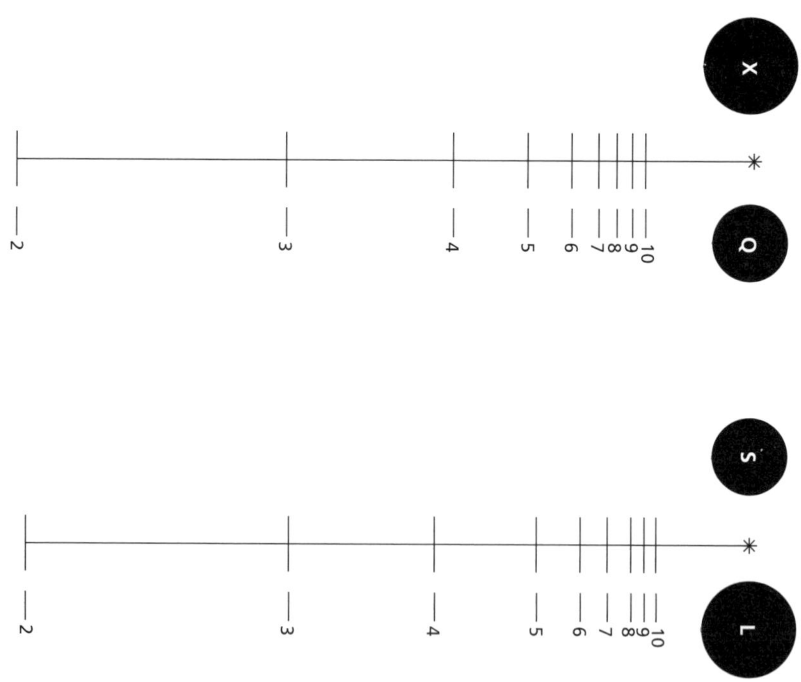

Figure 13.7 The method suggested by Benito Daza de Valdés for measuring the grade of, respectively, concave (top) and convex (bottom) lenses. See the text for an explanation. Reproduced from Daza de Valdés, B., *Uso de los antoios para todo genero de vistas*.... 1623, Diego Perez.

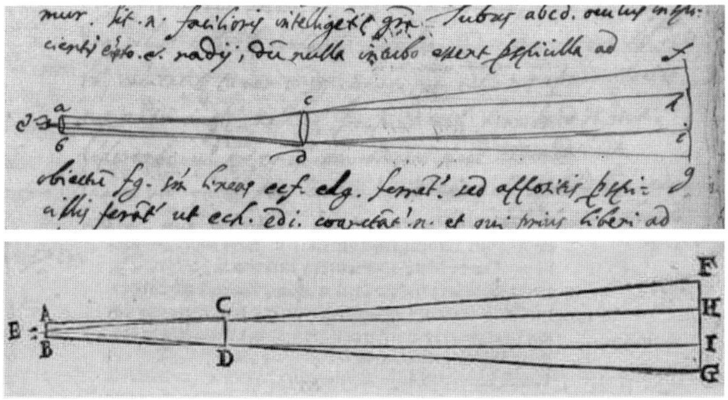

Figure 13.8 The diagram of *Sidereus nuncius* in the handwritten version (top) and published version (bottom) in which Galileo illustrates a phase of his method for ascertaining the magnifying power of the telescope. As in Daza de Valdés' procedure, two targets of different sizes should be looked at from a convenient distance, and at the same time, with, respectively, an unaided eye (the smaller one) and with the other eye through the telescope (the bigger one). The relative size of the targets should be adjusted to the required telescope magnification. In this diagram ABDC is the telescope, E the eye, FG is the target seen with the unaided eye, whereas, with the telescope HI would appear with the same size ad FB. Reproduced from, respectively, BNF GAL 48, F9R—© Biblioteca Nazionale of Florence, Italy and Galileo, G. *Sidereus nuncius*, 1610, p. 7.

expounded a somewhat similar method for calculating the magnification of the telescope (Figure 13.8).

As a matter of fact, most of Galileo's optical work was inspired by a comparable operational and pragmatic approach, which similarly did not require an optic theory of the eye's function. Moreover, as in the case of Daza de Valdés' procedure for ascertaining the optical power of the lenses, Galileo knew that within certain limits, the magnification produced by a convex lens increases by increasing the distance from the eye. This was indeed the optical background on which he elaborated his refractive theory of moon illusion expounded in both *Mauri* and *Saggiatore* (see Chapter 12). In both cases he attributed the stronger magnification of the sun or moon image at the horizon to the greater distance from the eye of the spherical surface of the terrestrial vapours in the horizontal view.

13.4 Galileo and Kepler's invitation to read his *Optics*

The efficacy of Galileo's approach to vision in an astronomical context (and his difference from Kepler) emerges in the measurement of the apparent size of stars. We will now try to examine the differences by following Kepler's analysis of Galileo's discoveries announced in *Sidereus*. This will allow widening our scope to consider the reasons that led the German astronomer to a detailed investigation of optics.

In his *Dissertatio cum nuncio sidereo*, Kepler commented on Galileo's remarks about the appearance of the (fixed) stars and particularly of their illusive magnification. In considering Kepler's comments, it must be noticed that in *Sidereus* the Italian scientist had not yet provided any definite hypothesis on the means whereby the apparent sizes of stars and small planets (that is all planets except the Moon) were overestimated. Indeed at that time he had not yet fully investigated the matter and had not performed the cord experiment to measure the 'true' angular size of their images. However, Galileo directed attention to the phenomenon in *Sidereus*. He did it in the context of a statement on the relatively poor magnification of the size of the stars and small planets by the telescope, with a first allusion to the adventitious rays capable of expanding their apparent size:

> The reason for this is that when the stars are observed with the naked eye, they do not show themselves, according to their simple and, so to speak, naked size but rather surrounded by a certain brightness and crowned by twinkling rays especially as the night is far advanced. Because of this they appear much larger than if they were stripped of these extraneous rays, for the visual angle is determined not by the primary body of the star but by the brightness that surrounds it. You will perhaps understand this more clearly from this: that stars emerging in the first twilight at sunset, even if they are of the first magnitude, appear very small and Venus herself, when she presents herself in broad daylight, is perceived so small that it hardly appears to equal a star of the last magnitude. Things are very different with other objects, and the Moon herself, which, whether she is observed in midday or in the deepest darkness, appears always of the same size to us. Stars are therefore seen unshorn in the midst of darkness, but daylight can shear them of their hair—and not only daylight but also a thin little cloud that that is interposed between the star and the eye of the observer. The same effect is also achieved by dark veils or and colored glasses, by the opposition and interposition of which the surrounding brightness will desert the star. The spyglass [*perspicillo*, i.e. the telescope] does the same thing, for it first takes away the borrowed and accidental brightness from the star and thereupon it enlarges the simple globes (if indeed their figures are globular), and therefore they appear increased by a much smaller ratio for stars of the fifth or sixth magnitude seen through the spyglass are shown as of the first magnitude. (SIDEREUS, p. 16; transl. pp. 70–71)

On his side, Kepler wrote that he agreed with Galileo, on the basis of his own 'long experience' of the reduction observed by Galileo in the apparent size of the stars occurring in various conditions, like 'twilight, daylight, a cloud, a veil, coloured glass'. Not seeing this as a real explanation of the phenomenon, Galileo was referred to Kepler's observations and theories expounded in his 1604 optical treatise, within the context of a discussion on the imperfections of image formation on the retina:

> I should like to ask you, Galileo, whether you are satisfied with the reasons for this effect, as presented by me in my discussion on the process of vision on page 217 and especially on page 221 of my 'Optics'. For if you find nothing amiss, you may thereafter discuss the matter correctly. Point sources of light transmit their cones to the crystalline lens. The refraction takes place, and behind the lens the cones again contract to a point. But this point does not touch the retina [*attingit retinam*], the light being widened once more, spreads over a small area of the retina, whereas it should impinge on a point. Hence the telescope, by introducing another refraction, makes this point coincide with the retina [*in retiformem competat*]. It is not true, then, that some rays come down to the eye from the brightness enveloping the stars from the outside. On the contrary, the rays which come down from the shining body itself are scattered, as a result of imperfection of refraction and the widening of the opening in the uvea at night. They brighten the area on the retina around the point which should represent the star. The telescope on earth does not remove anything from the stars in heaven, but it does take away from the retina whatever light is superfluous [*quantum eius redundat*]. (Kepler, 1610, pp. 21–22; transl. Rosen, 1965, pp. 33–34, revised)

Kepler's criticism of Galileo needs some qualifications. First, the German astronomer tries to explain the phenomenon by referring to a well-defined optical theory, based on a convergence of light rays inside the eye effected mainly by the crystalline lens. On his side, Galileo does not invoke any kind of process belonging to the field of geometrical optics. Second, Kepler implicitly assumes that Galileo has ascribed the excess of shining of the stars to an atmospheric phenomenon (or some process occurring outside the eye). Kepler's assumption can be understood, as Galileo made reference to a series of observations involving twilight, clouds, coloured glass, i.e. to natural or artificial effects belonging to the external space. This could have directed the reader to suppose that the magnifications were attributable to an extraocular basis. However, if we consider what Galileo says, there is no direct or indirect indication that the adventitious rays are produced outside the eye. Although in *Sidereus* he does not express himself on where the adventitious shining is supposed to take place (intra- versus extra-ocular), in subsequent works Galileo sides in a clear way for an intraocular mechanism (as we have seen in Chapter 8).

A third remark concerns how the telescope removes the adventitious rays and thus 'shear off' the extra shining from the small body of stars. In this regard, both Galileo and Kepler were largely wrong in their interpretations. Galileo says that the telescope operates like twilight, clouds, and glass, by removing 'from the stars their adventitious and accidental splendour before it enlarges their true disk'. Although Galileo's telescopic images were not particularly bright (mainly because of the artificial pupil to reduce optical aberrations), a telescope does indeed admit more light than the naked eye. Because of this characteristic, the telescope allowed Galileo to visualize the stars also in daylight (see, for instance, OG VIII, pp. 463–464). In his remarks on the reduction of the apparent size of the stars Galileo was conflating two phenomena. On the one hand, by invoking twilight he was involving the action of an external light: as we know now this acts by adapting the eye to light and thus reducing its sensitivity, and also by inducing a reflex reduction of pupil size and thus reducing optical aberrations. On the other hand, with the reference to clouds and coloured glasses, he was implying the reduction of the light reaching the eye due to the filtering effect of intervening matters.

Regarding Kepler's opinion, it is incorrect that a telescope acts by adding a new refraction capable of converging the cones of luminous rays onto the retina. A normal eye, accommodated for far distance, focuses rays coming from a potentially infinite distance without any other optical assistance. At the time of the *Dissertatio*, Kepler neither had the possibility of using Galileo's telescope nor of knowing how it was built. His remark was thus a purely hypothetical guess about how the device could influence the visibility of the stars. In all probability, it was dictated by the assumption (expounded in his 1604 treatise) that vision can focus on the moon but not on more distant stars (see section 13.5).

Kepler was nonetheless right in directing Galileo to his 1604 work on optics. This is because it contained a new and powerful theory of the formation of the image on the retina which could prove useful for Galileo in his attempt to explain the phenomenon of the magnification of the stars. In particular, this theory could account for why a point source of intense light could result in an expanded retinal image.

Kepler's volume is worthy of consideration not only due to its importance in the history of geometrical and physiological optics, but also, in the context of our book, because it helps to define the difference between the approaches of Galileo and Kepler. For this and other reasons we will now discuss how the German astronomer got interested in astronomy, and to what extent the *Astronomiae, Pars optica*, and particularly its chapter 5, could contribute to the understanding of the problem of the apparent magnification of the stars.

13.5 **Founding optics on the clarity of a demonstration by a perceptive astronomer**

Astronomiae, Pars optica represents a milestone in the history of optics, and particularly physiological optics. Despite its importance, however, at its time this book had a very limited readership, being restricted almost exclusively to a few specialists in the field. Kepler's method of developing his arguments was not straightforward nor was the language in which they were expressed; these could have been due to the problems he was encountering at the time, and to editorial difficulties. As the title shows, Kepler considered his book as the 'Optical part' of a new astronomy, having the intention to publish it as a first part of a fuller volume expounding his revolutionary reformation of astronomy. He was, however, forced to abandon his initial project and to publish his astronomical masterwork, containing the new theory of the elliptic orbits (*Astronomia Nova*) later in 1609. The haste in which he wrote *Optica* contributed to the complexity of its organization and the difficulties it posed for readers. Kepler wrote his book to mark at the same time his continuity and rupture with the tradition of the medieval perspectivists and in particular Alhazen and Witelo.

There were the two main differences between Kepler's theory of vision and those expounded by Alhazen and his Western followers. Contrary to conceptions based on emission of visual rays from the eye (extramission theories), Alhazen had formulated a geometrical theory of image formation in the retina based on the reception (or intromission) of light. The physical model for Alhazen was the *camera obscura*, the device that we have mentioned in Chapter 12 in connection with Castelli's optical demonstrations. The formation of the image in this device (often called a pinhole camera) depends on narrow beams of light passing through the small aperture to fall on a screen. In the eye the pupil diameter is relatively large which creates problems for applying the pinhole model to human vision. However, Alhazen assumed that only rays perpendicular to the cornea would affect vision. With this restriction the eye turned into a living *camera obscura*. In opposition to this view, Kepler indicated that the refracting power of the optical media of the eye (and notably the crystalline lens) would result in all the rays from any single point focusing the image on the sensitive part of the eye.

Another important difference concerned the site responsible for the visual process. According to the old theories this occurred on the anterior face of the crystalline lens which was referred to as the 'seat of vision'. It was so considered for geometrical and physiological reasons. Galen supported this conjecture by virtue of the blindness that results from cataracts and the sight that is restored when they are surgically removed. The other reason for this assumption was that, as perspectivists knew well, refraction at the crystalline lens would produce inverted and reversed images. Since vision was not inverted this was a difficult idea to endorse. For the old authors, this led to locating the crystalline centrally within the eye, and assuming some form of anatomical and functional continuity between the crystalline and the optical nerve.[2]

Kepler was impressed by the clear discontinuity between the crystalline lens and the retina in the dissections performed by the 'eminent man Felix Platter'. Platter illustrated the anatomy of the eye in *De corporis humani structura et usu* first published in 1583 and re-edited in 1603, when Kepler was writing his *Optica*. Kepler reprinted the whole plate (part of which is shown in Figure 13.9) in his *Optica*. Of particular relevance for Kepler was the section at the left indicating that the crystalline lens is not continuous with the retina, and is separated from the back of the eye by a large space filled with the vitreous humour. Notice that, unlike Descartes' scheme based on the work of Scheiner (see Figure 13.2), in this image the optical nerve is (incorrectly) assumed to exit from the centre of the posterior pole of the eyeball. Kepler remarked that Platter's book was 'deservedly reprinted in this year 1603', i.e. just while he was writing his new treatise.

2 Among the variations avoiding optical inversion of the image in the eye were those, endorsed among others by Leonardo, of a double inversion occurring within the eye, leading eventually to an upright image.

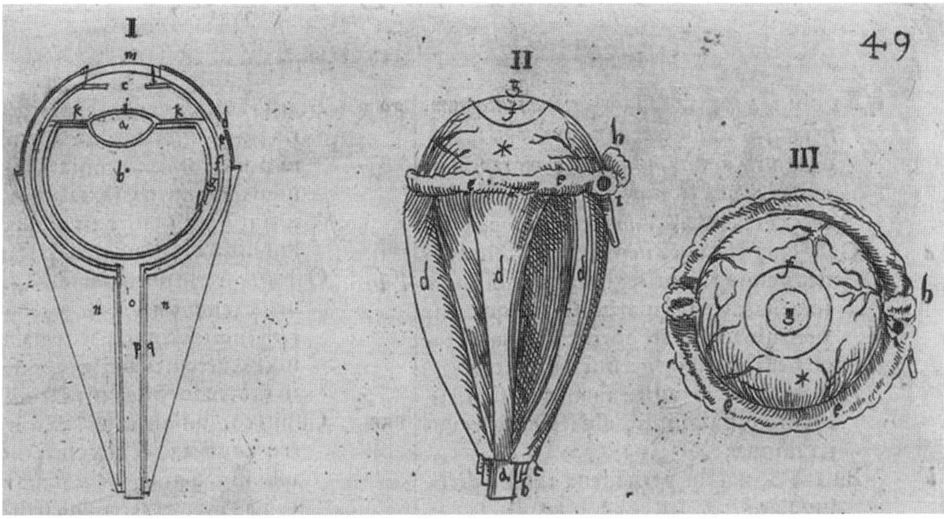

Figure 13.9 Some images from the plate illustrating the anatomy of the eye from the 1583 edition of Platter's anatomical treatise reprinted in Kepler's book. Unlike Scheiner's diagram (and similarly to the old anatomical conceptions) the optic nerve is situated on the optic axis on the eye. Reproduced from Platter, F., *De corporis humani structura et usu: libri III*, 1583, Basileae, ex Officina Frobeniana.

Kepler trusted Platter's anatomy and considered them preferable to those expounded by his friend Johannes Jessen in an anatomical book published in Prague in 1601. This was because he thought that Jessen, having been influenced by old authors and notably by Witelo, had insisted on a non-existent continuity between the crystalline lens and the retina (*retiformis*). Moreover, Platter suggested that the retina was the sensitive organ of vision and he was explicit in specifying the retina as the receptive organ:

> The principal organ of vision, namely the optic nerve, expands through the whole hemisphere of the retina as soon as it enters the eye. This receives and discriminates the form and colour of external objects which together with the light enter the eye through the opening of the pupil and are projected on it by the lens. (Platter, 1583, p. 187)

It should not be supposed, however, that Kepler started his revolutionary work on the basis of anatomical considerations on the mechanism of image formation in the eye. On the contrary, as he narrates in his dedicatory letter to his patron, the Emperor Rudolph II, his interest in vision derived from his astronomical work, and notably from some problems that had emerged from the observations of eclipses and from the alteration of the shape of and distance between celestial bodies due to atmospheric refraction. This is how he explained his commitment to optics and particularly his desire to bring a scientific precision to this discipline:

> For I thought it unworthy in optical science, since senses and instruments are required in astronomy, while in optics, geometrical certainty is not lacking, that optics be surpassed by astronomy, and that one cannot establish in the former by demonstrations what in the latter the eyes have comprehended; it is much more unworthy that when summoned by astronomers to assist them, optics does not appear, and is unable of itself to soften the fault of hindering the precision of astronomy, with which it is charged. (OPTICA, unnumbered; transl. p. 5)

The close connection between optics (considered as a general science of vision) and astronomy has a long history and it is not by chance, for example, that a great astronomer like Ptolemy wrote five books on optics (Lejeune, 1948, 1989; Smith, 1996). The relevance of optics to astronomy had increased considerably with improvement of the astronomical observations carried out by Tycho Brahe. This was particularly because the precision of the instruments used by the Danish astronomer had made intolerable the errors of measurement due to vision and optics.

Soon after his assertion about the need for more precise optics in astronomy, Kepler gives the impression that, in publishing his volume, he believed he had fulfilled his duty:

> And so I have considered no small honor if it might fall to me to undo the knots that have been in the way, by a good method and the clarity of demonstrations [*demonstrationum evidentia*], and lead the optical science through that degree of subtlety that might satisfy the astronomer. (OPTICA, unnumbered; transl. pp. 5–6)

There is indeed no doubt that Kepler was producing a momentous revolution in the history of optics considered as a science largely based on geometrical demonstration. It is less certain that the book represented immediately a similarly great advance in the understanding of vision in general, and particularly in its psychological dimensions. He wrote:

> I say that vision occurs when an image [*idolum*] of the whole hemisphere of the world that is before the eye, and a little more, is set up at the white wall, tinged with red, of the concave surface of the retina. How this image or picture is joined together with the visual spirits that reside in the retina and in the nerve, and whether it is arraigned within by the spirits into the caverns of the cerebrum to the tribunal of the soul or of the visual faculty; whether the visual faculty, like a magistrate given by the soul, descending from the headquarters of the cerebrum outside to the visual nerve itself and the retina, as to lower courts, might go forth to meet this image—this, I say, I leave to the natural philosophers [*physici*] to argue about. (OPTICA, p. 168; transl. p. 180)

This was the case for vision of small luminous bodies like stars, which is the main theme of this chapter.

13.6 The *camera obscura*, ambiguous appearances of eclipses, and a 'painting' in the eye

Eclipses have always attracted the attention of astronomers. This was not only because of the impressive character of these celestial events but also because—like comets and new stars –they disturbed the regularity of the heavens. Since the time of Aristarchus, Hipparchus, and Ptolemy, eclipses of the sun and moon have provided essential parameters for measuring cosmic distances and sizes. With increased interest in astronomy and the invention of more accurate instruments in the fifteenth century, correct predictions of the occurrence of eclipses, and precise measurements of the sun and moon images, could inform theories of planetary motion. After the publication of Copernicus' *De Revolutionibus*, the study of eclipses was pursued also in order to provide evidence for or against his cosmological conceptions.

In the second half of the sixteenth century the method favoured by astronomers for observing eclipses was one recommended by Erasmus Reinhold in his edition of Georg Peurbach's *Theoricae novae planetarum*, dated 1542, but published in 1544. This was based on an indirect observation of the images of the sun and the moon based on the use of a *camera obscura*. This method had already been applied to the observation of solar eclipses in the Middle Ages by the Jewish theologian and astronomer (living in the south of France) Levi ben Gerson (Gersonides) and by the French astronomer (probably of English origin) William (Guillaume) of Saint-Cloud (see Goldstein 1985, 1991; Mancha, 1992)

Tycho Brahe started his astronomical observations with such a device under the instructions given by Gemma Frisius in his *De radio astronomico et geometrico* published in 1545 (in turn Frisius said that he was following Reinhold's recommendations). Interestingly Frisius illustrated his book with a *camera obscura* image of an eclipse made in Louvain in 1544 (Figure 13.10).

Also Maestlin had been using a version of the *camera obscura* device in his observations of eclipses and young Kepler has been introduced to the use of this instrument by his teacher during his studentship in Tübingen (as Kepler, who had attended one of these observations, would relate in his 1604 volume).

A serious problem had, however, emerged from the astronomical studies involving instruments based on the *camera obscura*, as was noted by Brahe during his repeated observations of sun and moon eclipses. The diameter of the moon's shadow on the solar body observed with these instruments during the sun eclipse was smaller than that seen directly in the sky. Brahe was perplexed by this unexpected reduction in the measured size. Surprisingly, the moon seemed never to obscure the sun completely in the projected image. Since the phenomenon could not be accounted for astronomically, Brahe argued that it could be an artefact depending on the size of the aperture in the *camera obscura.* Accordingly, he introduced a correction to cope with the observations made with other astronomical methods. In a passage of his *Astronomiae instauratae progymnasmata* he suggested that 'by the force of the light of the sun its [i.e. moon's] boundaries are reduced, with some optical cause producing this result, so that about a fifth part of the moon disappears and does not present itself to the eye' (TOO II, p. 147). Among the possibilities invoked to account for the phenomenon was the idea that the 'optical cause' could be the existence of an atmosphere around the moon, shining together with the main part of its body when it was full, but transparent to the sunrays during the eclipse.

Kepler, who had started to keep records of eclipses with the projection method in the last decade of the sixteenth century, became aware of the problem of the aperture in the instruments used in astronomical observation through the correspondence between Brahe and Maestlin. Puzzled by what he considered an 'enigma', he decided to explore the matter during the solar eclipse expected for 10 July 1600. He set up an instrument, built according to Maestlin's directions and based on a projection method, in the market place at Graz (the Austrian town where he was teaching mathematics and astronomy) and waited for the eclipse. He recorded the measures accurately in

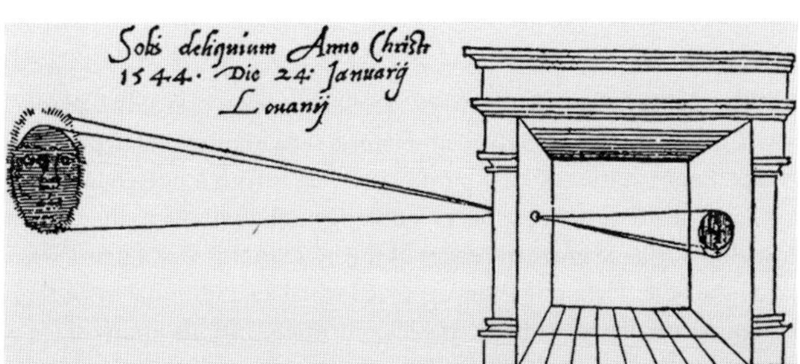

Figure 13.10 The illustration by Gemma Frisius of a sun eclipse observed on 24 January 1544 in Louvain with the help of a *camera obscura* according the method suggested by Erasmus Reinhold. This is the first printed image illustrating the use of the *camera obscura* in astronomical observations. Reproduced from Frisius, *De radio astronomico*, 1544, p. 32.

his notebook and made the important discovery that the inconsistencies between the measurements of the sun and moon diameter obtained with this method were reduced by decreasing the size of the aperture. Moreover, he noticed that with large apertures the reduction of the image of the moon on the sun body was paralleled by an increase of the size of the sun, compared to the standard values.

The problem emerging with the eclipses not only affected astronomical observation methods based on the projection of the images of celestial bodies but also the common techniques involving direct vision of stars or planets through viewing apertures. In order to find a compromise, various astronomers (notably Tycho Brahe) adopted, in the case of sighting instruments, apertures in the form of thin slits. The problem with a slit aperture was that precise localization was only possible along a direction of the visual space (the direction perpendicular to the length of the slit). Accordingly, in most of his astronomical instruments Brahe used pairs of slits oriented in orthogonal directions (vertical and horizontal), making observations alternatively with one then the other. Brahe's basic viewing system (a 'diopter' based on a modification of the old system attributed to Hipparchus) consisted of two horizontal and two vertical slits in the lamina near the observer's eye (ocular pinnule) and the same number and arrangement of slits in the lamina at the distant extremity of the instrument (objective pinnule; see, see Figure 13.11).[3]

On the basis of his observation of the eclipse in Graz, Kepler became aware that, in order to put astronomical observations on a firmer footing, it was necessary to understand the way the *camera obscura* works as well as to investigate how images are formed in the eye. He started studying the works of the medieval perspectivists and notably the *Perspectiva* of Witelo and the *Perspectiva communis* of Peckham where he could not find any clear explanation of image formation in a *camera obscura*. More generally, he could not find the reasons for the round shape of the projected image cast by a light beam passing 'any kind crack' [*quacumque rimulam*] as is seen—he says—'beneath the roofs that are split open, in shrines, in perforated windowpanes, and beneath a tree' (OPTICA, p. 37; transl. p. 55).

Being dissatisfied by the obscure explanations and 'twisting equivocations' that he found by previous authors, Kepler decided to investigate the problem starting from an experiment in which he attempted to model the geometry of image formation in a *camera obscura* without using real light. According to Stephen Straker, an American scholar who has investigated Kepler's optical studies, the experiment was inspired by a method suggested by Albrecht Dürer for drawing a lute in perspective; the woodcut, shown in Figure 13.12, is from *Underweysung der Messung*, first published in 1525 (Straker, 1981). This is how Kepler describes his non-optical imaging experiment in his 1604 volume:

> Several years ago, some light shone forth upon me out of the darkness of Pisanus. Since I was unable to understand the very obscure sense of the words from a diagram drawn in a plane, I had recourse to seeing with my own eyes in space [*aujtoψivan in solido*]. I set a book in a high place, which was to stand for a luminous body. Between this and the pavement a tablet with a polygonal hole was set up. Next, a thread was sent down from one corner of the book through the hole to the pavement, falling upon the pavement in such a way as to graze the edges of the hole. In this way a figure was created upon the pavement similar to the hole. The same thing occurred when an additional thread was added from the second, third, and fourth corner of the book, as well as from the infinite points of the edges. In this way,

[3] Brahe described and illustrated his diopter in a supplement to his *Astronomiae instauratae mechanica* (Brahe, 1602, no pagination; see also TOO, vol. 6, p. 154). For a discussion on the different viewing methods in pre-telescopic astronomy see particularly Strano, 2003, 2007 and also Roslund, 1989.

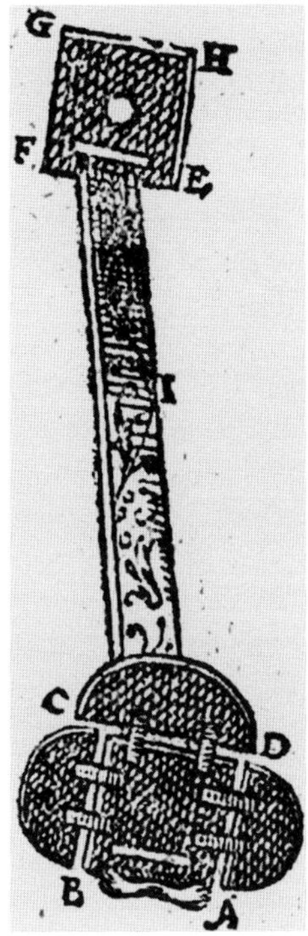

Figure 13.11 The diopter used by Tycho Brahe for many of his astronomical observations. The lower lamina (ABCD) corresponds to the ocular pinnule while the upper one is the objective pinnule. Both pinnules have four slits (two horizontal and two vertical, more clearly visible in the lower one). In the ocular pinnule the breadth of the two vertical slits, and of the upper horizontal slit, could be adjusted through a screw system (while the lower horizontal slit was of fixed size). The localization of the celestial body was achieved by collimating the star or planet through the two corresponding slits in the two pinnules. The hole in the upper pinnule (which has no correspondence in the lower pinnule) was used to project the image of sun in a way similar to a *camera obscura*. Reproduced from Brahe, T. *Opera Omnia,* 1913, vol. 6, p. 154.

> a narrow row of infinite figures of the hole outlined the large quadrangular figure of the book on the pavement. It was thus obvious that this was in agreement with the demonstration of the problem, that the round shape is not that of the visual ray but of the sun itself, not because this is the most perfect shape, but because this is generally the shape of a luminous body. This is the first success of this work. (OPTICA, p. 39; transl. p. 56)

For Kepler this was a crucial experiment inasmuch as it convinced him that, contrary to what was assumed by Witelo and Peckham, there was indeed nothing in the physical nature of light rays to make them naturally inclined to roundness in the course of their propagation. It was an indication that the laws of image formation in an optical system, including the human eye, could be studied with the application of geometrical methods. It then became necessary to pursue the optical investigations more precisely than the medieval perspectivists, and to correct and complete what Witelo (and Peckham) had left over (thus accounting for the phrase *Ad Vitellionem paralipomena* at the beginning of his 1604 treatise). This was the start of modern physiological optics.

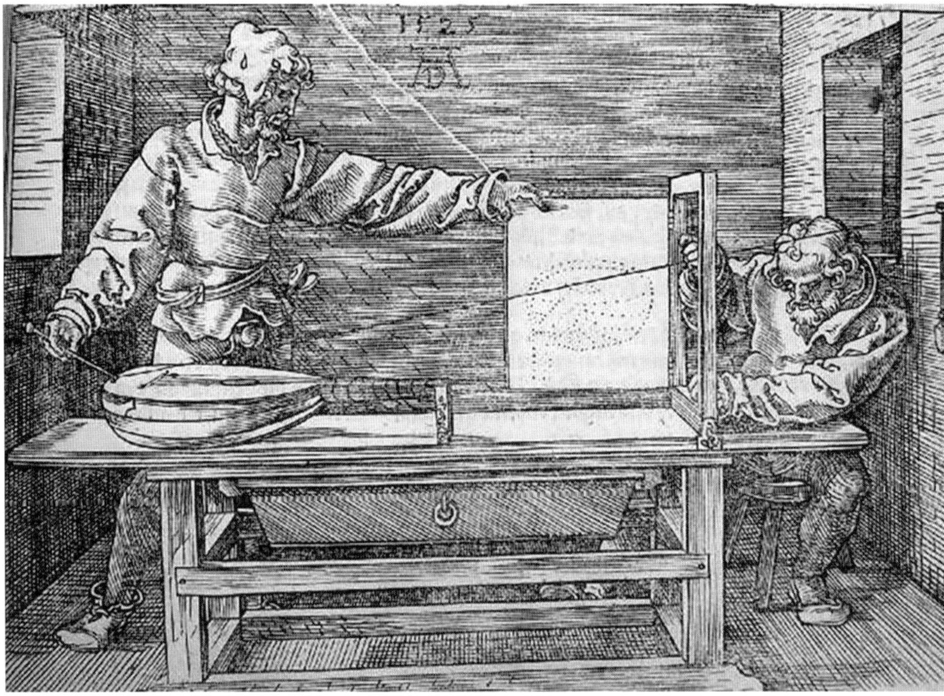

Figure 13.12 An illustration from the 1725 edition of the *Underweysung der messung* by Albrecht Dürer illustrating a mechanical method based on the use of a thread for drawing an object according to the rules of linear perspective. Reproduced from Dürer, A., *Underweysung der Messung, mit dem Zirckel unnd richt scheyt, in Linien ebnen unnd gantzen Corporen*, 1525.

Kepler would apply the rules of light refraction in spherical (or quasi spherical) surfaces within the anatomical framework of Platter's studies of the eye. He assumed that light rays are refracted at two main surfaces of the eye: the anterior surface of the cornea and the posterior surface of the crystalline lens, and he provided a geometrical solution to the problem based on this assumption. The prediction is that an inverted image of the external object would be formed on the back of the eye. After some hesitation, he accepted this possibility and defended its validity and plausibility on a conceptual basis against possible objections from the readers.

The proud statement by which he announces the conclusion of his study of image formation in the eye betrays an evident inspiration from the pictorial techniques, particularly for the use of the term *pictura* (meaning 'painting' or 'picture') rather than *imago* (image).[4] The word *pictura* is preferred—he says—because the projection on the retina is not akin to a fictitious entity (*Ens rationale*—'Entity of reason') to which the word *imago* is normally assigned. On the contrary it is

[4] About 60 years after Kepler, the English mathematician Isaac Barrow would make a clear distinction between real and virtual images in optical imagery, as respectively the point of convergence (for real images) or the point of divergence (for virtual images) of the refracted (or reflected) rays (Barrow, 1669).

something real, even capable of having an existence relatively independent of the external object that has produced it:

> Vision thus occurs through a picture of the visible object at the white of the retina and the concave wall; and those things that are on the right outside, are depicted at the left side of the wall, the left at the right, the top at the bottom, the bottom at the top. Further, green things are depicted in the color green, and in general any object whatever is pictured in its own color within. The result of this is that if it were possible for this picture on the retina to remain while the retina was taken out into the light, while those things out in front that were giving it form were removed, and if some person were to possess sufficient keenness of vision, that person would recognize the exact configuration of the hemisphere in the compass of the retina, small as it is. Moreover, that proportion is preserved, such that when straight lines are drawn from the individual points of objects that can be viewed to some particular point within the compass of the eye, the individual parts within are depicted at very nearly the same angle at which the lines will have come together, so much so that not even the smallest points are left out. And to such an extent that the fineness of this picture within the eye of any person you please is as great as the acuteness of vision in that person. (OPTICA, p. 180; transl. pp. 181–182)

13.7 **The imperfections of a painting and the vision of stars**

Through his optical investigations, not only had Kepler displaced the sensitive part of the eye away from the crystalline lens, but he had also succeeded in resolving another visual paradox that had perplexed the previous investigators. In the initial version proposed by Alhazen and endorsed by many of his Western followers, the *camera obscura* model eliminated all but one of the rays issuing from all points of the external object from vision process. Only the perpendicular ray that struck the cornea was assumed to pass through the ocular media and cast the *pictura*. Those who experimented with the *camera obscura* readily realized that making the aperture extremely small resulted in the image becoming very faint and eventually invisible. This was why relatively large apertures were used, with the unwanted consequence that the quality and dimensions of the projected image became worse. In the fifteenth century, several authors (like Barbaro, Maurolico, and Porta) noticed that a convex lens placed at the aperture of the *camera obscura* could sharpen the projected images, even if the aperture was rather wide. One of the motives leading Kepler to investigate the dioptric properties of the eye was probably a knowledge (through the optical works of Della Porta) of the effects of convex lenses on a *camera obscura* with a wide aperture.

With Kepler's model (mainly based on spherical lenses), the convergence properties of the ocular media focused *almost* all the rays from a single point of an external object on a single point of the retina. Not, however, the totality of the rays. This was because, as Kepler discovered with his geometrical calculations, with spherical lenses there was not a single locus for the totality of rays converging towards the image surface of the optical system (a paper screen in the model, the retina in the eye). The convergence occurred instead over a small area that increased in size when the incoming rays impinged on the most peripheral parts of the lenses.

Kepler considered the visual problems arising from the optical imperfections of the eye towards the end of last section of the fifth chapter of his book. He concentrates on the vision of luminous bodies and remarks that in general 'all things that are luminous appear greater in proportion to things placed nearby that are less luminous' (OPTICA, p. 217; transl. p. 232). After discussing various errors of visual estimation of celestial bodies attributable to this phenomenon and the individual variability in size judgements, he concludes by saying that 'all these things, and whatever others there are, draw their origin from the retina tunic, but in a different respect' (p. 218; transl. p. 233).

It is at this point that he starts considering vision of single luminous points:

> For the most distant bodies, such as the celestial bodies, gather the radiations from a single point, into a single point, before they touch upon the retiform, and, cutting each other at that point, they now strike

> spread out upon the retina. Thus it is not a single point that of the retina that is illuminated by a point of the object, but a small part of its surface [*superficiecula*] that is illuminated by a point of the object, and thus it is encircled by many points; white things, however, and bright things illuminate its surface strongly. They therefore bring it about that those things that are depicted less bright in the same place, where they themselves showed their own boundaries [...] become entirely invisible, and give way to the white things. (OPTICA, p. 218; transl. pp. 233–234)

For Kepler, the expansion of the image of a distant luminous point (like celestial bodies) would depend on the inability of the dioptric system of the eye to focus the cone of light emerging from the posterior surface of the crystalline lens.

After remarking that the effect might be worsened by the dilatation of the pupil which occurs at night-time, Kepler continues by saying:

> On this account, therefore, the visual picture [*pictura visoria*] is corrupted, which is a necessary consequence of defective vision. If all things were equally bright, vision would be confused; now, however, because the luminous things predominate, they are flawed in their quantity. And even if perchance the pictorial cone is spread out in all observers, nevertheless, not everyone uses so subtle a visual faculty as to perceive by means of all the radiations, but those alone who are affected by all radiations imagine for themselves that the luminous things are larger. Hence, those who have a conspicuous weakness of vision have double vision not of luminous things only, but also of dark ones, if they be narrow and exceedingly distant. (OPTICA, pp. 219–220; transl. p. 234)

Kepler considers these limitations in the vision of punctiform light sources attributable to geometrical optics effects, and afterwards goes on with other kinds of reflections which seems to adumbrate mechanisms belonging to a more physical and physiological dimension. To this purpose he invokes the different behaviour of two sheets of paper, one white the other black, exposed to an intense light beam concentrated through the action of 'a globe of water or crystal'. The illuminated surface would appear larger on the white paper and smaller on the black. Moreover, with a particularly intense light, the black paper would ignite more quickly than the white. These differences, Kepler says, cannot be interpreted as evidence that the optical laws are different for the two types of paper. They depend instead on some property of the retina, or perhaps of the visual spirit (*spiritum visorium*) connected to the sensory process within this membrane, by which the stimulating action of a small light beam falling on a tiny surface diffuses to the surrounding zones. In a marginal note inserted at this point Kepler explains that, with the phrase optical laws (*legibus opticis*), he means the laws of refraction, because 'at the origin "optical" means anything that pertains to vision' (p. 220; transl. p. 235).

To clarify the point he invokes another analogy, based on the difference in the lateral diffusion of a coloured drop falling on the surface of water or dust. In this context he also considers the lateral spreading of the afterimages of a brilliant image [*mora speciei lucidae*], a consequence in his opinion of the tendency of the visual system to avoid the excessive effect of intense brightness.

On this basis Kepler repeats a motif that characterizes the whole volume, that astronomers should be cautious about trusting vision. Deceptions might arise not only from the limits of geometrical optics but also from other, non-geometrical factors, and this is particularly true for the vision of bright, distant point sources of light.

Despite having elaborated a modern optical theory of the eye functioning, when it came to consider visual appearance of stars, Kepler was obliged to invoke extra-geometrical factors and make considerations which belong more to the approach of practical mathematicians (like Ausonio and the other operational opticians of the Renaissance).

13.8 The non-optical vision of an acute surveyor

Both Galileo and Kepler were motivated to investigate vision because of their interests in astronomical appearances but they approached them quite differently. Kepler's consideration of the illusory expansion of distant light sources amply justifies his remarks on the apparent magnification of stars expressed in *Dissertatio cum nuncio sidereo*. In his analysis of Galileo's telescopic observations, Kepler invited his correspondent to take into consideration those passages of his own *Optica* discussed earlier in this chapter. Although Kepler embraced non-geometrical factors to account for some aspects of visual magnification of bright points, there is no doubt that his text erected a magnificent edifice for the analysis of vision.

This notwithstanding, when he made his critical remarks to Galileo, Kepler still endorsed the measurement of star size following Tycho Brahe's method (despite assuming that the physical dimensions of the fixed star were much smaller than that of the sun). Despite the precision of the Danish scholar's measurements, his estimates of the sizes of stars were largely in excess of their true angular sizes (as we have mentioned in Chapter 8). It remained to Galileo to break with this tradition even though his ideas of optical functioning were still anchored in medieval conceptions, with little concern for intraocular refraction.

In Chapter 8 we discussed how Galileo showed that the luminous irradiation seen surrounding a star was largely a consequence of entoptic mechanisms. Based on the use of a cord to hide a star, this method did not rely on the sophisticated and expensive instruments contrived by Brahe. Moreover, it worked without any consideration of the dioptric properties of the eye. Indeed, it was based on a rather primitive conception of the functioning of the eye; this was more closely related to the Euclidean-Ptolemaic tradition and certainly not beyond the elaborations of Alhazen, Witelo, Peckham, and other medieval scholars. It would appear from various passages in Galileo's works and from his correspondence that he still endorsed a theory of vision based on the emission of visual rays. This is particularly evident in a letter addressed to him by Sagredo on 7 July 1612 (in response to a lost letter from Galileo). In this letter Sagredo also remarked on the inverted images of sun spots observed with the projection method commonly used by Castelli and Galileo for the observation of the sun; from this it is possible to argue that one of the reasons for Galileo's adherence to such an old doctrine was his difficulty in imagining how vision could work if the dioptric mechanism formed an inverted retinal image (OG XI, p. 356).[5]

As discussed earlier, Galileo's conception of the visual process was likely inspired by the perspective tradition of Renaissance artists and by the prospecting techniques of engineers and architects that he knew well and taught in his university classes. In Galileo's method of star measurement, the eye became simply an instrument of prospecting, a compass similar to the 'geometric and military compass' that he had invented in Padua in 1597 and described in a booklet published in 1606 (Figure 13.13). Galileo's compass was a rather sophisticated contrivance which could also be used in a variety of arithmetic computations for both military and civil purposes.

For measurement of the apparent size of the stars with the cord method, the eye was considered by Galileo only a device for angular size estimation, according to simple geometrical and

[5] In a previous letter dated 30 June, Sagredo asked Galileo's opinion on a theory of image formation in the retina that he (Sagredo) had been proposing based on the refraction of light at the crystalline lens (likely similar to that of Kepler). He mentioned a discussion involving Sarpi, Della Mula, and Marc'Antonio De Dominis, a prelate who had published in 1611 a treatise on vision in which he adhered to the traditional conception that the sensitive part of the eye is the crystalline lens.

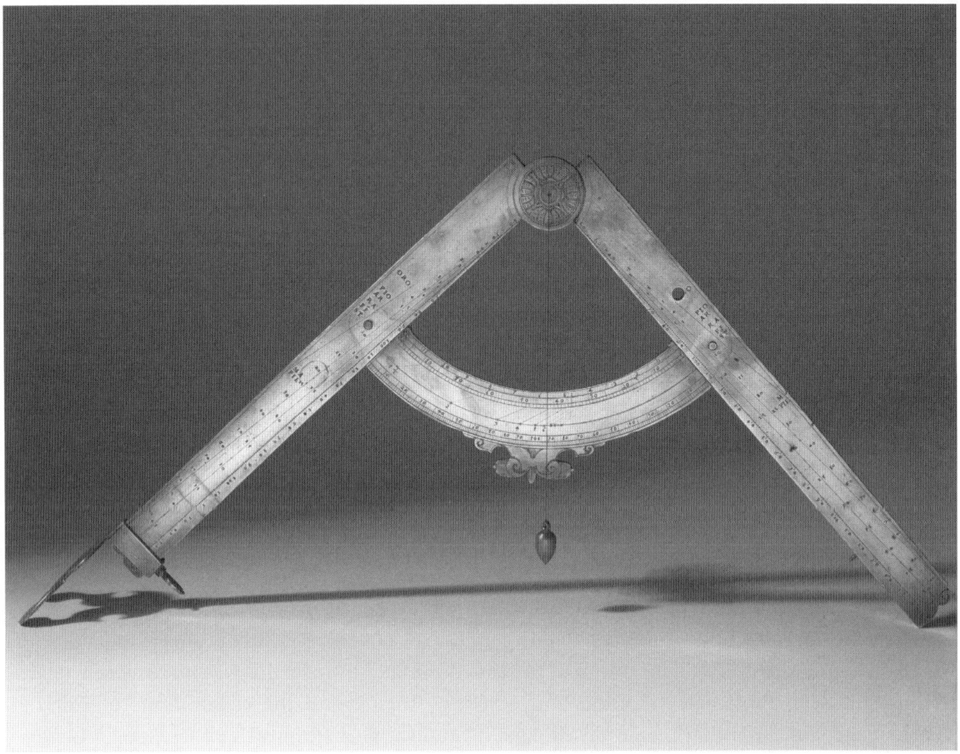

Figure 13.13 The geometric and military compass invented by Galileo in 1597. It was a multipurpose geometric and arithmetic computing device which somewhat anticipates the slide rules largely used by engineers and architect until the era of electronic computers. By courtesy of the Galileo Museum, Florence.

trigonometric laws, and with no other assistance than one (or two) cords or strips. Although simple, Galileo's star measurement implied, however, that there were some important conceptual difficulties connected to a problem of physiological optics. Irrespective of the particular technique used, a basic requirement of correct measures of the angular sizes of distant objects depends on a correct and precise knowledge of the site from which the measure is taken (i.e. the vertex of the angle to be measured). This requirement is relatively (but not completely) easy to fulfil with ordinary measuring devices but it was much less so in the case of the eye under the conditions of Galileo's experiments. This was because, as was known at least since the era of ancient Greek astronomy, the measurement cannot be taken from the anterior surface of the eye. Instead it requires a precise knowledge of the point within the eye where the rays would meet after passing through the dioptric media of the eye without being deviated. In the language of modern physiological optics, this crucial point corresponds to the optical centre of the eye or main nodal point, which is a fundamental parameter in any geometrical or arithmetic computation of the image forming process in the eye.

At the beginning of the sixteenth century a calculation of such an important locus in the eye was beyond the reach even of Kepler's sophisticated physiological optics. Accordingly, it would not be expected that Galileo, with his rather outdated optical knowledge, would endeavour to establish it. Moreover, there was the important problem that vision does not function in a simple geometrical way (as implied by the optics of Euclid and his followers until the Renaissance), that is, on the basis of the convergence of a single ray issuing from every individual point of the object. Kepler's optical investigations indicated that the image of any single point is focused in the eye by convergence of all rays issuing from the object point and passing through the pupil. This added a further complication and a possible source of error in Galileo's cord experiment.

13.9 Measuring the heavens: the precise calculation of a 'divine' sand-reckoner on the beach at Syracuse

Galileo applied to the stars a method that had been used many centuries earlier which is generally attributed to Archimedes, the great mathematician of Syracuse. The title of the work in which it was published, known in the Renaissance as *Arenarius* or *Harenarius*, is normally translated into English as *Sand-reckoner*. This is because in his book Archimedes pretends to show to the sovereign of his city, King Gelon, that despite the limitation inherent in the Greek system of numeration, it is nevertheless possible to write a number greater than the estimate of grains of sand existing in the world. To increase the difficulty, Archimedes says that he would write down a number greater even than the sand grains in the entire universe if it was composed only of sand.

A point of great importance for the history of astronomy is that the *Sand-reckoner* contains the most important allusion to the heliocentric system expounded by Aristarchus of Samos in a work that has been lost (Figure 13.14). This is because Archimedes decided to calculate the diameter of the sphere of the fixed stars, not following the geocentric system but on the basis of the system advocated by Aristarchus. As would happen many centuries later in the case of Copernicus, this system was based on the assumption of an annual revolution of the earth

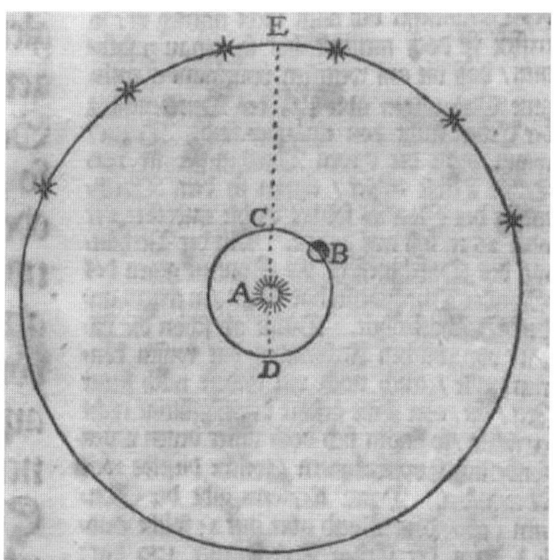

Figure 13.14 A diagram of the cosmological system of Aristarchus of Samos illustrated in a seventeenth-century German edition of the *Sand-reckoner* by Archimedes. A is the sun and B the earth. Reproduced from Archimedes, *Des unvergleichlichen Archimedis Sand-Rechnung, oder, Diessinnige Erfindung einer, mit verwunderlicher Leichtigkeit aussprechlicher*, Zahl, 1667, P. Fürstens.

around the sun. Archimedes' choice is justified by the fact that, for reasons similar to those that would be invoked afterwards by Copernicus, Aristarchus was obliged to assume that the distance of the earth from the fixed stars was much greater than that estimated by the supporters of the geocentric system.

One of the steps necessary for Archimedes to calculate the volume within the sphere of the fixed stars is to measure the size of the sun. To this end he develops a method that would be, many centuries later, an important source of inspiration for Galileo. Being conscious of the possibility of errors intrinsic in his method, Archimedes tries to estimate the possible range of the angular size of the sun. The method that he describes in detail to King Gelon is basically a method of occultation of the sun's image made by the interposition of an object of known size, a cylinder in this particular case:

> I have attempted to measure by means of instruments the angle subtended by the Sun and having its vertex at the eye in the following way. It is, however, not easy to measure this angle with precision, for neither the eye, nor the hands, nor the instruments for measuring it are reliable enough for determining it exactly; but this is scarcely the occasion to discuss this subject further, especially as this has often been pointed out. In order to demonstrate my proposition, it is sufficient for me to find an angle which is not greater than that which is subtended by the sun and has its vertex at the eye, and then to find another angle which is not smaller than that which is subtended by the sun and has its vertex at the eye. Having first placed a long, straight rod on a vertical stand, the stand was put in a position where the rising sun could be seen. A small cylinder, turned on a lathe, was placed vertically on the rod immediately after the rising of the sun. Then, when the sun was still near the horizon and could be looked at directly, the rod was directed towards the sun and the eye was placed at one end, while the cylinder, placed between the eye and the sun, concealed the sun. The cylinder was then shifted away from the eye, and when the sun showed slightly on each side of the cylinder it was set in place. (Archimedes, transl. in Shapiro, 1975, p. 82)

Although at the time of Archimedes, trigonometric methods were not available, there should have been no great difficulty in obtaining the necessary approximation of the angular size of the sun, on the basis of the diameter of the cylinder and its distance from the eye. However, as he immediately remarks, this would be straightforward only if it could safely be assumed that the distance to be calculated was that from the cylinder to the anterior surface of the eye. This assumption is, however, justified—he says—only 'if it were so that the eye sees from a single point'. But this assumption is not granted, because, in accordance with the optical theory of his time 'the eye does not see from a single point, but from a certain area', and the convergence point of the ray is a virtual locus whose distance from the anterior pole of the eyeball needs to be calculated.

At this point it becomes necessary for Archimedes to ascertain the extension of that 'certain area' through which the eye sees. According to the type of visual theory endorsed (intromission versus extramission) this area could be considered in two ways. Within an intromission framework, it would correspond to the surface admitting light rays into the eye. For extramission theory, it would be the area through which the visual rays generated inside the eye would exit through the anterior pole of the eyeball. The Greek term used by Archimedes to indicate this 'certain area', όψεις, has a very general meaning (vision, sight, appearance, and also—as we shall see—image) and it has been translated in various ways (pupil, eye, sight; see Lejeune, 1947, 1948, 1989). From the second step of Archimedes's sun-measurement procedure it seems that it corresponds to the pupillary foramen. It should be considered, however, that in Archimedes' time nobody seemed to be aware that the pupil size could vary according to the physiological conditions.

To measure the size of the όψεις (that we translate provisionally as pupil) Archimedes takes various pairs of cylinders with diameters in the range of the real pupil size, the two elements of each pair having exactly the same diameter (Figure 13.15). This is how he then proceeds:

> One takes two thin cylinders of the same thickness, one white, and the other not, and places them in front of the eye in such a way that the white one is removed from the eye, and the non-white one is brought as close as possible to the eye so that it touches the face. Then, if the cylinders chosen are smaller than the pupil, the closer cylinder is encompassed by the pupil and the white is seen behind it. If the cylinders are much smaller, the white is seen in full. If they are not much smaller, a part of the white is seen on each side of the cylinder nearer the eye. But, if cylinders of a suitable magnitude are chosen, then one covers the other without covering a larger area. It is therefore certain that a magnitude equal in size to the thickness of the cylinders which are determined in this way is not less than that of the pupil. (Archimedes, transl. in Shapiro, 1975, p. 82)

Having determined the size of the pupil (όψεις), Archimedes can obtain a lower estimate of the angular size of the sun on the basis of the previous measurement. With an analogous method he obtains next the upper estimate of the image size. The values are given as fractions of a right angle, respectively 1/164 and 1/200 (corresponding to 32′ 56″ and 27′ in the sexagesimal system). This is indeed a good estimate since, according to modern measurements, the angular size of the sun varies between 31′6″ and 32′7″. On the basis of the measurement of the sun, and of the available values of the astronomical distances, Archimedes calculates the relative size of the sphere of the fixed stars. This allows him to compute the extremely large number of sand grains that could be accommodated within this huge space.

We cannot go into the details of the entire calculation but, before leaving Archimedes while he writes down, with the old system of Greek numeration, this enormous figure (corresponding

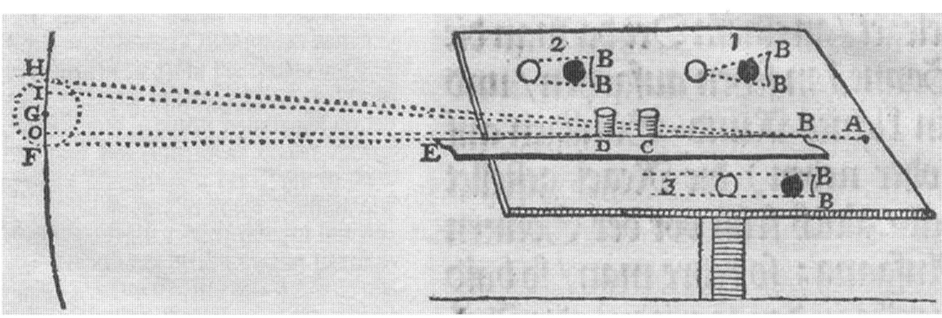

Figure 13.15 The apparatus used by Archimedes in his measurement of the angular size of the Sun according to the same seventeenth-century German edition of the *Sand-reckoner* as in Figure 13.13. In this figure, 1 to 3 indicate the experiment of measurement of the viewing surface (i.e. the pupil) based on the use of two small cylinders, with 1, 2, and 3 referring respectively to the conditions of cylinder size decidedly smaller, 'not much smaller', and almost equal to the viewing surface. The central diagram represents the experiment of sun occultation made by using one movable cylinder. The sun (HF) is on the left while B is the anterior pole of the eye. C and D correspond respectively to the position of complete (C) or partial (D) occultation. A is the point of calculated convergence of the rays coming from the external circumference of the sun and tangent to the external surface of the cylinder in the position of almost total occultation. Reproduced from Archimedes, *Des unvergleichlichen Archimedis Sand-Rechnung, oder, Diessinnige Erfindung einer, mit verwunderlicher Leichtigkeit aussprechlicher*, Zahl, 1667, P. Fürstens.

to about 10^{63} in Arabic numerals) we need to say how he measures the other essential element needed for the success of his calculation, the size of a grain of sand. He does this by assuming that a volume no greater than a poppy-seed contains no more than 10,000 sand grains. Afterwards he measures the size of a poppy-seed putting together, side by side, several of these seeds, and noting that 25 of them occupy a length more than a finger-breath. In such a way he can connect the microscopic measure of the sand grain to a more intuitive quantity useful for the final computation, the digit.

It should be noted that the problem of the ὄψεις in Archimedes' scheme was also essential for the further development of the method of astronomical observation described in the *Sand-reckoner* and notably in the diopter of Hipparchus and his successors. To reduce the difficulty connected to the size of the ὄψεις and to the precise localization of the convergence of visual rays, astronomers utilized a diopter with a lamina (or pinnule) located close to the observer's eye and a small hole aimed at narrowing the size of the ὄψεις. In some diopters the mobile cylinder was substituted with another, mobile, lamina with one (or more) circular apertures. Brahe's diopter illustrated in Figure 13.11 represented a sophisticated evolution of the diopter of Archimedes and his successors.

Having briefly described the method used by Archimedes in the measurement of the sun in the third century BC, we are now ready to compare it with that applied by Galileo to the measurement of the stars about two millennia later. We will discuss the problems intrinsic to both methods, and particularly that concerning the supposed angle of convergence of the light rays, after considering the way in which Galileo readapted to the vision of stars the method of his ancient predecessor.

13.10 The acute sight of a new Archimedes

In Chapter 8 we mentioned the method developed by Galileo to measure the angular size of the stars, and its importance within the framework of the discussion on the Copernican system. We have referred to the explanation given by Salviati in the *Dialogue*, and also to a passage of the *Discorso delle comete*. We have, moreover, mentioned a more detailed description of the method present in texts of the last years of Galileo's life, and particularly in an unfinished manuscript entitled *Operazioni astronomiche* of 1637, and in a report of a friend who visited him in 1638 (OG VIII, pp. 449–468). These texts indicate that the problem of the deceptive appearance of the stars' size occupied a large part of Galileo's life. Possibly preceding the period of his first telescopic observations, this interest was undoubtedly stimulated by his awareness of visual deceptions of previous observers, as is attested in a letter sent by Galileo to Sarpi on 8 February 1611 (i.e. less than one year after *Sidereus*); he wrote to his correspondent (with some exaggeration) that he has found a method which demonstrates that the size of the stars had been overestimated by previous authors 'and by someone of them more than by 6000 percent' (OG XI, p, 49).

In the second section of *Operazioni astronomiche* Galileo says that a convenient thickness of the cord useful for the measurement of a big star, like the Dog Star (Sirius), could be 'one digit' (*un dito*). This is a length which corresponds to about 1° at a distance of 1 metre. Since in various places he writes that the angular size of the stars of first magnitude is about 5″, this would imply that with a cord of this thickness there was a complete occultation of the star at a distance of about 60 metres. As in the case of Archimedes, Galileo is confronted with the problem of the site of convergence of the rays corresponding to the vision of the star (and of the cord hiding it). He makes reference to a purely geometrical theory, probably inspired by Euclid (as it seems from the use of an extramission-type terminology and particularly by his repeated allusion to 'visual rays'). In order to calculate the precise location of the point of reunion of the rays (point of convergence to, or divergence from, according to the theoretical framework), located somewhat behind the cornea, Galileo proceeds in a different way to Archimedes, and less dependent on assumptions on the extent of the visual area. In contrast to Archimedes, Galileo is confronted with another difficulty, dependent on his awareness that the size of the pupil foramen is not fixed, but a variable value.

The technique used to achieve this goal is described in both the *Dialogue* and in the first section of *Operazioni astronomiche*. In the *Dialogue*, before Salviati goes on to describe the method of the cord, Sagredo raises a preliminary question, specifically concerning the convergence of the visual rays when viewing stars. This is how Salviati puts it in the *Dialogue* in answering a question raised by Sagredo:

> SAGREDO. I see and I quite understand. But before going further I should like to propose the doubt that occurred to me about finding the meeting point of the visual rays included within very acute angles. My trouble arises from the impression that this intersection might vary in its location not on account of the greater or smaller size of the object looked at, but because of a certain other respect in which it seems to me that the meeting of the rays might be farther from or closer to the eye when looking at object of the same size. (DIALOGO, p. 355; transl. pp. 362–363)

In his response Salviati praises the perspicacity of his interlocutor and asks him if his doubt might concern the possible variation of pupil size during the attempts to measure the angular size of the stars (according to a 'doctrine'—he says—that he had learned from Sagredo himself).[6] Sagredo confirms that that was indeed the nature of his doubt, thus giving to Salviati the opportunity to expound the way he (i.e. Galileo himself) had faced the problem.

> SALVIATI. The method is very easy, and it is as follows. I take two strips of paper, one black and the other white, making the black strip half the wide of the white. I attach the white one to a wall, and fix the other at a distance of some 15 or 20 cubits [*braccia*] from it on a stick or some other support. Then I move away an equal distance from this in the same direction, and it is obvious enough that at this distance those straight lines intersect which, leaving from the edges of the white paper, would just touch in passing the edges of the strip placed midway between. From this it follows that the eye being placed at this intersection, the black strip in the center would just hide the white one, provided that vision took place in a single point. But if we should find that the edges of the white strip could still be seen, it would argue necessarily that the visual rays are not converging at one point alone. And to make the white strip stay hidden by the black one, the eye would have to be brought closer. This done so that the central strip hides the distant one, and the amount of the required approach being noted, this amount will be a safe measure of the distance from the eye of the true intersection of the visual rays in such operations. Moreover, we shall thus have the diameter of the pupil or rather of the hole from which the visual rays emerge. From its proportion to the width of the black paper will be that which is borne to the distance between the two papers by the distance from the intersection of the lines produced along the edges of the papers to the place where the eye was when it first saw the more distant paper hidden by the intermediate one. (DIALOGO, p. 356; transl. pp. 363–364, revised)

In the first and second section of the *Operazioni astronomiche*, Galileo describes the ways by which, on the basis of this measurement (that he does now with two strips rather than with two cords) he calculates the size of the pupil. What he is calculating is not the actual size of the pupil considered as the variable anatomic foramen encircled by the iris, but a rather abstract parameter

[6] As already remarked in Chapter 12 through Salviati's words Galileo was probably paying in an allusive and indirect way a tribute to Sarpi, the scholar from which he might have known about the pupillary reflex.

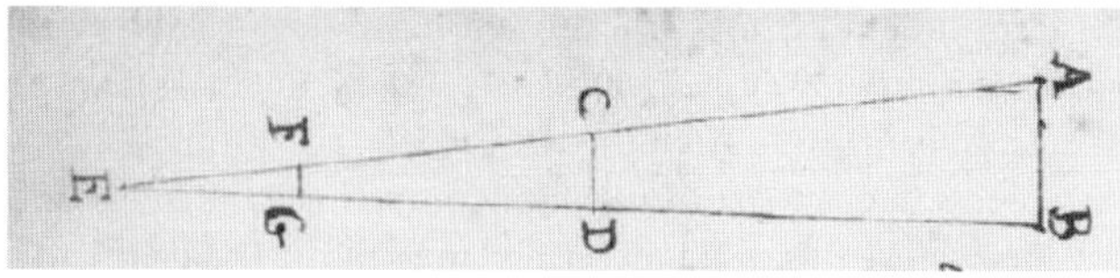

Figure 13.16 One of the figures by which in the *Operazioni astronomiche* Galileo illustrates his experiment aimed at determining the point of concurrence of the visual rays needed to measure the angular size of stars. AB and CD represent a section of the strips used in the occultation experiment (AB being white and CD black), CD being half AB. E is the geometric point of convergence of the straight line tangent to respectively A and C, and to B and D. FG is the place where the anterior pole of the eye should be located in order that CD might obscure AB (BNF GAL 70 f40v).

corresponding to the optical aperture of the eye; or, better, the equivalent in the living eye of the small hole pierced in the movable pinnule of one of the most common astronomical surveying instruments of the age, the diopter (the ancestor of the modern theodolite used nowadays by professional surveyors).

With reference to a diagram that we reproduce in Figure 13.16 he writes:

> Let us assume that the straight line AB is the width of the white strip, whose half CD is the width of the black. Let us draw parallel lines in whichever distance, that is from the extreme points A, B let us draw the straight lines passing through the points C,D, concurring in the point E. If the pupil were situated in the said point, and the sight would occur in a single point, AB would be occulted by CD. If this would not happen, let us move the eye toward CD, until AB is occulted by CD: let us assume for instance that this would occur in FG. It is manifest that FG is the diameter of the *visual power*, that is the pupil. Its size will be known by means of the three known lines CD, CE, EF; this is because the same proportion exists between CE and EF of that there is between CD and EF. (OG VII, p. 457, our emphasis)

In the *Operazioni astronomiche* Galileo gives no value for the actual distance of E from EG, that is, of the separation of the putative concurrence point of the visual rays from the anterior surface of the eye corresponding to the site of the pupil or 'visual power'. He does this in the *Dialogue* with the words that Salviati pronounces soon after describing the two cords experiment, with relation to a possible measurement of the star diameter.

> SALVIATI. [...] having found e.g. that the diameter of the cord to be quadruple than that of the pupil, and being by example the distance between the eye and the cord 30 cubits [*braccia*], we should say that the true intersection of the lines traced from the extremes of the diameter of the star, and passing at the extremes of the diameter of the cord, would occur far from the cord by 40 cubits. In this way the ratio between the distance from the cord of the intersection to the location of the eye will properly be in the proportion that that exists between the diameter of the cord and the pupil. (DIALOGO, pp. 356–357; transl. 364, revised)

What Salviati says here is really surprising if we consider that, at least from the linguistic point of view, here (and in many others passages of his writings) Galileo seems to endorse an extramission theory of vision. To say that the concurrence point of the visual rays can be 10 cubits (that is about six metres) behind the eye would amount to saying, within an extramission framework, that the locus of the eye from which the visual rays are virtually emitted is largely outside the eye.

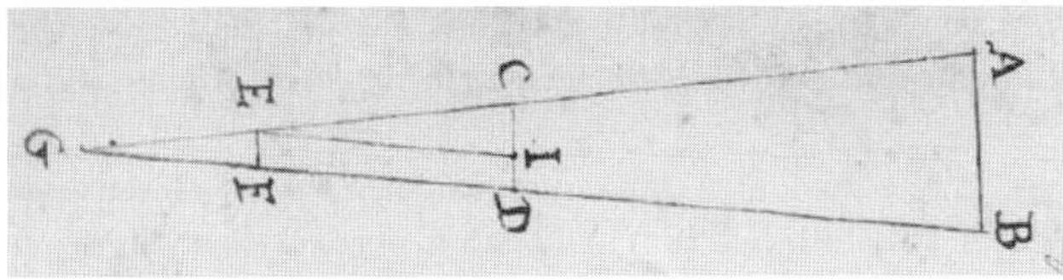

Figure 13.17 The diagram by which in his *Operazioni astronomiche* Galileo illustrates the method for calculating the concurrence point of the visual rays (G) and the size of the pupil (EF). As indicated in the text, AB represents the star, and CD the cord occulting it. The triangle CEG is a geometrical construction necessary for the calculation of the convergence point (BNF GAL 70, F41v).

We have another indication even more striking of the paradoxical consequences of Galileo's perspectivist approach to the cord experiment. This appears from Figure 13.17, derived from the second of his astronomical operations, which illustrates schematically the cord experiment in the case of the actual occultation of the star. Without going into the details of Galileo's geometrical construction we need to consider that in this diagram AB represents the star, CD the cord occluding it, EF the pupil, and G the concurrence point of the rays tangent to the image of the star and to the cord. The paradox of this diagram is that the angular size of the pupil would be in this case or the order of seconds of arcs if we assume that concurrence point of the rays is somewhere within the eye. Since the diameter of the actual, anatomical pupillary hole in a human eye varies between 2 and 8 mm, in order that the linear measure of the segment EF could correspond to these values we should situate the concurrence point of the rays behind the eye, at a distance of more than 300 metres (330.023 metres in the case of a star of 5″ angular size)! The difficulty might perhaps come from the ambiguity of the meaning of the word (and of the concept) of 'pupil' in Galileo's case (as well of the corresponding Greek term at Archimedes's era, όψεις, see later).

It is worth noticing in this context that even though Galileo seemed to adhere to an extramission theory of vision, he was intellectually free from the strictures of this theory. He was not necessarily assuming that what he called visual rays were something else than rays of light entering into the eye. Indeed for Galileo, as for other perspectivists of his age, vision was a purely geometrical and non-optical affair when it came to the task of calculating distances or sizes, and the phrase 'visual rays' was just meaning a geometrical and not physical entity. What is sure is that, with an approach diametrically opposite to that of Kepler, Galileo was simply neglecting what could occur to the rays entering into the eye (or exiting from it) through the refraction occurring across the dioptric media of the eyeball. Whatever Galileo's actual conception of the vision mechanism might have been, we must also consider that, within a conception that assumed that the vision was effected on the anterior face of the crystalline lens, it mattered relatively little if the prolongation of the visual rays converged within the eye or much beyond the eye fundus.

The source of the paradoxes leading Galileo to localize, in his cord experiments, the convergence point of visual rays behind the eye has to do in part with his interpretation of the concept of 'visual area' or 'pupil' in Archimedes' experiments (the όψεις, which Galileo tended to identify with the actual pupil). Although, as remarked in Chapter 8, the image of a luminous point can increase when the pupil gets larger due to optical aberrations, there is no simple relation between the dimension of the (real) pupil and the size of the image in the eye as implied by the faulty identification of Archimedes' όψεις with the anatomical pupil. We could remark here that a diagram like Figure 13.17 would be impossible to draw if EF was the actual pupil. This is because the rays issuing from a visual object of angular size in the range of the seconds of arc could not meet the border of the human pupillary size in their convergence path towards the eye. Despite its physiological variations, the pupil always subtends a visual angle of several degrees and the luminous rays coming from a star would be necessarily divergent when passing tangential to the pupillary border.[7]

Coming to Galileo's inspiration for the cord experiment, we have already remarked that Archimedes (the 'divine Archimedes' as Galileo calls him in a Latin treatise on the motion—OG, I p. 303) was a fundamental reference for his research in various fields (notably those on motion, gravity, floating bodies). There is indeed little doubt that he was an attentive reader of the work of the great mathematician of Syracuse. He owned a copy of the works of Archimedes published in Basel in 1544, which unfortunately has been lost (Archimedes, 1544). We know nonetheless that he annotated it because the marginal notes to Archimedes' treatise *On the sphere and cylinder* were transcribed and are now extant among Galileo's manuscripts at the National Library of Florence (see OG VII, p. 612).

There is thus little doubt that Galileo was acquainted with the version of *Sand-reckoner* which was inserted in the Basel edition. In all probability, he had also read this small opus of Archimedes in the edition of his selected works commented on by Federico Commandino and published in Venice in 1558 (an edition also quoted by Kepler in his *Optica*). The similarities between the measurement methods of the *Sand-reckoner* and those used by Galileo in his estimation of star sizes go beyond the step of the specific astronomical observation. Indeed even the method by which Galileo measured the diameter of the cord used in some of the star occultation experiments may have been inspired by Archimedes and notably by the way in which he establishes, with relation to the size of poppy-seeds, that '25 of them occupy a length more than a finger-breath'.

In the *Dialogue* Salviati says that in order to establish 'with very great precision' the thickness of such a cord, he puts 'many pieces of the said cord on a table so they touch each other' and afterwards he determines the 'entire space occupied by 15 or 20 of them'.[8]

Afterwards he comments on the success of the measurement method with words that betray Galileo's proudness in having overturned the supposedly precise estimates of previous and contemporary astronomers.

> SALVIATI. By this very precise operation I find that that the apparent diameter of a star of the first magnitude (commonly believed to be two minutes, and even put at three by Tycho in his *Astronomical Letters*, p. 167) is no more than five seconds, which is one twenty-fourth or one thirty-sixth of what they thought. Now you see what a serious mistake their doctrine was based upon! (DIALOGO, p. 355; transl. p. 362)

The pride is justified if we consider that by using a simple method with cords or strips, Galileo has succeeded, not only in correcting the astronomers' errors, but also in supporting the revolutionary conception of the world advocated by Copernicus.

In another respect, we cannot but be amazed there could exist continuity through the complex meanders of the history of scientific ideas. This could be between the numerical lucubrations of an acute mathematician and the astronomical perspicacity of an inquisitive observer noting how wide the splendour of a distant torch could appear in the darkness of the night.

---

[7] In the old Euclidean conception of vision (to which Galileo seems to adhere) the only reasonable meaning that can be attributed to the ὄψεις of Archimedes is that of the angular extension of the image of the object at the level of the receptive surface of the eye (anterior to the convergence point and generally assumed to correspond to the anterior surface of the crystalline lens: see Lindberg, 1976).

[8] It is likely that in the measurement of the star size alluded to by Salviati in the *Dialogue* Galileo was using a cord much smaller than that indicated in the *Operazioni astronomiche*. This is suggested by the term *cordicella* (small cord) used by Salviati and, moreover, accounts for the need to put several pieces together in order to accurately determine the thickness.

Chapter 14

Galileo's visions

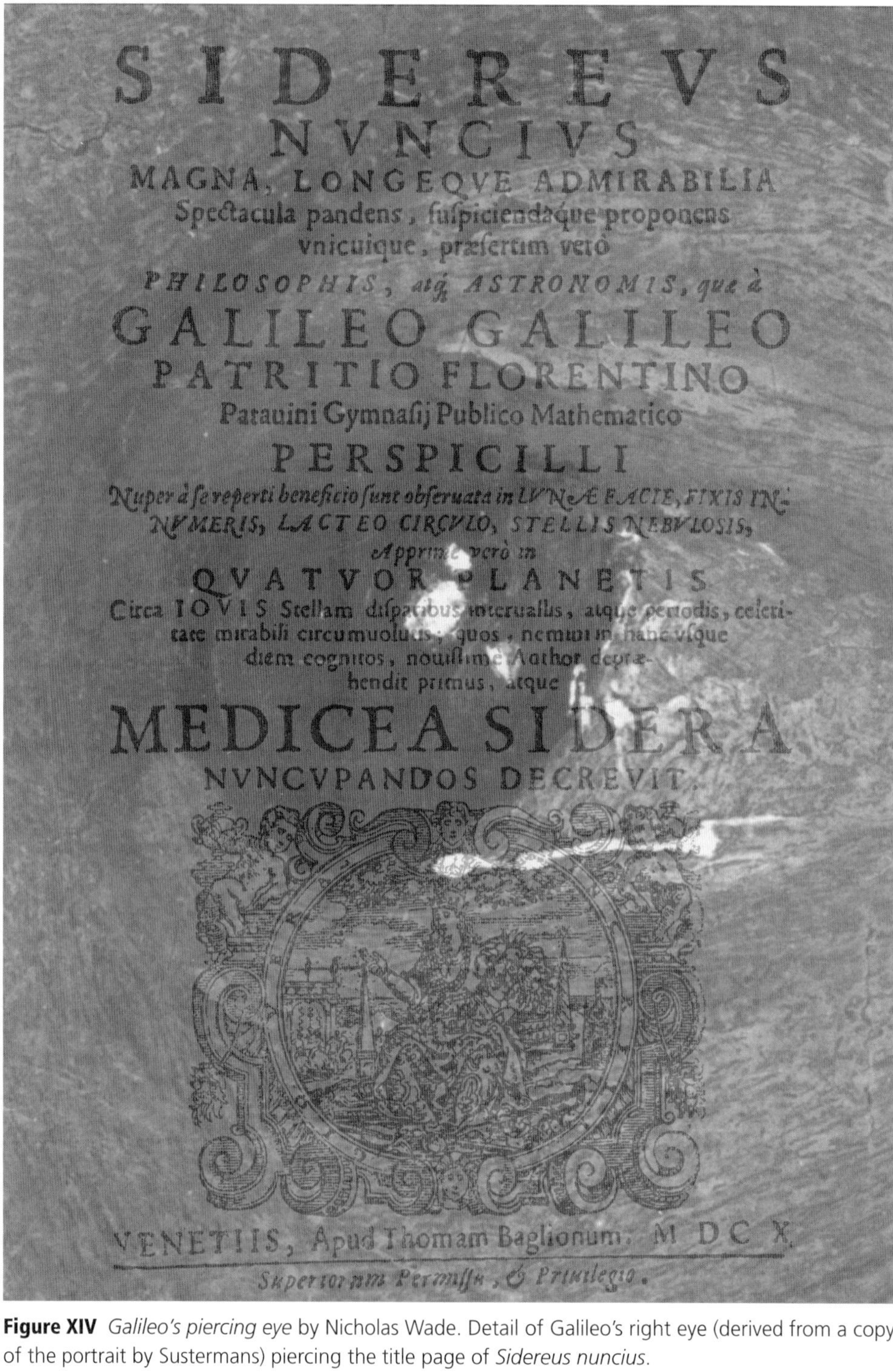

Figure XIV *Galileo's piercing eye* by Nicholas Wade. Detail of Galileo's right eye (derived from a copy of the portrait by Sustermans) piercing the title page of *Sidereus nuncius*.

In the last part of Chapter 13 we dealt with the method developed by Galileo to measure the angular size of stars. Using this method he was able to reduce to 5″ of a degree (or less) the angular size of the most prominent stars, from the traditionally accepted values of 2–3′. By doing so Galileo succeeded in undermining an important objection against the Copernican system based on the supposedly excessive dimensions of the cosmos (see Chapter 8). Despite being successful, Galileo's method was confronted with several difficulties due to the lack of a proper conception of image formation in the eye, and also the limits of the contemporary knowledge on the physical nature of light. Concerning this second point it should be noted that any method of measurement of the angular size of a distant object based on purely visual cues is faced with the limits imposed by the oscillatory nature of light. These limits apply particularly to small angular sizes. The first kind of difficulty came into play when Galileo faced the problem of the convergence point of the visual rays when establishing the size of the 'pupil' or 'visual power' (a problem that has a long history having emerged since at least the time of Archimedes' *Sand-reckoner*). A paradoxical consequence of Galileo's way of facing the problem was that he was obliged to locate the convergence point (or origin) of the light (or visual) rays behind the posterior pole of the eye.

14.1 **A complex path to the vision of the stars**

Despite these (and other) difficulties, the fact that Galileo arrived at a measure of the angular size of the stars which was much more precise than those accepted in his day is important and impressive. It is likely that his occultation experiments were guided by the common observation (also present in Kepler's 1604 *Optica*) that in the sky, bright objects appear much larger than expected on the basis of purely geometrical considerations. This observation was for him an important intellectual tool in the period of the first telescopic investigations, when he encountered the problem of the minimal telescopic magnification of the stars. The problem was puzzling at first, but eventually its solution, achieved by Galileo through a complex intellectual and experimental path, also entailed a better comprehension of an important aspect of the vision process with significant astronomical implications.

The theme of the vision of the stars was among Galileo's reflections since the period of his considerations of the new stars of 1604. It had various dimensions inasmuch as it was connected to the discussion of the reason for the twinkling of the stars, and—more generally—to the problem of the intrinsic versus extrinsic nature of the luminosity of the celestial bodies. Among the notes concerning the new star of 1604 there is a critical remark addressing the way Kepler interpreted the mechanism of the scintillation of stars. One of the causes invoked by the German astronomer in his 1606 treatise *De stella nova* to account for the bright shining and intense twinkling of the star was the idea that its body was continuously rotating in order to enjoy the illumination of the sun from all sides. Within the framework of the Copernican conception Kepler assumed that the earth, all planets, as well as the fixed stars reflected the light of the sun which was located at the centre of the cosmos. The scintillation would be produced in the same way as could occur with a rotating diamond illuminated by an external light.

The idea that stars could reflect the light of the sun was, however, fraught with a difficulty. As we know from previous chapters (and particularly Chapter 8) Copernicus had been obliged to assume that fixed stars were situated at an immense distance from the earth and sun in order to face the problem of an annual parallax of the fixed stars. Kepler recognized that a consequence of this was that the sun would be hardly visible for an observer located on one of the fixed stars. It was because of this that Galileo criticized Kepler's opinion with these words:

> In the Stella Nova, at the page 95, with regard to the scintillation Kepler says that it can be caused by the rotation of the fixed stars.; and even though the Sun would in no way be perceptible from them (such as that we could not see it if we imagined to be on them) nevertheless it is not devoid of natural effects. One should consider that the illumination produced by a natural body loses its effectiveness much more rapidly than its visibility; it is in this way that we see from a great distance a burning torch that is, however, not capable of illuminating the bodies around us. (OG II, p. 280)

In other words, Galileo believed that if the sun was hardly visible from the fixed stars, it was unlikely that it could exercise some significant effect on them, similar to what happens to the flame of a torch that keeps its visibility at distances from which it cannot have an effective illuminating effect. Although Galileo did not own a copy of Kepler's *Stella nova* until 1610, he could have had the chance to read the text much earlier, because there were copies of it in libraries in Padua. This could explain why the remark is among the manuscript notes on the 1604 new star.

It is certain, however, that the problem of the peculiar visual behaviour of intensely luminous bodies situated afar acquired a particular importance in the period of the first telescopic observations. As it comes out from Galileo's writings (see Dupré, 2002, 2005; see also Bucciantini, Camerota, & Giudice, 2012), there is abundant evidence to suggest that Galileo was familiar with the techniques of production of optical instruments and lenses; he made lenses in his home laboratory (with the assistance of a technician) to correct sight problems, and/or acted as an intermediary for their sale between producers and customers. In his practice with the lenses, and in his knowledge of the optical principles exploited by practitioners in order to produce optical instruments, Galileo was surely aware of the common changes of vision occurring in a person upon correction with appropriate lenses. Besides becoming sharper and defined in its details, the image of the object usually appears smaller. This occurs in the vision of small luminous objects on a dark background as is the case for most of the celestial bodies. Kepler was also familiar with this as he was myopic and could only see the moon when looking at the sky with unaided eyes. On his side Galileo, who periodically suffered with some form of eye inflammation [*flussione*], noticed that the halo that surrounded the image of a candle flame or a star became enlarged in the periods in which his eyes were more irritated and moist. Another possible source of Galileo's idea that the image of a small luminous source is magnified by a phenomenon occurring within the eye could have derived from his practice with lenses and optical devices. In his long experience with lenses, Galileo had surely noticed that the halo and irradiations visible around the image of a luminous source were particularly evident when using imperfectly ground lenses, and decreased while the polishing of their surface was improved.

It is very likely that these observations directed Galileo's attention to the eye, and to its possibly defective performance (also in normally sighted individuals), as the cause of the apparent magnification of small distant lights (like the stars). At the time of his telescopic observations, he was led to suppose that the general magnifying effect of the instrument went together with a somewhat opposite action, which tended to make the image smaller, as it rendered it sharper and richer in details. This occurred, for instance, with Venus, Jupiter, and Saturn, which were poorly magnified by the telescope but showed various specific features suggestive of a better visualization: the phases in the case of Venus, the small satellites in the case of Jupiter, and the 'tricorporeal' aspect in the case of Saturn (due—as we know now—to its rings). The association of a relatively low magnification and better visualization was particularly evident in the case of the best telescopes, a consideration that emerged

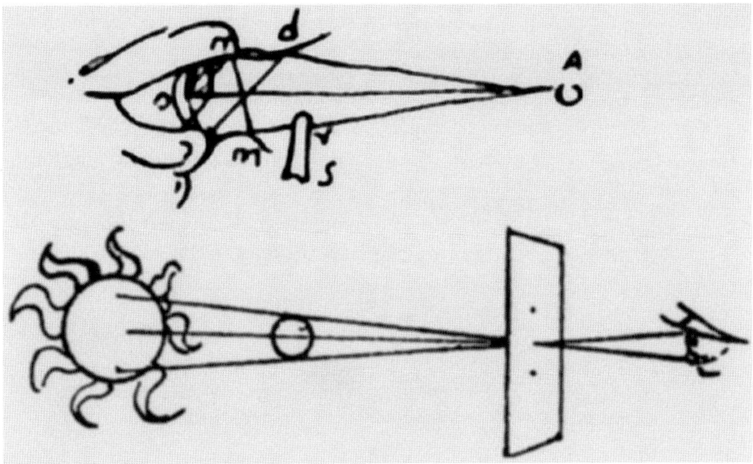

Figure 14.1 Two images from Leonardo's manuscripts illustrating respectively the reflection of light rays on the eyelids supposed to be responsible for the irradiations seen around luminous bodies (top figure), and (on the bottom) a method of looking to the sun through a small hole which removes the peripheral irradiation from the periphery of its image. The idea of Leonardo that the irradiation visible around the image of a luminous body might be due to reflections at the eyelids could have been for Galileo one of the sources of his idea that the 'adventitious rays' are produced in the eye. From, respectively, Manuscript F of the National Library of France, f. 30r (reproduced from Ravaisson-Mollien, C. - 1889 - *Le Manuscrits de Léonardo de Vinci, Manuscrits F et I*. Paris, Quantin), and Codex Trivulziano 6b. (reproduced from Leonardo da Vinci - 1970 - *The notebooks of Leonardo da Vinci*, vol II / compiled and edited from the original manuscripts by Jean Paul Richter, para. 891, Dover Publications).

particularly at the time in which Galileo was improving the performance of his instruments by using a diaphragm (or stop aperture) to occult the peripheral area of the objective lens. This procedure was probably inspired by some observations of Leonardo who tended to attribute the phenomenon of the enlargement of the image of bright objects to a reflection occurring at the eyelids (Dupré, 2002: see Figure 14.1). Leonardo was aware that an enlarged pupil produced less distinct vision and a deceptive magnification, particularly evident in the case of stars or intensely luminous bodies seen against a dark background. Moreover, in Manuscript D, now at the Institut de France, he wrote:

> If you look at the stars, cutting off the rays (as may be done by looking through a very small hole made with the extreme point of a very fine needle [*agucchia*] placed so as almost to touch the eye), you will see those stars so minute that it would seem as though nothing could be smaller, it is in fact their great distance which is the reason of their diminution, for many of them are very many times larger than the star which is the earth with the water. (LNB II, para. 879, p. 148)

In the case of the telescope, the application of the diaphragm (which Galileo tended to use in the form of an oval aperture) improved the visual performance by making the image less blurred and indistinct but, at the same time, of a smaller size.

Besides being an acute observer and expert of practical optics (and having a direct or indirect knowledge of Leonardo's texts), Galileo might have arrived at his conclusion of eye localization of the adventitious rays responsible for the apparent magnification of the size of luminous object by reading Della Porta's more mature treatise on optical phenomena, *De refractione*, first published in 1593 (Figure 14.2).

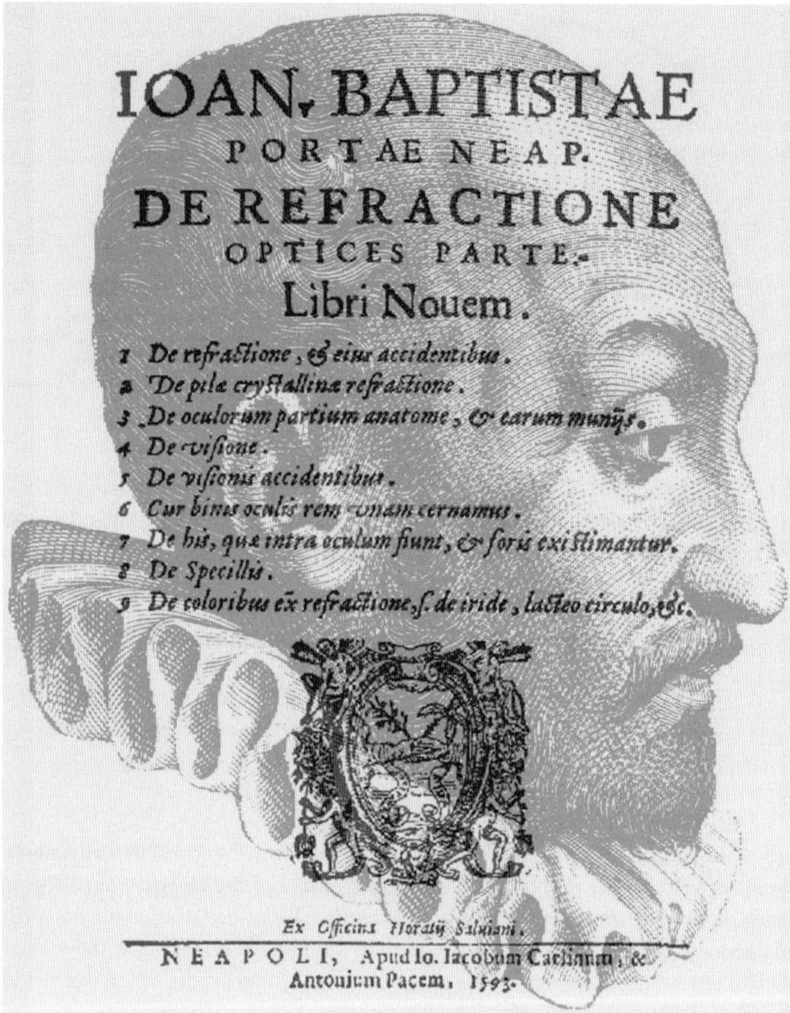

Figure 14.2 *Della Porta's De Refractione* by Nicholas Wade. An engraved portrait of Giovanibattista Della Porta (derived from Mach, 1926) is combined with the title page of his *De Refractione optices parte libri novem* published in 1593.

In proposition 4 of the book VI of this text (see Figure 14.3), Della Porta deals with the appearance of a halo [*iris*] around the flame of a candle particularly evident—as noticed by Aristotle in his *Meteorologica*—during the cold season for people 'having humid eyes'. He discounts the opinion of the Greek philosopher who considered the halo as the consequence of atmospheric phenomenon located in the proximity of the flame and he claims that it is instead due to the some process intrinsic to the eye. These are the first three considerations in his list:

> First, if the flame [*lumen*] of the candle is oblong, or pyramidal, why is the halo not oblong or pyramidal, given that from any part of the flame the rays are emitted in the same way [*ab omni luminis parte aequales lineae proiiciuntur*] are emitted? Second, if it is near the candle, why [the rays] does it decrease

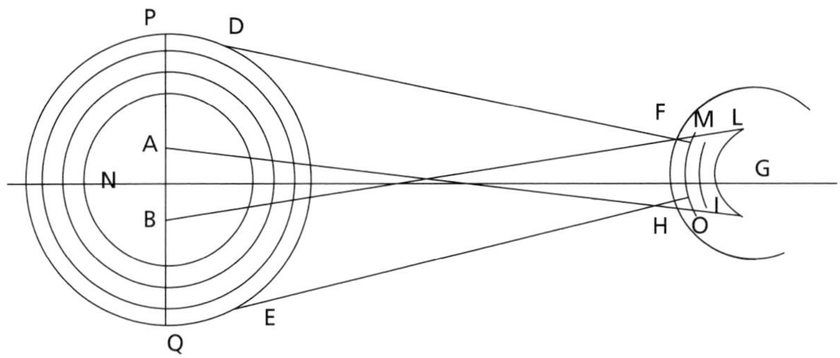

Figure 14.3 The optical diagram by which in his *De refractione* Della Porta accounts for the appearance of a wide halo around the flame of a candle. In this diagram, AB represents the flame, BL and AI the rays issuing from the border of the flame and hitting the periphery of the cornea at, respectively, F and H. G is the crystalline lens, considered as the seat of the visual power. The limits of the halo's image are at P and Q on the basis of the traditional 'rule of cathetus', expounded in the *Catoptrics* of the pseudo-Euclid for reflecting mirrors, and largely followed by the Medieval perspectivists also in image formation due to refraction processes. This rule stipulates that an image is seen at the intersection of the reflected (or refracted) ray and the 'cathetus', i.e. the perpendicular drawn from the object to the reflecting (or refracting) surface. In his 1604 optical treatise Kepler proved the cathetus rule to be unsatisfactory and criticized Della Porta's image formation conceptions. He assumed instead that the localization of the image in the visual world was due mainly to a triangulation mechanism involving the two eyes, and, in the case of monocular vision, to the divergence of the rays coming from the object and hitting the pupil. Reproduced from Della Porta, G. D., *De Refractione optices parte libri novem*, Apud J. J. Carlinum et A. Pacem, 1593.

> when one comes near, and increase when going far? The matter should be the opposite, since the things that are farther should look smaller. Third, if we make a hole in a paper and put the flame of the candle before us, and put the paper in between the eye and the candle, then we will see the halo on the paper and not near the candle. (Della Porta, 1593, p. 164)

This experiment (to which Della Porta claims priority) is easy to reproduce and rather impressive when performed under appropriate viewing conditions (looking at a concentrated light source in an otherwise dark room): the rays issuing from the core of the light seem capable of piercing the paper. They disappear only when the border of the hole occults the central core of the light source.

Galileo owned a copy of *De refractione* as documented by the inventory made by his son Vincenzio Galilei junior and his wife Sestilia Bucchinieri. It is very likely that he had been consulting it at the time he was improving the telescope and looking for an explanation of the problem of the vision of stars. That he had being reading Della Porta's text is made even more probable if one considers another important correspondence between his method of the cord for the stars and a method described in proposition 4 of Book III in *De refractione*. Della Porta's procedure, explicitly inspired by Archimedes' measurement of the sun diameter and illustrated by a diagram (Figure 14.4), aims at evaluating the effects of changes of pupil size on the estimations of the size of the objects.

After inviting the reader to notice the decrease of the pupil size in 'the opened eye of a friend' upon exposition to the sunlight, and to its increase in a dark room, Della Porta describes his occultation method, based on a modification of those of the *Sand-reckoner*, using two cylinders

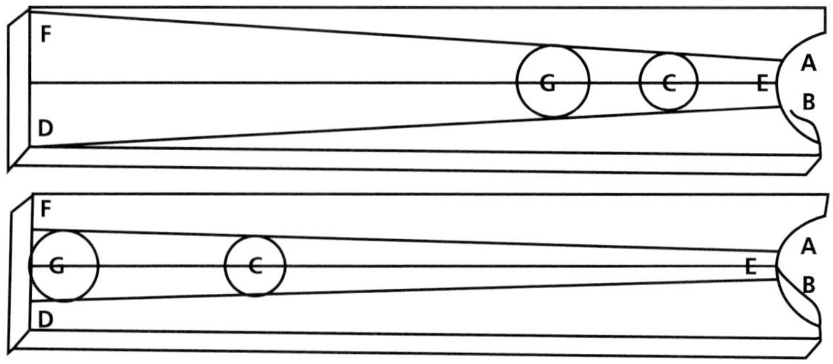

Figure 14.4 The figure from Della Porta's *De refractione* illustrating his experiment aimed at verifying the change of pupil size on a two cylinders occultation experiments inspired from Archimedes's method. Reproduced from Della Porta, G. D., *De Refractione optices parte libri novem*, Apud J.J. Carlinum et A. Pacem, 1593.

of different sizes. The experiment consists in finding the location of the two cylinders in which the smaller one, situated nearer to the eye, occludes the vision of the larger one. The procedure, carried out with only one eye open, is first done with the eye exposed to sunlight. Having drawn the lines tangent to the external borders of the circles of the two cylinders, the observer should repeat it 'in a dark place'. What happens—Della Porta says—is that 'in the dark the lines tangent to the circles are wider'.

Following these considerations, it is not difficult to envision the way by which Galileo was led to the winning trick that completely overturned the classical approaches to the estimation of star sizes based on variations of the diopter of Hipparchus. As mentioned in Chapter 13, these methods were generally founded on the attempt to measure the star size 'from outside', for instance, by moving a sliding rule bearing a hole, up to the point that the luminous globe of the star was just encircled by the circumference of the hole.[1] Galileo was led to conceive that much of the apparent luminosity of the stars was indeed produced inside the eye. Within this framework, it was evident that a method similar to that of the diopter provided a measure of a physiological phenomenon rather than of a physical object.

The success of the occultation method used by Galileo in the measurement of the size of stars depended on the fact that it relied only to a small extent on knowledge of the eye dioptrics. This was because, in the process of obscuring the star by the cord, the observer was required only to detect any light from the star; no other judgement about the appearance or intensity of this light was required. It could be said that this is a seen versus unseen procedure, involving what can be considered the most elementary visual task of light detection. Judgments of the presence or absence of a target are less demanding that those requiring a discrimination difference in its intensity. The same considerations on the difference between a detection or discrimination process apply to all sensory systems. In a rather amazing way, it is because of its elementary nature

[1] It is somewhat paradoxical that Tycho Brahe, the main authority on the measurement of the apparent size of the stars at Galileo's time, did not provide any detail of the method he used in his measurements. This is so despite the fact that in his *Progymnasmata*, in the place in which he lists the stars of different magnitudes, Tycho says that he measured the stars with great consideration ('diligenti adhibita consideratione': TOO, vol. 2, pp. 430–431). Some hint to the methods he used can be gathered, however, from his works (see Croslund, 1989; Strano, 2003).

that Galileo's experiment of stars measurement with a cord was successful, despite the many experimental drawbacks and the inappropriate theoretical framework of Galileo's optics.

14.2 An enduring and unshakable interest in vision

As we saw in Chapter 4, Galileo's interest in vision within an astronomical context continued until the last years of his life. His last published text was a long letter dealing with the dark light of the moon, or 'lunar candour'. This letter, originating from a discussion with the peripatetic philosopher Fortunio Liceti, was addressed in 1640 by Galileo to Prince Leopold of Tuscany and printed by Liceti in 1642 (the year of Galileo's death). Liceti inserted Galileo's text inside a book entitled *De lunae subobscura luce prope coniunctiones, & in Eclipsibus observata* ('On the dark light of the moon observed near conjunctions and in the Eclipses').

The dim light of the moon was not Galileo's only interest concerning observation and astronomy in his last years, as we have mentioned *en passant* in Chapter 13, with relation to the unpublished manuscript on the *Operazioni astronomiche*. He had started composing these texts after the last months of 1637, as we know particularly from a letter he sent on 5 November 1637 to Fulgenzio Micanzio, Sarpi's disciple and successor. From another letter dated 23 January of the following year and addressed by Galileo to Elia Diodati we are informed that he had been progressing in this task. However, the *Operazioni* were eventually left unfinished, with a blank page containing only the heading *Operazione settima* ('Seventh operation') after the sixth one (see Figure 14.5).

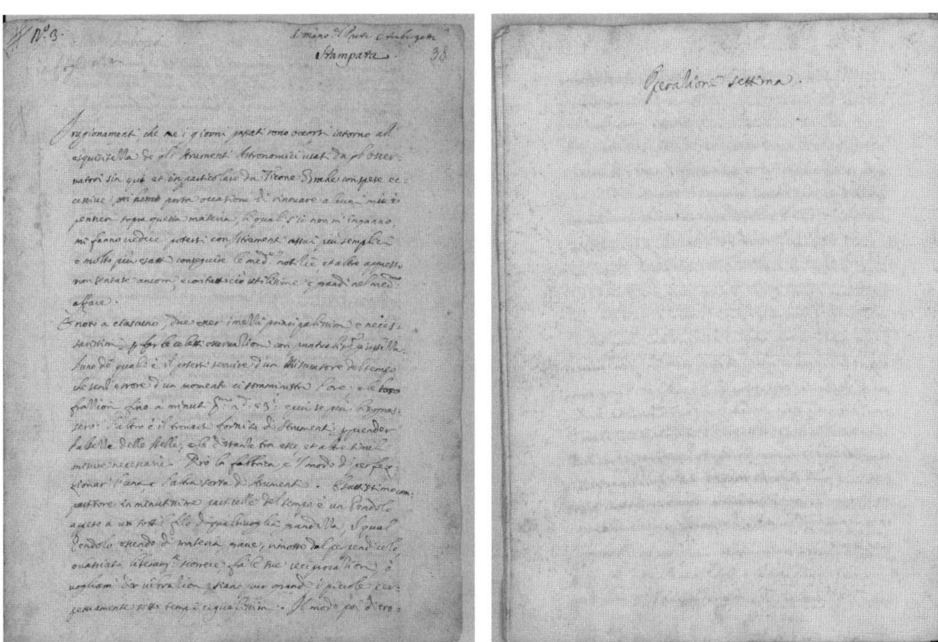

Figure 14.5 The first and last page of Galileo's manuscript *Operazioni astronomiche* with a blank page on the right corresponding to the seventh operation. The manuscript is a seventeenth-century transcription, not in Galileo's hand (BNF GAL 70, F38r and F46v; © Biblioteca Nazionale of Florence, Italy).

It is likely that the text of the *Operazioni* was conceived as material to be included in the Fifth Day (*Quinta giornata)* of the last masterpiece by Galileo, the *Discorsi e dimostrazioni matematiche intorno a due nuove scienze* ('Discourses and mathematical demonstrations concerning two new sciences') published in Leyden in 1638. This work is written in the form of a dialogue between the same three discussants, Salviati, Sagredo, and Simplicio, as in the 1632 *Dialogue concerning the two chief systems of the world.*

In Chapter 13 we have mentioned the *Operazioni astronomiche* with relation to the method used by Galileo for measuring the angular size of stars. It is worth considering the entire text of the *Operazioni*, and also the related writings extant among Galileo's manuscripts at the National Library of Florence. This is not only for their intrinsic importance but also because they show that in his approach to visual astronomy, Galileo persisted in an attitude largely independent on optical considerations even as Descartes was publishing his *Dioptrique* (and many years after Kepler's *Optica*).

Galileo's *Operazioni* were, however, far from being an outdated text by a scholar adhering to an old scientific methodology because of the difficulties he was experiencing in following the *nouvelle vague* of then current geometrical optics. On the contrary, with his text he was laying the foundations of a novel approach to astronomical observations—an approach potentially capable of exploiting fully the new possibilities offered by the telescope. It was based on the combination of the much finer visual resolution allowed by the new instrument with more precise techniques for the measurement of time. This approach would dominate observational astronomy after Galileo, and it is therefore unfortunate that he was unable to complete and publish his manuscript. His work may have been lost to scientific progress but it remains of interest to historians of science.

In the context of the historicity and factuality of the experiments and observations proposed by Galileo in his *Operazioni astronomiche* it must be said that very likely he was even unable to verify the feasibility of most of what he was proposing. This is because, while he was ruminating about the possibility of 'renewing some of [his] thoughts on this matter' his sight was declining in a very serious way. He announced 'the bad news of [his] imminent blindness' in the same letter in which he communicated to Micanzio his intention to write about the new astronomical operations he was contriving. These operations were conceived in order to achieve 'very subtle precisions, as to measure not only one degree or a prime or second minute of a degree, but even of a third or a fourth minute'. The bad news of his imminent blindness was, on the other hand, mitigated by the awareness of an otherwise general healthy body, with the consequent hope of being able 'to go along by putting down in writing various problems of mine and annotations [*postille*] in response to the main criticisms [*opposizioni*] written against me, and perhaps some other thoughts that by chance could come to my mind' (OG VIII, pp. 211–212).

14.3 **Two exact dividers of time and angles in minute particles**

Before proposing various methods of 'making celestial observations with a very punctual exactitude', Galileo describes how time could be measured with the precision needed for these observations. To such purpose it is first necessary to arrange a pendulum 'of length say of half a cubit or a palm [i.e. about 29 cm in Florentine units] and let it go by numbering patiently, for just one time, the oscillations elapsing during one natural day' (OG VIII, p. 454). A convenient way to do so is to use a 'very exquisite telescope' and point it at a fixed star when it is near the meridian, while the pendulum oscillates, and, with the telescope completely still, wait until the star exits from sight. At this precise instant the observer should start counting the oscillations, and continue to do so until the next night, waiting for the reappearance of the same star within the field of the telescope. He should stop counting exactly at the moment that the star exits again from the telescope field.

Galileo writes that, as an example, the number of oscillations (that he indicates usually as *vibrazioni*) 'in the time of the 24 natural hours might have been 280536'. This might indeed correspond to that of a pendulum of a palm length because, in standard conditions, the number of oscillations of a 1-metre pendulum is 86400, and to a good approximation the period of a pendulum is proportional to its length. We do not know, however, if he (or one of his collaborators) really carried out to completion this long and painstaking count; or simply he applied to his case the knowledge about the duration of the day and the laws of the pendulum that he had personally discovered.

Taking into account the number of oscillations in a day, it would have been simple—Galileo says—to find the difference of the right ascension between two stars, i.e. the angular distance between the two stars along the celestial equator. It sufficed to take into account (with the same pendulum) the time elapsing from the passage of the first star within the field of the telescope pointed towards the celestial meridian, until the passage of the second star.

A second instrument that Galileo proposes for performing very exact astronomical operations (with instruments which are at the same time 'considerably more simple and much more exact' than those currently performed with expensive tools) is a modified version of common astronomical devices like the sextant or quadrant. The modification should consist in greatly increasing the number of partitions existing within an angle of a degree, by using 'a small rod of the shape of a triangular prism' around which one should 'coil up a thin cord of a cither' or better 'a cord of a golden thread drawn through an extremely thin die' (p. 455). According to Galileo, with this method the resolution of the sextant or quadrant could be made very thin such as to allow the measurement of angular sizes in the order of the third minutes of a degree (i.e. less than 1/20,000 parts of a degree).

14.4 An astronomical operation among agricultural, economic, and domestic matters

In Chapter 8 we mentioned that some of the astronomical operations that Galileo proposed towards the end of his life were annotated outside the manuscript of the *Operazioni astronomiche*. Galileo probably wished to put some of them in the pages left blank in his notebook. Two descriptions of a method for measuring the angular size of the stars that was different from using the cord (to which the first and second sections of the *Operazioni* are dedicated) are worthy of note. As alluded to in the heading of the initial page, one of the descriptions of this alternative method was transcribed starting from an original contained in a bound collection of papers (now apparently lost) bearing the title: *Questo libro è di Niccolò di Francesco Arrighetti, sul quale farà alcuni ricordi in materia d'agricultura e d'economia e d'altre occorrenze domestiche* ('This is the book of Niccolò of Francesco Arrighetti, in which he will be writing some recollections on the subject of farming, economics and other domestic matters').

On 10 October 1638 Arrighetti writes:

> This day, I had the occasion to visit Sig. Galileo Galilei, supreme philosopher and mathematician and my friend, to whom I am very much obliged for that manner of discoursing that I have learned from him; finding myself, as I told, with this very great mind, he taught me a method [*problema*] found by him, of which I think it is necessary to make a record. This is to avoid the chance that, not being recorded by others, it could be lost. And despite that it does not concern matters of agriculture or

> economics, but exclusively of astronomy, nevertheless it would be here like a rose of diamonds or other precious gems could be in a vase containing flowers or natural fruits [*pomi naturali*], a rose that would stand among them in a way that it would be valued more than all. The problem is that: a very exquisite way to measure the diameter of the fixed stars. (OG VIII, pp. 464–465)

The way Galileo wishes to determine the angular size of a star is in fact a variation of the method based on the association of time and telescopic observations already suggested as a useful way to determine the angular separation of stars along the celestial equator. Basically it consists of measuring a phase of the transit of the star; it is the time the star is obscured behind an appropriate small board of rectangular shape (*una tavoletta*), located at an appropriate distance between the observer and the sky. From Arrighetti we know that a possible width of this screen could be 'a quarter of a cubit' (i.e. 14.54 cm). From him we also know that it is necessary to use a *cannoncino* (i.e. 'small cannon'), i.e. a telescope, possibly one of small magnification.

In describing the new method proposed by Galileo reference will be made mainly to the other extant description, that transcribed by Vincenzo Viviani, a student (and first biographer) of Galileo. This was derived from an original (also apparently lost) then in the possession of Galileo's son Vincenzio. It is likely that this is a more faithful rendering of Galileo's own words.

The particular interest of this second description is that it contains a figure useful for better understanding Galileo's proposal (see Figure 14.6). Interestingly, there is no mention at all in Viviani's transcription of the need for a telescope. Another difference is that in this second version there is the indication (absent in Arrighetti's account) that the pendulum should be 'adjusted such as to mark the prime minutes, the seconds etc'. This was evidently dictated by the brevity of the time to be measured, and suggests that Galileo might have been trying to contrive some device capable of measuring sub-seconds. We do not know what success he achieved, but let us now assume that he had a time measuring instrument endowed with the necessary precision and resolution.

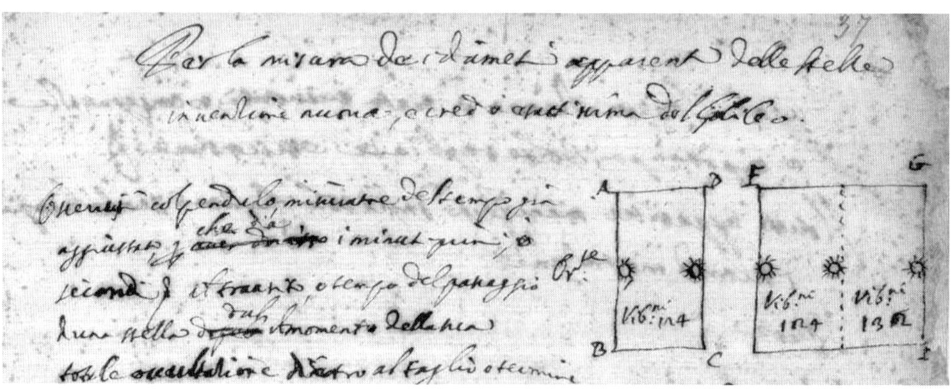

Figure 14.6 The beginning of one of the pages describing the method of the transit time contrived by Galileo to measure the angular size of a star. In the figure at the right of the page, ABCD and EGI are two small boards used for measuring the time that the star remains occulted during its transit, the width of the board on the right being exactly twice that on the left. The annotation inside the rectangles are abbreviations indicating, respectively Vibrations: 124, Vibrations: 124, and Vibrations: 132. On the left of the small rectangle is the abbreviation of *Oriente* (East). The dotted line cuts the rectangle at the right just at the middle, dividing it in two halves exactly equal in their width to the rectangle at the left (BNF GAL 70, F37r; © Biblioteca Nazionale of Florence, Italy).

Before translating in its entirety Viviani's transcription, it is noteworthy that a leitmotiv in Galileo's astronomical propositions during his last years was to consider the complete occultation of the celestial body to be investigated. In the case of the cord method this was achieved by finding out by trial and error the greatest separation of the eye from the cord in which the star disappeared completely. In the case of the experiments that we are considering now, a fundamental requirement to start counting the beats of the pendulum exactly when the star, approaching the target from the oriental side, is completely obscured, and to stop counting exactly at the moment of its first appearance on the occidental side.

But let us now read Galileo's words in Viviani's transcription which starts with the title, probably added by Viviani himself 'For the measurement of the apparent diameters of stars; a new invention, and I believe very exact of Galileo':

> Let one observe with the pendulum adjusted such as to mark the prime minutes, the seconds etc, the transit or passage time of a star from the moment of its total occultation behind the cut or extremity AB of the small board AC until the time of its first apparition out of the cut DC of the same small board, exposed to the air and distant from the eye always for the same length; let it be, for example, such passage time 124 vibrations of the pendulum. Afterwards, with another small board EF, exposed to the air at the same distance from the eye, but wider exactly by twice, let one observe again the passage time from the total occultation of the same star until the first apparition at the cut FG. One would find out that the number of the vibrations would be more than the double of the first number 124; and it would be, by example, 256, that is 8 vibrations in excess to the double. This number 8 will be the measure of the passage time of just the naked body of that star; having converted that time to a measure of angles, we will find the apparent diameter of the said star to be so many prime minutes or seconds etc. And if the small board would be triple or quadruple etc. than the first, the passage [of the star] through it would be more than triple and quadruple than the passage through the first; and such an excess will be the measure of the apparent diameter of the said star, taken so many times as is the multiplication factor of the said small board, with always the subtraction of one: that is, if the tablet is the triple of the first, the said excess would be two diameters [of the star]; if quadruple, it would give three, if quintuple, four, etc.; and as the multiplication factor ill increase until that given step, as much more exact will be the observation; and of that curiosity and consequence we could have more times the possibility of replicating and ascertaining. All appears manifest from the figure alone, without any need of other demonstration. (p. 466)

The page ends in an abrupt and somewhat enigmatic way, with a words '*Pure*', that can be have multiple meanings depending on the context ('nevertheless', 'on the other hand', or simply 'well').

Compared to the experiment with the cord, the new method contrived by Galileo was even less dependent on assumptions concerning the dioptrics of the eye. It depended on the most elementary aspect of vision, the process of detection of the presence or absence of a light (a process that in its essential dimensions can be effected even by a photoreceptor—natural or artificial—completely devoid of dioptric media). Galileo's new method was also less dependent on the quality of visual performance of the observer and on the exact state of focusing of the eye. This would be so provided that the small board used for the occultation was at a considerable distance from the observer, such as that the eye could be assumed to be accommodated to infinity (typically taken now as 6 metres). Moreover, the possibility of replicating the measure using boards of width larger than the unitary one by various multiplicative factors allowed for an averaging process capable of progressively reducing the statistical error of the measure at any reiteration.

The main difficulty with the new 'operation' concerned the resolution of the timing device. A simple calculation shows that it takes about 4 seconds for a star to move by 1 prime minute angular distance in the vault of the heavens along the equatorial direction. No doubt therefore that with this method Galileo could demonstrate that the currently accepted values of angular sizes for stars were greater than the real ones. This is because his pendulum was surely capable of resolving times of something less than 1 second. It is less granted though, that Galileo could arrive at angular resolutions of a few seconds of a degree. This is because the luminous image of a star would take about 60 milliseconds to make an angular displacement of one second of a degree. A time of 60 milliseconds was very likely beyond the reach of Galileo's 'very exquisite' method of measuring time. He could perhaps have approached, and possibly passed the resolution limit of the cord method, inasmuch an angular size of 5″ would correspond to a transit time of about 1/3 of a second.

Although Galileo concluded the description of his new 'operation' with the statement: 'all appears manifest from the figure alone, without any need of other demonstration', the fact that he terminated with the word *pure* suggests that he had perhaps doubts about the feasibility of the 'operation'.

We would like to imagine that this last and enigmatic word was indicating Galileo's intention to return to the subject, an intention that he could not put into effect probably because of the final decline of his sight.

14.5 **Investigating the constitution of the world by looking at the pyramid of a campanile**

Despite his declining sight (or perhaps because of it) in his last years Galileo was conceiving far-sighted 'astronomical operations' capable of providing information as to 'very great conclusions which draw with them greater consequences [*conclusioni massime, e che dietro si tirano conseguenze maggiori*]', as he wrote at the beginning of his *Operazione terza* ('Third operation'). (OG VIII, pp. 459–460). In this section he devises methods of observations of the sky basically similar to those already considered, but differing in the object used for occultation. Instead of a cord or a small board, he proposes the use of objects situated 'at very big distances [*lontananze massime*]'.

A first possibility—he writes—is 'to arrange on the top of a certain high mountain, some big [wooden] beam, situated at four, five cubits from the ground, and placed orthogonally with respect to the [celestial] meridian' (p. 459). This beam should be observed, from below on a plain at the south of the mountain, by observers who should wait until a star 'of those which revolve around the North pole' would happen to be obscured by the beam. They should then observe the star with a telescope at different times, possibly from a small shelter [*piccolo ricetto*]. If by chance the beam were to exactly hide the star, then the method would enable measurement of its angular size (following the same procedure of the cord experiment, but with the better precision offered by the telescopic observation). It could happen instead that from such a distance the wooden beam 'would intersect the disk of the star leaving a part above and a part below' (p. 459). In this was the case, by replicating the observations at different times they could possibly establish if there were 'some minimal titubation of the starred sphere'.

If, on the other hand, the angular size of the wooden beam were such as to exceed the angular size of the star, 'so that for a while it would remain hidden', then—Galileo says—we could arrive at the same important conclusion about possible movements in the sky through another way. This would be because 'our very precise measurer of time would show us whether the times of occultation of that [star] are always the same' (p. 459).

Probably inspired by the panorama of Florence, Galileo says that the same operations could be realized by finding 'a site where one could see some fixed star crossing the pyramid of some campanile' or perhaps 'the pinnacle of our Dome'.[2] Also in this case one could establish if there was some minimal change in the celestial appearances, by repeating at different moments the measurement of the occultation time of the star (starting always from the beginning of the total occultation and ending at the moment of the first reappearance).

In the *Operazione quarta* ('Fourth operation') Galileo suggests that comparable methods could be used to measure the time of occultation of the sun and moon and also of planets. In his opinion, this would allow the gathering of important information on their relative distances in various periods of time and thus the ability to follow their orbits. Very likely, his secret desire was that with these methods one could obtain useful indications to support the Copernican system.

14.6 **Looking at the oval sun at the horizon with a cord**

Galileo's virtuoso attitude in dealing with optics without invoking geometrical laws emerges in the *Operazione quinta* ('Fifth operation') devoted to the astronomical problem of refractions. As mentioned in Chapter 13, this was one of the main problems confronting astronomers of the time when trying to determine the position of celestial bodies, even though its history was much more ancient. Tycho Brahe had become particularly interested in them, and Kepler had written in his *Optica* that this was one of the reasons that led him to study vision and optics. In the sixteenth century the study of refractions had contributed to undermine the idea of the existence of solid, crystalline spheres.

Galileo himself was interested in the problem and he had correctly attributed the oval appearance of the sun at sunset to refractions. The method he proposed to resolve the problem of refractions was, however, totally independent of optical principles. At the outset of the 'Fifth operation', following the themes of a cosmological discussion dating at least since the debates between Brahe and the German astronomer Christoph Rothmann, Galileo remarks that two types of refractions could possibly interfere with the observation of stars and planets. One is due to the earth's atmosphere being responsible for the lightness of the sky before sunrise and after sunset. This type of refraction tends to be relatively constant. The other is due to 'more thick vapours that to a lesser altitude spread themselves in some particular part of the terrestrial globe' probably not arriving at the elevation where clouds, rains and winds are produced. A possibility to ascertain the role of these thick and low vapours would be to have, near the time of sunset, 'two observers, one on the top of a very high tower, or at the peak of an extremely high rock, and the other at the foot of the said tower or rock' (p. 462). With the use of the precise timing device, each of the two observers should measure the time needed for the sun to complete its disappearance below the horizon. If the thick and low vapours were to have an important role in the vision of sunset, the time of the disappearance could possibly be longer for the observer in the low location than for the other in the elevated position. 'And it could perhaps happen that the Sun showed itself plunged below the horizon first to the [observer] situated in a high position than to that situated in a low one' (pp. 462–463).

He also suggests that an accurate method for quantifying the effect of refraction at sunset could be to arrange one or more cords, aligned parallel to the line of horizon, one or more degrees above

[2] The original for 'pinnacle' in the manuscript (and in the printed text of Galileo's works) is *pergamena* (i.e. *parchemin*). This is very likely a wrong transcription of *pergamo* a word generically used in the Middle Ages to indicate an elevated site, and afterwards employed to indicate especially the monumental pulpit in historical cathedrals.

it, and calculate the time needed for the sun to pass across these cords in its movement leading eventually to its complete disappearance below the horizon.

14.7 The impossible final vision of an inquisitive and restless mind

Galileo could still imagine new visions of the world and 'see' the sky better than a normal-sighted peripatetic philosopher of his age. An example was Fortunio Liceti who—as repeatedly mentioned—in the very last years of Galileo's life engaged him in a debate on the cause of the dark light in the unilluminated face of the moon.

Galileo eventually accepted that, because of his declining sight, he could not personally perform experiments that depended on visual assessments. He had thus to abandon the ambitious proposals to investigate with a 'very exquisite precision' the sidereal spaces. We can see this from the *Proposizione sesta* ('Sixth proposition') where he suggests a method aimed at ascertaining the relative position of the stars and sun during the day, based on the fact that stars could be seen even during daytime with the telescope.[3] He goes on by saying that in the next *proposizione* (the seventh of the series) he will expound a method suitable for this task, that of establishing the position of 'a very exact meridian line'. However, as it appears from Figure 14.5, the page where the *Proposizione settima* should have been written, remained blank.

Galileo was still ruminating on new astronomical operations capable of providing, with simple methods, 'very admirable news' useful for understanding the real constitution of the cosmos. This was around October 1638 when he received the visit of his beloved former student, Benedetto Castelli.

These are the words that Castelli would write about one year later with relation to the 'eye of Galileo', in his *Discorso della visione*, within the context of a discussion on the diseases of vision and particularly blindness:

> Of that disease I cannot treat, nor discourse, but with a feeling of very deep pain, because nowadays it has struck the noblest eye which nature ever made. I say the eye of Signor Galileo Galilei, first Philosopher of the Most Serene Grand Duke of Tuscany; an eye so privileged, and gifted with such rare powers, that it may be said with truth to have seen more than the eyes of all that are gone; and to have opened the eyes of all that are to come. Because it was only to him to make all the celestial discoveries to be admired in the future centuries in the Milky Way, in the nebulae, in the Medicean planets, in Saturn, in Jupiter, in Mars, in Venus, in the Moon and in the Sun itself. It is therefore to be preserved for ever, as a precious gem; and more so because it was the minister of his wonderful mind, exciting him to speculate so highly about the things, whereby he has exceeded any human intelligence, which until now has been involved in penetrating the most recondite secrets of Nature; a loss so pernicious, and to be deplored with the universal tears of all human eyes, and particularly of the legitimate investigators of truth. (Castelli, 1669, pp. 11–12)

If we were allowed to borrow the words by which, at the end of the First Day of the *Dialogue*, Sagredo concludes the praise of the 'admirable human inventions', arriving to this point we could perhaps say:

Let Castelli's praise of Galileo's eye be the ending to our book.

---

[3] This method was based on the fact that a telescope admits more light than the eye, and also on the possibility of restricting the field of view and thus avoid the light adaptation caused by peripheral light extraneous to the observation field.

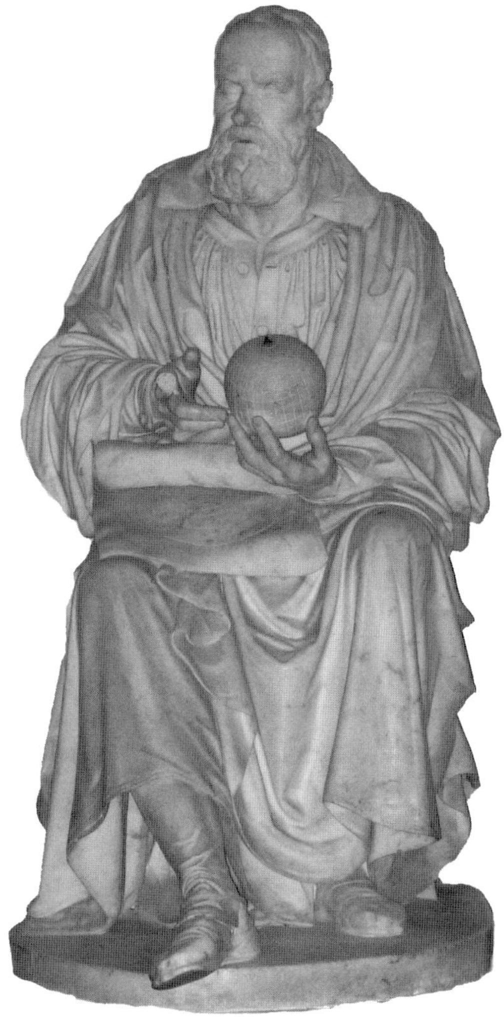

Figure 14.7 *Solidity and chiaroscuro in Galileo* by Nicholas Wade. A photograph of Emilio Demi's statue of Galileo which stands at the rear of the Aula Magna Storica, University of Pisa. Galileo is holding a globe in his left hand with a scroll of astronomical designs on his lap. This statue was realized following a public fund-raising on the occasion of the 'First Meeting of Italian Scientists' held in Pisa in 1839.

References

Accolti, P. (1625). *Lo inganno degl'occhi, prospettiva pratica*. Firenze, Cecconcelli.

Adams, W. (1932). A note on Galileo's determination of the height of lunar mountains. *Isis* **17**: 427–429.

Aguilonius, F. (1613). *Opticorum libri sex, philosophis iuxta ac mathematicis utiles*. Antverpiæ, ex offina Plantiniana apud viduam et filios Io. Moreti.

Airy, G. B. (1835). On the diffraction of an object-glass with circular aperture. *Transactions of the Cambridge Philosophical Society* **5**: 283–291.

Alberti, L. B. (1980). *Ludi matematici*. R. Rinaldi ed. Milano, Guanda.

Albertus De Saxonia. (1497). *Questiones subtilissime Alberti de Saxonia in libros de celo et mundo*. Venetiis, Otinus de Luna, Papiensis.

Aquapendente, F. ab (1600). *De Visione, voce, auditu*. Venetiis, apud F. Bolzettam.

Archimedes. (1544). *Archimedis Syracvsani Opera quæ quidem extant....* Basileae, Ioannes Heruagius excudi fecit.

Archimedes. (1667). *Des unvergleichlichen Archimedis Sand-Rechnung, oder, Diessinnige Erfindung einer, mit verwunderlicher Leichtigkeit aussprechlicher Zahl*. J. C. Sturm & P. Fürst trans. Nürnberg, In Verlegung P. Fürstens.

Arago, F. (1856). *Astronomie populaire*, Vol. 3. Paris, Gide et J. Baudry.

Ariotti, P. E. (1973). A little known early seventeenth century treatise on vision: Benedetto Castelli's Discorso sopra la vista. *Annals of Science* **30**: 1–30.

Ausonio, E. Theorica Speculi Concavi Sphaerici, Manuscript, Biblioteca Nazionale di Firenze, Gal. 83, f. 4r. (Reprinted and translated in Dupré, S. (2002). *Galileo, the telescope, and the science of optics in the sixteenth century, a case study of instrumental practice in art and science*. Thesis, University of Ghent.)

Babuchin, A. I. (1876). Uebersicht der neueren Untersuchungen über Entwicklung, Bau und physiologische Verhältnisse der elektrischen und pseudoelektrischen Organe. *Archiv für Anatomie, Physiologie und wissenschaftliche Medicin* 501–542.

Bacon, F. (1609). *De sapientia veterum*. Londini, Robertus Bakerus.

Barbaro, D. (1569). *La pratica della perspettiva... opera molto utile a pittori, a scultori, & ad architetti*. Venetia, Camillo & Rutilio Borgominieri.

Barrow, I. (1669) *Lectiones XVIII, Cantabrigiæ in Scholis Publicis Habitæ...* Londini, Typis Gulielmi Godbid.

Beare, J. I. (1906). *Greek theories of elementary cognition from Alcmaeon to Aristotle*. Oxford, Clarendon.

Bell, C. (1811). *Idea of a new anatomy of the brain; submitted for the observations of his friends*. London, published by the author; printed by Strahan and Preston. (Reprinted in N. J. Wade ed. (2000). *The emergence of neuroscience in the nineteenth century*. Vol. 1. London, Routledge/Thoemmes Press.)

Bethune, J. E. D. (1829). *The life of Galileo Galilei*: with illustrations of the advancement of experimental philosophy. London, Clowes.

Bettini, M. (1642). *Apiaria universae philosophiae mathematicae....* Bononiae, Ferronius.

Brahe, T. (1913). *Tychonis Brahe Dani Opera omnia*. J. L. E. Dreyer, ed. Hauniæ, in Libraria Gyldendaliana.

Brecht, B. (1955). *Leben des Galilei*. Berlin, Suhrkamp Verlag. (English edition by Desmond I. Vesey in Brecht, B. (1967). *The life of Galileo*. London, Methuen.)

Bredekamp, H. (2009). *Galileis "Sidereus Nuncius" unter dem Mikroskop jüngste Forschungen zu einem enigmatischen Buch*. Heidelberg, Universitätsverwaltung.

Bredekamp, H., Brüle, I., & Needham, P. (2011). *Galileo's O.* Berlin, Akademie Verlag.

Bucciantini, M., Camerota, M., & Giudice, F. (2012). *Il telescopio di Galileo, Una storia europea.* Torino, Einaudi.

Cahan, D. ed. (1994). *Hermann von Helmholtz and the foundations of nineteenth-century science.* Berkeley, CA, University of California Press.

Cajori, F. (1929). History of determinations of the heights of mountains. *Isis* **12**: 482–514.

Calvino, I. (1988). *Lezioni americane, Sei proposte per il prossimo millennio.* Milano, Garzanti.

Camerota, F. (2010). *Linear perspective in the age of Galileo Ludovico Cigoli's Prospettiva pratica.* Firenze, L. S. Olschki.

Campbell, F. W. & Gubisch, R. W. (1966). Optical quality of the human eye. *Journal of Physiology* (London) **186**: 558–578.

Campani, G. (1664). *Ragguaglio di due nuove osservazioni, una celeste in ordine alla stella di Saturno, e terrestre l'altra, in ordine a gl' istrumenti medesimi, co' quali s'è fatta l'una e l'altra osservazione....* Roma, F. de Falco.

Casseri, G. C. (1600–1601). *De vocis auditusque organis historia anatomica singulari fide methodo ac industria concinnata....* Ferrariae, Excudebat Victorius Baldinus, typographus Cameralis.

Castelli, B. (1669). *Alcuni opuscoli filosofici del padre abbate D. Benedetto Castelli da Brescia... non più stampati.* Bologna, Per gli Heredi del Dozza.

Cellarius, A. (1661). *Harmonia macrocosmica, seu Atlas universalis et novis.* Amstelodami, apud Joannem Janssonium.

Cigoli [Ludovico Cardi] (*c.*1610). *Prospettiva pratica di fra Lodovico Cardi... dimostrata con tre regole...* [Manuscript]. Gabinetto disegni e stampe degli Uffizi, Firenze, ms. 2660A.

Clavius, C. (1581). *Gnomonices libri octo.* Romae, Apud Franciscum Zanettum.

Clavius, C. (1593). *Astrolabium.* Romae, impensis Bartholomaei Grassi, ex typographia Gabiana.

Clavius, C. (1602). *Christophori Clauii Bamb. ex Societate Iesu, in sphæram Ioannis de Sacro Bosco, commentarius.* Lugduni, Sumptibus Joannis de Gabiano.

Commandino, F. (1558). *Archimedis Opera non nulla.* Venetiis, Apud Paulum Manutium.

Commandino, F. (1566). *Apollonii Pergaei Conicorvm libri qvattvor.* Bononiae, ex officina A. Benatii.

Conti, L. (1990). *Francesco Stelluti, Il copernicanesimo dei Lincei e la teoria galileiana delle maree,* in *Galileo e Copernico,* Alle origini del pensiero scientifico moderno, C. Vinti ed. Assisi, Porziuncola.

Copernicus, N. (1543). *De revolutionibus orbium coelestium, libri VI.* Norimbergæ, Apud Ioh. Petreium.

Cusanus, N. (1990). *Nicholas of Cusa, On learned ignorance: a translation and an appraisal of De docta ignorantia.* J. Hopkins, ed. Minneapolis, MN, Arthur J. Benning Press.

Danti, E. (1573). *La Prospettiva Di Evclide nella quale si tratta di quelle cose, che per raggi diritti si veggono....* Fiorenza, Giunti.

Daxecker, F. (2004). *The physicist and astronomer Christopher Scheiner : biography, letters, works.* Innsbruck, Leopold-Franzens-University of Innsbruck.

Daza De Valdés, B. (1623). *Uso de los antoios para todo genero de vistas....* Sevilla, Diego Perez.

De Dominis, M. A. (1611). *De radiis visus et lucis in vitris perspectiuis et iride.* Venetiis, Thomas Baglionum.

Della Porta, G. D. (1593). *De Refractione optices parte libri novem.* Neapoli, Apud J. J. Carlinum et A. Pacem.

Delle Colombe, L. (1606). *Discorso di Lodovico delle Colombe nel quale si dimostra, che la nuoua stella apparita l'ottobre passato 1604...* Firenze, Nella stamperia de' Givnti.

Descartes, R. (1637). *Discours de la methode pour bien conduire sa raison, & chercher la verité dans les sciences: plus la dioptriqve; les meteores; et la geometrie; qui sont des essais de cete methode.* A Leyde, De l'imprimerie de Ian Maire.

Devalois, R. L., Morgan, H., & Snodderly, D. M. (1974). Physiological studies of monkey vision. III. Spatial luminance contrast sensitivity tests of macaque and human observers. *Vision Research* **14**: 75–81.

Digges, L. & Digges, T. (1576). *A prognostication euerlasting of right good effect fruitfully augmented by the auctor, contayning plaine, brief, pleasaunt, chosen rules to iudge the weather by the sunne, moone, starres, cometes, rainebow, thunder, cloudes.* Aldbrough, St John Publications. (The appendix contains Thomas Digges's *A Perfit Description of the Cælestiall Orbes.. .*)

Drake, S. & O'Malley, C. D. eds. (1960). *The controversy of the comets of 1618.* Philadelphia, PA, University of Pennsylvania Press,

Duhem, P. M. M. (1913–1959). *Le système du monde; histoire des doctrines cosmologiques de Platon à Copernic.* 10 vols. Paris, A. Hermann.

Duhem, P. M. M.. (1985). *Medieval cosmology: theories of infinity, place, time, void, and the plurality of worlds.* R. Ariew transl. & ed. Chicago, IL, University of Chicago Press.

Dupré, S. (2002). *Galileo, the telescope, and the science of optics in the sixteenth century, a case study of instrumental practice in art and science.* Thesis, University of Ghent.

Dupré, S. (2005). Ausonio's mirrors and Galileo's lenses: the telescope and sixteenth-century practical optical knowledge. *Galilaeana* **2**: 145–180.

Dürer, A. (1525). *Underweysung der Messung, mit dem Zirckel unnd richt scheyt, in Linien ebnen unnd gantzen Corporen.* Nuremberg [s.n.].

Fahie, J. J. (1926). Memorials of Galileo Galilei, 1564–1642. Portraits and paintings, medals and medallions, busts and statues, monuments and mural inscriptions. Leamington and London, Printed for the author.

Faraday, M. (1861). A course of six lectures on the chemical history of a candle. London, Griffin, Bohn.

Finger, S. & Piccolino, M. (2011). *The shocking history of electric fishes: from ancient epochs to the birth of modern neurophysiology.* New York, Oxford University Press.

Finger, S. & Wade, N. J. (2002a). The neuroscience of Helmholtz and the theories of Johannes Müller. Part I: Nerve cell structure, vitalism, and the nerve impulse. *Journal of the History of the Neurosciences* **11**: 136–155.

Finger, S. & Wade, N. J. (2002b). The neuroscience of Helmholtz and the theories of Johannes Müller. Part 2: Sensation and perception. *Journal of the History of the Neurosciences* **11**: 234–254.

Finocchiaro, M. A. (1989). *The Galileo affair a documentary history.* Berkeley, CA, University of California Press.

Galilei, G. (1605). *Dialogo de Cecco di Ronchitti da Bruzene in perpuosito de la stella nuova.* Padova, Tozzi.

Galilei, G. (and possibly Spinelli, G.) (1605). *Dialogo de Cecco di Ronchitti… in perpuosito de la stella nuova….* Padova, Appresso Pietro Paulo Tozzi.

Galilei, G. (1606a). *Considerazioni d' Alimberto Mauri sopra alcuni luoghi del discorso di Lodovico delle Colombe intorno alla stella apparita 1604.* Firenze, appresso Gio. Antonio Caneo.

Galilei, G. (1606b). *Le operazioni del compasso geometrico et militare.* Padova, In casa dell'Autore, per P. Marinelli.

Galilei, G. (1612). *Discorso al serenissimo don Cosimo II, gran duca di Toscana: intorno alle cose, che stanno in sù l'acqua: ò che in quella si muovono.* Firenze, Apresso Cosimo Giunti.

Galilei, G. (1613). *Istoria e dimostrazioni intorno alle macchie solari e loro accidenti: comprese in tre lettere scrite all' illustrissimo signor Marco Velseri linceo, duumviro d'Augusta, consigliero di sua Maestà Cesarea.* Roma, Appresso Giacomo Mascardi.

Galilei, G. (1623). *Il Saggiatore: nel quale con bilancia esquisita e giusta si ponderano le cose contenute nella libra astronomica e filosofica di Lotario Sarsi.* Roma, Appresso Giacomo Mascardi.

Galilei, G. (1632). *Dialogo… sopra i due massimi sistemi del mondo Tolemaico, e Copernicano….* Fiorenza, Per Gio: Batista Landini.

Galilei, G. (1638). *Discorsi e dimostrazioni matematiche: intorno à due nuove scienze attenenti alla mecanica & i movimenti locali….* Leida, Appresso gli Elsevirii.

Galilei, G. (1890–1909). *Le opere di Galileo Galilei. Edizione nazionale sotto gli auspicii di Sua Maestà il re d'Italia.* A. Favaro ed., 20 vols. Firenze, Tip. di G. Barbèra.

Galileo, G. & Guiducci, M. (1619). *Discorso delle comete di Mario Guiducci*. Firenze, Cecconcelli.

Galluzzi, P. (2011). *Tra atomi e indivisibili: la materia ambigua di Galileo*. Firenze, L. S. Olschki.

Gardner, E. P. &. Martin, J. H. (2000). Coding of sensory information. In *Principles of neural science*, 4th ed. E. R. Kandel, J. H. Schwartz, & T. M. Jessell eds. New York, McGraw-Hill, pp. 411–429.

Garin, E. (1961). Il problema delle fonti del pensiero di Leonardo. In *La cultura filosofica del Rinascimento italiano*. Firenze, Sansoni, pp. 388–401.

Gemma Frisius, R. (1545). *Gemmae Frisii Medici et Mathematici, De Radio Astronomico & Geometrico....* Antuerpiae, Gregorius Bontius.

Gilchrist, A. (2006). *Seeing black & white*. New York, Oxford University Press

Goldstein, B. R. (1985). *The astronomy of Levi ben Gerson (1288-1344): a critical edition of chapters 1-20 with translation and commentary*. New York, Springer-Verlag.

Goldstein, B. R. (1987). *Remarks on Gemma Frisius's De Radio Astronomico et Geometrico*. In *From Ancient Omens to Statistical Mechanics: Essays on the Exact Sciences Presented to Asger Aaboe*, J. L. Berggren and Bernhard R. Goldstein. edrs. *Copenhagen*, University Library.

Goldstein, B. R (1991). Levi Ben Gerson: on astronomy and physical experiments. In *Physics, Cosmology and Astronomy, 1300-1700: Tension and Accommodation*. S. Unguru Ed. Dordrecht, Kluwer Academic Publishers, pp. 75–82.

Grassi, O. (1619a). *De tribus cometis anni M. DC. XVIII: disputatio astronomica publice habita in Collegio Romano Societatis Iesv*. Romae, Ex typographia Iacobi Mascardi.

Grassi, O. (1619b). *Libra astronomica ac philosophica....* Perusiæ, Ex typographia M. Naccarini.

Gregory, R. L. (2005). *Eye and brain. The psychology of seeing*, 5th ed. New York, Oxford University Press.

Grienberger, C. (1612). *Catalogus veteres affixarum longitudines ac latitudines conferens cum novis*. Romae, apud B. Zannettum.

Grisellini, F. (1761). *Memorie anedote spettanti alla vita ed agli studi del sommo filosofo e giureconsulto f. Paolo [Sarpi] Servita*. Helmstat, Jacopo Mulleri.

Grisellini, F. (1785). *Del genio di f. Paolo Sarpi in ogni facoltà scientifica e nelle dottrine* 2. vols. Venezia, appresso Leonardo Bassaglia al Segno della nuova salamandra.

Gualdo, P. (1607). *Vita Joannis Vincentii Pinelli patricii Genuensis*. Augustae Vindelicorum, Christophorus Mangus.

Haskell, P. T. (1960). Sound production. In *The physiology of insects*. M. Rockstein ed. New York, Academic Press, pp. 563–608.

Hatfield, G. (2011). *Kant and Helmholtz on Primary and Secondary Qualities*. In *Primary and secondary qualities: the historical and ongoing debate*. L. Nolan ed. New York, Oxford University, pp. 304–337.

Helmholtz, H. (1867). *Handbuch der physiologischen Optik*. Leipzig, Voss.

Helmholtz, H. (1895). Popular lectures on scientific subjects. London, Longmans, Green.

Helmholtz, H. (1896). Handbuch der physiologischen Optik. 2nd ed. Hamburg, Voss.

Helmholtz, H. (1924). Helmholtz's Treatise on physiological optics.Vol. 2. J. P. C. Southall trans. New York, Optical Society of America.

Helmholtz, H. (1925). *Helmholtz's Treatise on physiological optics*. Vol. 3. J. P. C. Southall trans. New York: Optical Society of America.

Kant, I. (1787). *Critik der reinen Vernunft*. Riga, Hartknoch.

Kemp, M. (1990). *The science of art. Optical themes in Western Art from Brunelleschi to Seurat*. New Haven, CT, Yale University Press.

Kepler, J. (1606). *De stella nova in pede Serpentarii*. Pragae, typis P. Sessli, impensis authoris.

Kepler, J. (1610). *Dissertatio cum Nuncio sidereo nuper ad mortales misso Galilaeo Galilaeo*. Florentiae, Antonium Caneum.

Kepler, J. (1634). *Somnium, seu Opus posthumum De astronomia lunari*. Sagani Silesiorum, absolutum, Francofurti, Sumptibus haeredum Authoris.

Knight, C. (1834). The gallery of portraits with memoirs. Vol. 3. London, Knight.

La Galla, G. C. (1612). *De phoenomenis in orbe lunae novi telescopii usu a D. Gallil. Gallileo nunc iterum suscitatis physica disputatio: necnon de luce et lumine, Altera disputatio*. Venetiis, apud Thomas Balionum.

Lejeune, A. (1947). La dioptre d' Archimede. *Annates de la Société Scientifique de Bruxelles*, series 1, **61**: 27–47.

Lejeune, A. (1948). *Euclide et Ptolémée: deux stades de l'optique géométrique grecque*. Louvain, Bibliothéque de l'Université, Bureaux du "Recueil".

Lejeune, A. (1989). *L'Optique de Claude Ptolémée dans la version Latine d'après l'Arabe de l´Émir Eugène de Sicile*. Leiden, Brill.

Leonardo. (1956). *Treatise on painting [Codex urbinas latinus 1270]*. A. P. Mcmahon ed. Princeton, NJ, Princeton University Press.

Leopardi, G. (1827). *Crestomazia italiana, cioè, Scelta di luoghi insigni o per sentimento o per locuzione raccolti dagli scritti italiani in prosa*. Milano, Stella.

Liceti, F. (1640). *Litheosphorus, sive de lapide Bononiensi lucem in se conceptam ab ambiente claro mox in tenebris mire conservante: liber*. Utini, Ex Typographia Nicolai Schiratti.

Liceti, F. (1642). *De lunae subobscura luce prope coniunctiones, & in eclipsibus obseruata libros tres: in quibus ad opticen, astronomiam, physiologiam, & alias disciplinas attinentia plurima dogmata pulchra & difficilia diligenter explicantur*. Utini, Typis Nicolai Schiratii.

Lindberg, D. C. (1970). *John Pecham and the science of optics: Perspectiva communis*. Madison, WI, University of Wisconsin Press.

Lindberg, D. C. (1976). *Theories of vision from al-Kindi to Kepler*. Chicago, IL, University of Chicago Press.

Lissmann, H. W. (1951). Continuous electric signals from the tail of a fish, *Gymnarchus niloticus* Cuv. *Nature* **167**: 201.

Lissmann, H. W. & Machin, K. E. (1958). The mechanism of object location in Gymnarchus niloticus and similar fish. *Journal of the Experimental Biology* **35**: 451–486.

Locke, J. (1690). *An essay concerning humane understanding in four books*. London: Printed for Tho. Basset, and sold by Edw. Mory.

Lohrmann, W. G. & Schmidt, J. F. J. (1878). *Mondcharte in 25 Sectionen und 2 Erläuterungstafeln: mit Erläuterungen und selenographischen Ortsbestimmungen*.... Leipzig, Barth.

Lomazzo, G. P. (1585). *Trattato dell'arte della pittura, scoltura, et architettura*. Milano, per Paolo Gottardo Pontio...a instantia di Pietro Tini.

Lucretius, T. C. (2004). *On the nature of things*. W. E. Leonard trans. New York, Dover.

Lupicini, A. (1582). *Discorso sopra la fabrica: e uso delle nuove verghe astronomiche*. Fiorenza, appresso Giorgio Marescotti.

Mach, E. (1926). *The principles of physical optics; an historical and philosophical treatment*. John S. Anderson & A. F. A. Young transl. London, Methuen & Co.

Macrobius, A. T. (1848). *Macrobii Ambrosii Theodosii Commentarii in Ciceronis somnium Scipionis*. Ludovicus Ianus ed. Quedlinburgi et Lipsiae, Typis et sumptibus, Godofredi Bassii.

Maestlin, M. (1596). *Disputatio de eclipsibus solis et lunae, quam; divina favente gratia: praeside clarissimo viro*. Tubingae, Apud Georgium Gruppenbachium.

Mancha, J. L. (1992). Astronomical use of pinhole images in William of Saint-Cloud's Almanach Planetarum (1292). *Archive for History of Exact Sciences* **43**: 275–298.

Maurolico, F. (1611). *Photismi de lumine, & umbra ad perspectivam, & radiorum incidentiam facientes*. Neapoli, Longus.

Maurolico, F. (1613). *Theoremata de lumine, et umbra, ad perspectiuam, & radiorum incidentiam facientia. Diaphanorum partes, seu, Libri tres... Problemata ad perspectivam & iridem pertinentia*. Lugduni, Apud Ludouicum Hurillion.

May, M. T. (1968). *Galen, On the usefulness of the parts of the body.* Ithaca, NY, Cornell University Press.

McMurrich, J. P. (1930). Leonardo da Vinci the anatomist (1452–1519). Baltimore, Williams & Wilkins.

Micanzio, F. (1646). *Vita del Padre Paolo dell'Ordine de' Servi e theologo della Serenissima.* Leidaa [s.n.]

Millosevich, E. (1919). Leonardo e la luce cinerea. In *Per il IV centenario della morte di Leonardo da Vinci.* M. Cermenati ed. Bergamo, Istituto italiano d'arti grafiche, pp. 17–19.

Moller, P. (1995). *Electric fishes, history and behaviour.* London, Chapman & Hall.

Müller, J. (1840). *Handbuch der Physiologie des Menschen für Vorlesungen,* 3 vol. Coblenz, Hölscher.

Newton, I. (1671/1672). A letter of Mr. Isaac Newton, Professor of the Mathematicks in the University of Cambridge; containing his new theory about light and colors. *Philosophical Transactions of the Royal Society of London* **6**: 3075–3087.

Newton, I. (1704). Opticks: or, A treatise on the reflections, refractions, inflections and colours of light. London, Smith and Walford.

Panofsky, E. (1954). *Galileo as a critic of the arts.* The Hague, M. Nijhoff.

Parronchi, A. (1964). Della prospettiva di Paolo del Pozzo Toscanelli. In *Studi su la Dolce Prospettiva.* Milano: Aldo Martello Editore, pp. 533–641.

Pena, J. (1557). *Euclidis Optica & catoptrica.* Parisiis, Ex officina Andreae Wecheli.

Peurbach, G. V., Reinhold, E., & Ptolemy. (1542). *Theoricae novae planetarum Georgii Purbacchii Germani.* Impressus hic theoricarum libellus Vitembergae, Per Ioannem Lufft.

Piccolino, M. (2003). *The taming of the ray: electric fish research in the Enlightenment from John Walsh to Alessandro Volta.* Firenze, L. S. Olschki.

Piccolino, M. & Bresadola, M. (2003). *Rane, torpedini e scintille: Galvani, Volta e l'elettricità animale.* Torino, Bollati Boringhieri.

Piccolino, M. & Bresadola, M. (2013). *Shocking frogs, Galvani, Volta and the electric origins of neuroscience.* N. J. Wade transl. Oxford, Oxford University Press.

Platter, F. (1583). *De corporis humani structura et usu: libri III.* Basileae, ex Officina Frobeniana.

Plutarch. (1968). *Plutarch's Moralia: in fifteen volumes.* vol. 12. H. Cherniss & W. C. Helmbold transl. & ed. London: W. Heinemann.

Prickard, A. O. (1911). Plutarch on the face which appears on the orb of the moon. London, Simpkin.

Ravaisson-Mollien, C. (1889). Les Manuscrits de Léonardo de Vinci, Manuscrits F et I de la Bibliothèque de l'Institut. Paris, Quantin.

Reeves, E. A. (1997). *Painting the heavens: art and science in the age of Galileo.* Princeton, NJ, Princeton University Press.

Reeves, E. A. & Van Helden, A. (2010). *On sunspots.* Chicago, IL, University of Chicago Press.

Riccioli, G. B. (1651). *Almagestum novum astronomiam veterem novamque complectens.* Bononiae, Typographia haeredis Victorii Benatii.

Rippa Bonati, M. & Pardo-Tomás, J. eds. (2004). *Il teatro dei corpi. Le pitture colorate d'anatomia di Girolamo Fabrici d'Acquapendente.* Milano, MediaMed.

Risner, F. (1572). *Opticae thesaurus.* Basileae, Per Episcopios.

Robin, C. (1865). Mémoir sur la démonstration expérimentale de la production d'électricité par un appareil propre aux poissons du genre des raies. *Journal de l'Anatomie et de la Physiologie* **23** : 577–645.

Rodieck, R. W. (1998). *The first steps in seeing.* Sunderland, MA, Sinauer Associates.

Rosen, E. (1965). *Kepler's conversation with Galileo's Sidereal Messenger: first complete translation.* New York, Johnson Reprint Corporation.

Roslund, C. (1989). Tycho Brahe's innovations in instrument design. *Bulletin of the Scientific Instrument Society* **22**: 2–4.

Ross, D. W. (1931). *The works of Aristotle.*Vol. 3. Oxford, Oxford University Press.

Ross, H. & Plug, C. (2002). *The mystery of the moon illusion.* Oxford, Oxford University Press.

Sabra, A. I. (1967). The authorship of the *Liber de crepusculis*, an eleventh-century work on atmospheric refraction. *Isis* **58**: 77–85.

Sabra, A. I. ed. & trans. (1989). *The Optics of Alhazen. Books I-III. On direct vision.* London, The Warburg Institute.

Sarpi, P. (1619). *Historia del Concilio Tridentino.* Londra, Appresso Giovan, Billio.

Sarpi, P. (1961). *Lettere ai Gallicani.* B. Ulianich ed. Wiesbaden, F. Steiner.

Sarpi, P. (1996). *Pensieri naturali, metafisici e matematici.* L. Cozzi & L. Sosio eds. Milano, Ricciardi.

Scheiner, C. (1612a). *Tres epistolæ de maculis solaribus: scriptæ ad Marcum Velserum.* Augustae Vindelicorum, Ad Insigne Pinus.

Scheiner, C. (1612b). *De maculis solaribus et stellis circa Iovem errantibus, accuratior disqvisitio ad Marcum Velserum.* Augustae Vindelicorum, Ad Insigne Pinus.

Scheiner, C. (1619). *Oculus hoc est: fundamentum opticum....* Oeniponti, Apud Danielem Agricolam.

Scheiner, C. (1630). *Rosa Ursina sive sol: ex admirando facularum & macularum suarum phaenomeno varius, necnon circa centrum suum & axem fixum... mobilis ostensus.* Bracciani, Phaeus.

Scheiner, C. & Locher, J. G. (1614). *Disquisitiones mathematicæ, de controuersiis et nouitatibus astronomicis.* Igolstadii, Ex Typographeo Ederiano apud Elisabetham Angermariam.

Shapiro, E. (1975). Archimedes's measurement of the sun's apparent diameter. *Journal of the History of Astronomy* **6**: 75–83.

Schmitz, E.-H. (1981). Handbuch der Geschichte der Optik. Vol. 1. Bonn, Wayerborgh.

Smith, A. M. ed. & transl. (1996). *Ptolemy's theory of visual perception: An English translation of the Optics with introduction and commentary.* Philadelphia, PA, American Philosophical Society.

Smith, A. M. (2001). *Alhacen's theory of visual perception.* Philadelphia, PA, American Philosophical Society.

Smith, L. P. (1907). *The life and letters of Sir Henry Wotton.* Oxford, Clarendon Press.

Snellius, W. (1621). *Willebrordi Snellii... Cyclometricus, de circuli dimensione secundum logistarum abacos et ad mechanicem accuratissima.* Lugduni Batavorum, ex officina Elzeviriana.

Stark. J. (1844). On the existence of an electrical apparatus in the flapper skate and other rays. *Proceedings of the Royal Society of Edinburgh* **25** (Vol. 2): 1–3.

Straker, S. (1981). Kepler, Tycho, and the 'Optical Part of Astronomy': the Genesis of Kepler's Theory of Pinhole Images. *Archives for the History of Exact Sciences* **24**: 267–293.

Strano, G. (2003). *Claudio Tolomeo e Tycho Brahe: tradizione e innovazione negli strumenti per l'osservazione astronomica.* PhD Dissertation, University of Florence.

Strano, G. (2007). Strumenti alessandrini per l'osservazione astronomica: Tolomeo e la Mathematiké syntaxis. *Automata* **2**:79–92.

Stratton, G. M. (1917). *Theophrastus and the Greek physiological psychology before Aristotle.* Amsterdam, E. J. Bonset, P. Schippers.

Tarde, J. (1984). *A la rencontre de Galilée: deux voyages en Italie.* F. Moureau & M. Tetel eds. Genève, Slatkine.

Tongiorgi Tomasi, L. (2005). Capitolo contro il portar la toga di Galileo Galilei. Pisa, Edizioni ETS.

Vignola, G. B., *da.* & Danti, I. (1611). *Le due regole della prospettiva practica.* Roma, nella Stamperia camerale.

Wade, N. J. (2003). The search for a sixth sense: The cases for vestibular, muscle, and temperature senses. *Journal of the History of the Neurosciences* **12**: 175–202.

Wallace, E. (1882). *Peri psyches; Aristotle's psychology.* E. Wallace ed. Cambridge, Cambridge University press.

Witelo. (1535). *Vitellionis... Peri optikēs, id est de natura, ratione, & proiectione radiorum uisus, luminum, colorum atq[ue] formarum, quam uulgo perspectiuam vocant, libri X.* Norimbergæ, Apud Io. Petreium.

Wood, E. ed. (1885). *Portraits of the one hundred greatest men in history.* London, Samson Low, Marston, Searle, & Rivington.

Young, D. & Bennet-Clark, H. C. (1995). The role of the tymbal in cicada sound production. *The Journal of Experimental Biology* **198**: 1001–1019.

Suggested readings

Artal, P. & Tabernero, J. (2010). Optics of the human eye: 400 years of exploration from Galileo's time. *Applied Optics* **49**: D123–D130.

Battistini, A. (2000). *Galileo e i gesuiti: miti letterari e retorica della scienza*. Milano, Vita e pensiero.

Bellini, E. (1997). *Umanisti e lincei: letteratura e scienza a Roma nell'età di Galileo*. Padova, Antenore.

Biagioli, M. (2006). *Galileo's instruments of credit: telescopes, images, secrecy*. Chicago, IL, The University of Chicago Press.

Boring, E. G. (1942). *Sensation and perception in the history of experimental psychology*. New York, Appleton-Century.

Brewster, D. (1841). *Martyrs of science; or the lives of Galileo, Tycho Brahe, and Kepler*. New York, Harper.

Bucciantini, M. (2003). *Galileo e Keplero. Filosofia, cosmologia e teologia nell'Età della Controriforma*. Einaudi, Torino.

Bucciantini, M. & Camerota, M. (2009). *Scienza e religione: scritti copernicani*. Roma, Donzelli.

Buyse, F. (2013). *The Distinction between Primary Properties and Secondary Qualities in Galileo Galilei's Natural Philosophy*. Cahiers du Séminaire québécois en philosophie moderne/Working Papers of the Quebec Seminar in Early Modern Philosophy, vol. 1.

Camerota, F. (2004). Galileo's eye: linear perspective and visual astronomy. *Galilaeana* **1**: 143–170.

Camerota, F. & Kemp, M. (2006). *La prospettiva del Rinascimento: arte, architettura, scienza. Architetti e architetture*, 19. Milano, Electa.

Camerota, M. (2004). *Galileo Galilei e la cultura scientifica nell'Età della Controriforma*. Salerno, Roma.

Casini, P. (1983). *Il Dialogo di Galileo e la Luna di Plutarco, in Novità celesti e crisi del sapere*. P. Galluzzi ed. Firenze, Giunti Barbèra.

Cozzi, G. (1978). *Paolo Sarpi tra Venezia e l'Europa*. Torino, G. Einaudi.

Crombie, A. C. (1952). *Augustine to Galileo. The history of science A.D. 400–1650*. London: Falcon.

Crombie, A. C. (1967). The primary properties and secondary qualities in Galileo Galilei's Natural Philosophy. In *Saggi su Galileo Galilei*. C. Maccagni ed. Florence, G. Barbera, pp. 72–91.

Crombie, A. C. (1990). *Science, optics, and music in medieval and early modern thought*. London, Hambledon Press.

Dijksterhuis, E. J. (1956). *The Arenarius of Archimedes: with glossary*. Leiden, E.J. Brill.

Dijksterhuis, E. J. (1987). *Archimedes*. Princeton, NJ, Princeton University Press.

Dreyer, J. L. E. (1953). *A history of astronomy from Thales to Kepler, formerly titled History of the planetary systems from Thales to Kepler*. New York, Dover Publications.

Edgerton, S. Y. (1984). Galileo: Florentine disegno, and the strange spottednesse of the moon. *Art Journal* **44**: 225–232.

Edgerton, S. Y. (1991). *The heritage of Giotto's geometry: art and science on the eve of the scientific revolution*. Ithaca, NY, Cornell University Press.

Edgerton, S. Y. (2009). *The mirror, the window, and the telescope: how Renaissance linear perspective changed our vision of the universe*. Ithaca, NY, Cornell University Press.

Fabbri, N. (2012). The moon as another earth: what Galileo owes to Plutarch. *Galilaeana* **9**: 103–135.

Freedberg, D. (2002). The eye of the Lynx: Galileo, his friends, and the beginnings of modern natural history. Chicago, IL, University of Chicago Press.

Galluzzi, P. (2006). *The mind of Leonardo: the universal genius at work*. Firenze, Giunti.

Grant, E. & Grant, E. (2009). *Planets, stars and orbs: the medieval cosmos, 1200–1687*. Cambridge, Cambridge University Press.

Hallyn, F. (1994). Le regard pictural de Galilée sur la lune. *Créis* **2**: 25–41.

Hamou, P. (1999). *La mutation du visible: essai sur la portée épistémologique des instruments d'optique au XVIIe siècle. Vol. 1, du Sidereus Nuncius de Galilée à la Dioptrique cartésienne*. Villeneuve d'Ascq, Presses universitaires du Septentrion.

Heilbron, J. L. (2010). *Galileo*. Oxford, Oxford University Press.

Ilardi, V. (2007). *Renaissance vision from spectacles to telescopes*. Philadelphia, PA, American Philosophical Society.

Istituto Veneto Di Scienze, Lettere Ed Arti. (1995). *Galileo e la cultura Veneziana: convegno a cura dell'Istituto Veneto di Scienze Lettere ed Arti, Venezia, 18–20 giugno 1992*. Trieste, Edizioni LINT.

Kepler, J. & Pantin, I. (1993). *Dissertatio cum nuncio sidereo; narratio de observatis Jovis satellitibus*. Paris, Les Belles Lettres.

Lerner, M. -P. (1997). *Le monde des sphères*. 2 vols. Paris, Les Belles Lettres.

Müller, J. (1826). *Zur vergleichenden Physiologie des Gesichtssinnes des Menschen und der Thiere, nebst einen Versuch über die Bewegung der Augen und über den menschlichen Blick*. Leipzig: Cnobloch.

O'Leary, De L. (1949). *How Greek science passed to the Arabs*. London, Routledge and Kegan Paul.

Pantin, I. (1992). *Galileo Galilei, Sidereus nuncius—Le messager céleste*. Paris, Les Belles Lettres.

Piccolino, M. (2005). *Lo zufolo e la cicala: divagazioni galileiane tra la scienza e la sua storia*. Torino, Bollati Boringhieri.

Piccolino, M. & Wade, N. J. (2007). *Insegne ambigue: percorsi obliqui tra storia, scienza e arte da Galileo a Magritte*. Pisa, ETS.

Piccolino, M. & Wade, N. J. (2008a). Galileo Galilei's vision of the senses. *Trends in Neurosciences* **31** (11): 585–590.

Piccolino, M. & Wade, N. J. (2008b). Galileo's eye: a new vision of the senses in the work of Galileo Galilei. *Perception* **37** (9): 1312–1340.

Polyak, S. (1957). *The vertebrate visual system*. Chicago, IL, University of Chicago Press.

Rossi, P. (1970). *Philosophy, technology, and the arts in the early modern era*. B. Nelson, transl. New York, Harper & Row.

Reeves, E. (2008). *Galileo's glassworks: the telescope and the mirror*. Cambridge, MA, Harvard University Press.

Ronchi, V. (1964). *Galileo e il suo cannocchiale*. Torino, Boringhieri.

Ronchi, V. ed. (1968). *Scritti di ottica*. Milano: Ed. Il Polifilo.

Ronchi, V. (1970). *The nature of light: an historical survey*. V. Barocas transl. Cambridge, MA, Harvard University Press.

Settle, T. B. (1971). Ostilio Ricci, a bridge between Alberti and Galileo. *Science et Philosophie* **III/B**: 121–126.

Strano, G. (2008). *Il telescopio di Galileo*. Firenze, Giunti.

Strong, D. S. (1979). *Leonardo on the eye*. New York, Garland.

Valleriani, M. (2010). *Galileo engineer*. Dordrecht, Springer.

Van Helden, A. (1977). *The invention of the telescope*. Philadelphia, PA, American Philosophical Society.

Van Helden, A. (1985). *Measuring the universe: cosmic dimensions from Aristarchus to Halley*. Chicago, IL, University of Chicago Press.

Wolf, A. (1935). *A history of science, technology, and philosophy in the 16th & 17th centuries*. London, Allen & Unwin.

Ziggelaar, A. (1983). *François de Aguilón S. J. (1567–1617) Scientist and architect*. Rome, Institutum Historicum Societatis Iesus.

Name index

Subject index